W9-BUA-855

TEACHING CHILDREN
WITH AUTISM:

Strategies to Enhance Communication and Socialization

Teaching Children With Autism:

Strategies to Enhance Communication and Socialization

Edited by
Kathleen Ann Quill, Ed. D.

Delmar Publishers' Online Services
To access Delmar on the World Wide Web, point your browser to:
http://www.delmar.com/delmar.html
To access through Gopher: gopher://gopher.delmar.com
(Delmar Online is part of "thomson.com", an Internet site with information on
more than 30 publishers of the International Thomson Publishing organization.)
For information on our products and services:
email: info@delmar.com
or call 800-347-7707

Delmar Publishers Inc.™
I(T)P An International Thomson Publishing Company

New York • London • Bonn • Detroit • Madrid • Melbourne • Mexico City • Paris
Singapore • Tokyo • Toronto • Washington • Albany NY • Belmont CA • Cincinnati OH

NOTICE TO THE READER

Publisher does not warrant or guarantee any of the products described herein or perform any independent analysis in connection with any of the product information contained herein. Publisher does not assume, and expressly disclaims, any obligation to obtain and include information other than that provided to it by the manufacturer.

The reader is expressly warned to consider and adopt all safety precautions that might be indicated by the activities described herein and to avoid all potential hazards. By following the instructions contained herein, the reader willingly assumes all risks in connection with such instructions.

The publisher makes no representations or warranties of any kind, including but not limited to, the warranties of fitness for particular purpose or merchantability, nor are any such representations implied with respect to the material set forth herein, and the publisher takes no responsibility with respect to such material. The publisher shall not be liable for any special, consequential or exemplary damages resulting, in whole or in part, form the readers' use of, or reliance upon, this materials.

Publishing Team:
Senior Acquisitions Editor: Bill Burgower
Project Editor: Megan A. Terry
Art & Design Coordinators: Timothy J. Conners

Assistant Editor: Debra M. Flis
Production Coordinator: Mary Ellen Black

Copyright © 1995 by Delmar Publishers Inc., an International Thomson Publishing Company
The ITP trademark is used under license.

Printed in the United States of America
For more information, contact:

Delmar Publishers Inc.
Box 15015
3 Columbia Circle
Albany, NY 12212-5015

International Thomson Publishing
Berkshire House
168-173 High Holborn
London, WC1V7AA
England

Thomas Nelson Australia
102 Dodds Street
South Melbourne 3205
Victoria, Australia

Nelson Canada
1120 Birchmont Road
Scarborough, Ontario
M1K 5G4, Canada

International Thomson Publishing
GmbH
Konigswinterer Str. 418
53227 Bonn
Germany

International Thomson Publishing
Asia
221 Henderson Bldg. #05-10
Singapore 0315

International Thomson Publishing
Japan
Kyowa Building, 3F
2-2-1 Hirakawa-cho
Chiyoda-ku, Tokyo 102
Japan

All rights reserved. No part of this book covered by the copyright hereon may be reproduced or used in any form, or by any means—graphic, electronic, or mechanical, including photocopying, recording, taping, or information storage and retrieval systems—without the written permission of the publisher.

Printed in the United States of America
10 11 XXX 01 00 99

Library of Congress Cataloging-in-Publication Data
Teaching children with autism: strategies to enhance communication and socialization / edited by Kathleen Ann Quill.
    p. cm.
    Includes bibliographical references and index.
    ISBN 0-8273-6269-2
    1. Autistic children—Education—United States. 2. Communication—Study and teaching—United States.
3. Socialization—Study and teaching—United States. I. Quill, Kathleen Ann, 1952-
LC4718.T43 1995
371.94—dc20

94-10644
CIP

*This book is dedicated to
children with autism.
They have filled my mind,
my heart, and my soul
with much understanding,
joy, and sensitivity.*

Contributors

Nancy J. Dalrymple, M.A., Child Evaluation Center, University of Louisville, Louisville, Kentucky

Temple Grandin, Ph.D., Department of Animal Science, Colorado State University, Fort Collins, Colorado

Carol A. Gray, B.S., Jenison Public Schools, Jenison, Michigan

June Groden, Ph.D., The Groden Center, Providence, Rhode Island

Charles A. Hart, Ph.D. candidate, Seattle, Washington

Linda Quirk Hodgdon, M.Ed., CCC-SLP, Macomb Intermediate School District, Troy, Michigan

Thomas L. Layton, Ph.D., Division of Speech and Hearing Sciences, University of North Carolina at Chapel Hill, Chapel Hill, North Carolina

Patricia LeVasseur, M.Ed., The Groden Center, Providence, Rhode Island

Barry M. Prizant, Ph.D., Department of Communication Disorders, Emerson College, Boston, Massachusetts

Kathleen A. Quill, Ed.D., The Autism Institute, Manchester, Massachusetts

Patrick J. Rydell, Ed.D., Autism Communication Services, Lakewood, Colorado

Adriana L. Schuler, Ph.D., Department of Special Education, San Francisco State University, San Francisco, California

Diane D. Twachtman, M.A., CCC-SLP, Autism and Developmental Disabilities Consultation Center, Cromwell, Connecticut

Linda R. Watson, Ed.D., Division of Speech and Hearing Sciences, University of North Carolina at Chapel Hill, Chapel Hill, North Carolina

Pamela Wolfberg, Ph.D., Consultant, San Francisco, California

Contents

Part 3 Promoting Socialization

Foreword

The history of educational practice for children with autism and other pervasive developmental disorders has been characterized by disparate and sometimes contradictory approaches. Significant differences in educational philosophy and approach remain, often causing confusion for parents and recent graduates in education, communication disorders, and other related fields. Differences in practice have their basis in different philosophies about how children learn (e.g., behavioral versus developmental approaches) and different beliefs about the most significant challenges faced by children with autism and pervasive developmental disorders (PDD) and their families (e.g., communicative limitations, sensory integration deficits, and so on).

In recent years, educational approaches have become less constrained by philosophical dogma and are more eclectic in theoretical basis and practice. "Best practices" are now characterized by a number of themes. First, it is now widely accepted that a major focus of education must be on enhancing communication and socialization abilities that will enable children with autism to exercise a maximum degree of social control, make decisions, and participate actively with their peers. Second, education should focus on the acquisition of functional skills that will to the extent possible enable children to learn in settings that are integrated and normalized. Third, professionals and families must form partnerships in enhancing children's communication and socioemotional development and their membership in the extended family and community. Finally, it is clearly recognized that best practices in education involve the development of individualized approaches. That is, each student's—and indeed, each family's—strengths and needs must be incorporated and addressed in educational practices.

Although articles and chapters that reflect these practices have recently appeared, there has been a significant need for an integrated volume designed primarily for practitioners and parents. This book will help fill this need. Kathleen Quill has compiled a volume that clearly reflects, and will contribute to, best practices in the education of children. First, the volume clearly focuses on communication and socialization in the broadest sense of the terms. Verbal as well as nonverbal and augmentative approaches to communication are addressed, as is emotional as well as instrumental communication. Socialization within classroom settings, home settings, and community settings is also addressed. The chapter authors include not only professionals from a variety of disciplines, but also a parent, Charles Hart, and a highly respected person with autism whose insights have contributed greatly to educational practices, Temple Grandin, Ph.D. The volume's central message is that we must understand how children with autism and PDD think, learn, and organize information about the social and nonsocial world. Thus the creative approaches and practices espoused herein are strongly influenced by our knowledge of the learning styles most closely associated with autism and our awareness of how individual strengths and weaknesses must be addressed in appropriate education and treatment. Dr. Quill's anthology provides a much-needed complement to the literature in that its information and strategies can be applied "on Monday morning." Clinicians, educators, and parents will find an absolute wealth of relevant and creative suggestions for the full range of children with autism and related disabilities.

Kathleen Quill is to be congratulated for her achievement. It no surprise that she has accomplished this goal, for Dr. Quill has been driven by her observations of the needs of children and families through years of front-line hands-on work. This book should be kept within close reach; it will be a frequently used resource and will be enjoyed and valued by both professionals and parents. I have no doubt that it will have a significant impact in further advancing the implementation of "best practices" in the education of children with autism.

Barry M. Prizant, Ph.D., CCC-SLP
Professor, Division of Communication Disorders
Emerson College
Boston, Massachussetts

Preface

It has been more than fifty years since the social and communication differences characteristic of autism were first described by Leo Kanner. During that time, research has produced a wealth of knowledge about the complex developmental processes involved in autism symptomatology. The triad of impairments in social relationships, communication, and imagination appear closely intertwined with an idiosyncratic profile of cognitive strengths and weaknesses. This current perspective on autism has opened doors to new and diverse treatment options.

Teaching Children With Autism provides a framework for understanding these developmental differences and applying this knowledge to treatment efforts to promote the children's communication and socialization abilities. The reader is guided through a discussion of the child's cognitive and social perspectives, presented strategies to enhance communication and interpersonal relationships, and offered guidelines to assist children with autism through the social maze.

Part 1, Perspectives on Autism, presents one theoretical and two autobiographical perspectives on the nature of the disorder and educational methodology. The subsequent sections of the volume are devoted to strategies that promote communication and social development, the hallmarks of autism. Assessment and treatment are addressed concurrently. Informal measures for observing and assessing communicative competence and social behaviors are described, and specific assessment guidelines are provided in chapter appendices. Part 2, Communication Enhancement, presents intervention strategies for children who are nonverbal and verbal. The discussions include considerations for using augmentative communication, the treatment of echolalia, and methods that improve the quality of social-communicative interactions. Part 3, Promoting Socialization, covers strategies to foster play, social understanding, independence, flexibility, and self-control.

Teaching Children With Autism is intended for educators, clinicians, parents, and students in education, communication disorders, and related fields. It is hoped that this volume will expand and refine the reader's approach to intervention, and that these ideas will interface with other treatment options currently available for children with autism.

In the preparation of this book, I am grateful to many people at Delmar Publishers and Beckwith-Clark, Inc. who provided invaluable support throughout the process. The contributing authors were cooperative and enthusiastic about the book, making this formidable task manageable. A number of colleagues, especially Barry Prizant and June Fox, offered encouragement and kindness that I sincerely appreciated. My family and friends shared my frustrations, worries, accomplishments, and joy, and showered me with an abundance of love and emotional support. Finally, I am most grateful to the many children with autism who touch my life every day and teach me so much about life, love, and the human spirit. If this volume of work makes a difference in the life of one child, then the effort has been worthwhile.

Kathleen A. Quill, Ed.D.

Introduction

Kathleen A. Quill

Teaching children with autism is a challenging endeavor for educators and parents. The children present a unique array of problems that are perplexing because they often seem inconsistent with what is understood about human learning and behavior. It is generally assumed, particularly in education, that all children follow a similar developmental path, albeit at various rates. Yet children with autism display peculiar styles of social, communicative, and interpersonal relationships that seem to follow a different path. An understanding of these developmental differences must be incorporated into intervention in order to embrace the children's social perspective fully, to develop and use strategies that promote communication and socialization, and to assist children with autism through the maze of interpersonal relationships.

HISTORICAL OVERVIEW

It has been more than fifty years since the social and communication differences characteristic of autism were first described by Leo Kanner (1943). The wealth of his information and the profoundness of his insights are only now being recognized. In his seminal paper, Kanner addressed the pervasiveness of the children's interpersonal difficulties:

> There is from the start an extreme autistic aloneness (p. 33) . . . . these children have come into the world with innate inability to form the usual, biologically provided affective contact with people, just as other children come into the world with innate physical or intellectual handicaps (pp. 42–43).

From the onset, Kanner recognized the primacy of the social difficulties. He also reported about the children's purposeful abilities with objects, further noting the distinction between their people-oriented and object-oriented relationships. In addition to describing the severe social problems, Kanner provided astute descriptions of the language and communication idiocyncracies in autism. His attention to the children's ineffective use of language was noted in his descriptions of echolalia, repetitions, and pronoun reversal. Still, it has taken a half century of research efforts for Kanner's hypothesis to be scientifically understood and the clinical significance of his work to be fully realized.

Educational practices follow the lead of science. The treatment of autism in the 1950s and 1960s evolved from theories that prescribed an emotional etiology. The psychodynamic theory, most noted in the work of Bettelheim (1967), resulted in treatment aimed at "breaking through the emotional shell of autism." Once the hope of "emotional recovery" faded, the research of the 1970s shifted to regarding autism as a cognitive and linguistic impairment (Rutter and Schopler, 1978; Wing, 1976), opening the door to behavioral intervention (Lovaas, 1977) and related models of structured teaching. This theory assumed that the interpersonal difficulties in autism arose as a result of the cognitive and language impairments, and treatment focused on children's acquisition of discrete cognitive and language skills in a highly organized and precise instructional style. Even when the most successful behavioral interventions report impressive outcomes, judgments are based on IQ and academic achievements (Lovaas, 1987) with little attention to the social and emotional growth of the children.

Research in the past decade has revisited Kanner's original work, and discussions about the nature of autism emphasize the complex interdependence of cognitive learning style, social understanding, language learning, and communication patterns (Dawson, 1989; Frith, 1989). Explanations of autism no longer focus on a singular abnormality, whether cognitive, linguistic, or social. Today's views are more multifaceted and holistic and take into account the interplay of different developmental systems. The core symptoms of autism—that is, social-communicative relationships—are examined within their natural context, social understanding and social-communicative interactions. As a result, treatment can now apply this information by adding strategies that consider the children's perspective and the social context to the already successful intervention options for teaching children with autism.

PURPOSE OF THE BOOK

The purpose of this book is to provide educators, students, and parents with a framework for applying knowledge of current theoretical perspec-

tives on autism to their ongoing treatment efforts to promote communication and socialization abilities in the children. The book reflects the increase
in knowledge about the communication and social differences of children
with autism and the application of this knowledge to educational practice.
The authors are largely clinicians and educators who work directly with
children, families, and schools and appreciate the realities and challenges
of the classroom, home, and community. The authors recognize the complexity of deficits in autism, and they describe innovative teaching strategies to address these needs. The teaching strategies are based on clinical
research and clinical practices that utilize the inherent perspective and abilities of the child as a means to promote social-communicative competence
in natural settings. Two fundamental principles are central to the discussion: first, education and treatment must respect and accommodate the
unique and individual learning styles of children with autism; second, education and treatment must support children's participation with adults and
peers in integrated school and community settings.

A recent focus of intervention—and the principle theme of the book—
is an emphasis on instructional strategies that accommodate the learning
style of children with autism. The instructional strategies described in this
volume support children's exploration of the world of people, and by
doing so, make it easier for them to communicate and interact. Strategies to
support social and communicative success include augmentative instructional materials, environmental predictability, and modifications in adult-
child and peer-child social-communicative interactions. Each author
describes various techniques that incorporate these basic supports to
enhance communication, social behavior, and self-control in children with
autism.

A second focus of intervention, and secondary theme of the book, is the
emphasis on social context as instrumental to learning. A major goal of
education today is to enhance communication and socialization abilities
that support children's participation with adults and peers in integrated
school and community settings. The strategies outlined in each chapter
take into the account the social context in which the acquisition of communication and social skills occurs, and the authors describe the roles of
adults and typical peers in fostering this development.

The book is divided into three sections: Perspectives on Autism,
Strategies for Communication Enhancement, and Strategies for Promoting
Socialization.

PERSPECTIVES ON AUTISM

In 1988, Temple Grandin, a highly successful woman with autism, was lec-
turing in Massachusetts about her personal experiences living with the dis-

order. Grandin's descriptions of her thoughts, feelings, and learning style have had profound influence on the growing understanding of autism's complexity. That evening, however, her slide presentation was particularly meaningful. She showed a slide of an airplane and said, "This is here to remind me to talk about my perseverativeness." Next there was a slide picturing cement, and she said, "This is here to remind me about my concrete thinking." Some of the audience laughed at the slide, while others were transfixed by her message. In that moment, Grandin demonstrated very clearly one of her valuable strategies for organizing and sharing information: that is, having formed a concept by encoding an experience into a visual image, she uses the image as a retrieval cue! Her thinking appeared to be a series of visual associations, a learning style that she now describes in her writings.

After the lecture, I reread Temple Grandin's autobiography (Grandin & Scariano, 1986) in which she describes her use of visual similes as a means to understand abstract concepts such as social relationships. It seemed that she used logic, rather than emotion, to guide her understanding of the social world. Grandin shares this most personal and profound insight about her social perceptions and the strategies she uses for social adaptation in the first section of the book. Her important contribution has supplemented advancements in research, expanding and refining the possibilities of intervention to take into account individual learning styles and the children's perception of their environment.

The first section of this book includes three current perspectives on autism: one theoretical, one autobiographical, and one familial. In Chapter 1, Adriana Schuler presents a highly integrative overview of developmental research. Schuler examines the constellation of abilities and difficulties in autism and describes how cognitive patterns are closely intertwined with differences in communication, language learning, social understanding and emotional development. Reflecting on the work of Kanner (1943) she explains the developmental incongruencies as differences between "object- and people-referenced thinking." A diminished capacity to think about people as opposed to thinking about the physical world seems to account for the atypical profile characteristic of autism. Through a case study, the reader is guided through the idiosyncracies of thinking, learning, and development in autism, and is provided a framework for understanding the teaching strategies described in the remaining sections of the book.

An understanding of this developmental discrepancy becomes further illuminated as Temple Grandin relates her experiences with autism in Chapter 2. Grandin describes her "visual thinking," communication frustrations, sensory sensitivities, and social-emotional issues with honesty and sensitivity. These personal insights into the nature of autism are invaluable to all readers.

Because parents carry the major responsibility for supporting their child's development, any discussion about intervention must take into account the family's perspective on education. Today families have a wealth of treament options from which to choose, but this also means they have difficult decisions to make. Charles Hart shares one parent's view of educational philosophy in Chapter 3. Hart is a parent of an adult son with autism, a professional, an author, and an advocate for persons with autism. In a stimulating and candid discussion, Hart reflects on his experiences moving through the special education maze with his son. He shares the frustrations and emotional challenges surrounding the broad and often perplexing treatment options made available to him and other families over the past three decades. What parents want is respect for their child and a strong parent-professional partnership.

Thus equipped with a context for thinking about autism, the reader is prepared to turn to educational implications and methodological issues. Four chapters on strategies to enhance communication are followed by five chapters on strategies to enhance socialization. Throughout these discussions, it becomes evident that intervention is changing significantly.

Social-communicative competence is a dynamic phenomenon and strategies to promote the skills must be equally dynamic. Language, communication, and social skills do not emerge as a series of isolated behaviors. It is clear that the context of social interaction, the child's own perception of the social dynamic, and the strategies used by the interactant play a fundamental role in the success of any interaction and skill acquisition program. This recognition has reshaped approaches to assessment and intervention. The authors of these chapters explore creative ways to assess complex issues and support children through the maze of communication and socialization, yet they maintain the necessary qualities of objectivity and accountability in their work.

COMMUNICATION ENHANCEMENT

The second section of the book, Communication Enhancement, addresses the broad spectrum of abilities and challenges observed in both verbal and nonverbal children. In Chapter 4, Tom Layton and Linda Watson pursue the use of alternative and augmentative communication supports to enhance communication in nonverbal children. A description of early communicative behaviors is provided along with guidelines for assessing the nonverbal child's communicative repertoire. The reader is guided through an examination of the augmentative communication options, criteria for selecting augmentative systems for a child, and strategies to foster communication. The augmentative systems include sign language, communication boards, written language, and computers. As there has been significant attention given to the technology of facilitated communication in the past few years, the authors provide a current review of the literature on this topic. Layton and Watson recognize that access to a linguistic system is a necessary but not sufficient means to promote communication, thus they emphasize the child's development of intentionality and functionality.

Echolalic language in children with autism remains a fascinating and poorly understood aspect of their communicative behavior. In Chapter 5, Patrick Rydell and Barry Prizant shape our understanding of the specific patterns of echolalia and the contextual and interactive factors associated with it. Careful attention is given to assessment tools that identify the functional usage of echolalic messages and approaches to intervention that consider how such patterns contribute to the child's linguistic and communicative growth.

In Chapter 6, Diane Twachtman describes strategies to enhance communication in the more verbal children. The disparity between the often verbose language they exhibit and the paucity of effective social competencies gives rise to new challenges. Twachtman relates several approaches to promote the children's social use of language that take into account their social perspective and the multidimensional process of communication.

In Chapter 7, I focus in more detail on the nature of reciprocal social interaction and strategies to build social-comunicative interactions in children, regardless of their level of linguistic competence. The assessment of social-communicative interactions, the complexity of social relationships and communication, and the multiple factors that must be considered when interacting with a child are emphasized. A combination of interactive routines, modified adult/peer communication style, and the use of environmental supports are offered as strategies that can help children through the social maze. This chapter synthesizes our understanding of the contextual and interactive factors that promote communication and interpersonal relationships.

PROMOTING SOCIALIZATION

Although the fundamental aspect of autism is impaired development of social relationships, the social deficits have received little attention in the area of curriculum and instruction. As a result, the section entitled Promoting Socialization offers new and exciting opportunities for treatment.

This section begins by addressing the very fabric of young children's social development: play. Play is the means by which children make sense of the world through shared experiences. In Chapter 8, Pamela Wolfberg presents a model for promoting play skills in integrated settings. The integrated play groups model emphasizes the social nature of play and provides opportunities for children with autism to learn to play along with experienced peers. A social support system for peer play is achieved through careful assessment and adult guided participation within carefully designed play environments. Wolfberg's work takes an important step in assessing and designing opportunities for children's social growth and learning through play.

The remaining chapters describe various ways in which environmental supports can be used to enhance social understanding, social skills, social flexibility, and self-control. Environmental supports are teaching materials that assist the child's ability to organize and integrate information more readily. The premise behind the use of environmental supports is that they provide social clarity for the child, allow for self-monitoring and self-regulation, and increase independence at making social decisions.

In Chapter 9, Carol Gray describes an innovative technique to teach children with autism to "read" social situations through the use of "social reading." Social Reading is a term given to instructional materials that present social information and teach social skills. Individually designed books, audio tapes, and videotaped stories are developed as a means to improve a child's social skills through improved social understanding. Gray's technique uses environmental supports and interactive clarity through a medium that many children understand and enjoy.

In Chapter 10, Nancy Dalrymple details the many uses of environmental supports to promote independence and flexibility in children. Numerous ideas are provided to support the child's understanding of time, spatial organization, choices, and social rules. Parents and professionals will find that the work of both Gray and Dalrymple has enormous applicability across children and social contexts.

The communicative function of social and behavioral problems has been well researched in the past decaade. In Chapter 11, Linda Quirk Hodgdon takes this information and offers educators and parents concrete tools to support the child's development of communication skills as a means to reduce opportunities for social-behavioral problems. The recommended strategies reinforce the benefits of environmental supports in helping children understand and interpret the demands of their social world and support socially appropriate behaviors.

Another use of visually supported instruction is prescribed in Chapter 12 by June Groden and Patricia LeVasseur. Groden and LeVasseur developed a cognitive picture rehearsal procedure to teach appropriate social behaviors and self-control. Through repeated practice of pictorial scenes, children with autism are taught to identify stressful events and learn to use coping strategies. The use of imagery-based procedures to develop self-control incorporates all the elements of effective teaching advocated throughout the book.

SUMMARY

There is a growing awareness and respect for the obstacles facing children with autism in their efforts to communicate, socialize, and make sense of interpersonal relationships. Relationships are complex and do not lend themselves to simple remedies, but with each new idea or proposed treatment, additional insights are possible. It is hoped that this volume of work will shed new light on assessment and intervention options, will open doors for the children, and will stimulate new ideas about teaching children with autism.

REFERENCES

Bettelheim, B. (1967). *The empty fortress*. New York: Free Press.

Dawson, G. (1989). *Autism: Nature, diagnosis and treatment*. New York: Guilford.

Frith, U. (1989). *Autism: Explaining the enigma*. Oxford, England: Blackwell.

Grandin, T. and Scariano, M. (1986). *Emergence: Labeled autistic*. Novato, CA: Arena.

Kanner, L. (1943). Autistic disturbances of affective contact. *Nervous Child, 2,* 217–250.

Lovaas, O. I. (1977). *The autistic child: Language development through behavior modification*. New York: Irvington.

Lovaas, O. I. (1987). Behavioral treatment and normal educational and intellectual functioning in young autistic children. *Journal of Consulting and Clinical Psychology, 55,* 3–9.

Rutter, M., & Schopler, E. (Eds.) (1978). *Autism: A reappraisal of concept and treatment*. New York: Plenum.

Wing, L. (Ed.) (1976). *Early childhood autism* (2nd ed.). Oxford, England: Pergamon.

P A R T 1

Perspectives on Autism

1

Thinking in Autism: Differences in Learning and Development

Adriana L. Schuler

The confusion and controversy that surrounds the syndrome of early childhood autism has turned the jobs of teaching and parenting children with autism into an extraordinary challenge. It is argued that Kanner's remarkably astute clinical observations were not properly interpreted due to limited knowledge of early social development. Now, half a century later, the accumulated clinical profile is more readily described as a unique profile of strengths and weaknesses that jeopardize those forms of learning that are dependent on interaction with relevant others within the cultural context. Congruent with Kanner's early speculations, these differences can be explained as a discrepancy between object- and people-referenced thinking.

Guided by a quest for commonality and applied relevance, this chapter provides a summary of research findings that cuts across professional disciplines and research methodologies. It will point out that cognitive idiosyncracies are closely intertwined with differences in social interaction, affect, communication and language learning. A prototypical case profile will be presented to illustrate how discrepant the developmental profile of individuals with autism can be, explain how the disrepancies encountered can be explained as a difference between object- and people-referenced thinking, and discuss the implications in terms of educational and clinical practices. Specific recommendations will be made to help parents and practitioners capitalize on individual strengths and learning styles to support their children's and student's explorations of the world of people. By doing so they will make it easier for them to learn to interact and communicate with others.

THE NATURE OF AUTISM

Controversies have surrounded the syndrome of autism ever since it was first reported in the literature. More than fifty years have passed since child psychiatrist Leo Kanner (1943) first described eleven children who exhibited a shared group of unusual characteristics. Those characteristics, which continue to intrigue parents as well as professionals, have produced an unusual potpourri of theories and speculations. Autism has been viewed as primarily an affective, a perceptual, a linguistic, a cognitive, and a communicative disorder. Explanatory constructs have vacillated among psychogenic, biological, behavioral, and interactional models of causation.

While autism was initially attributed to aloof parenting, biological models of causation have now become widely accepted, and there is a growing recognition that many different causes may be involved. Autism may be better described as a conglomerate of subsyndromes that share a symptomatology of severe problems in social relating and related developmental dissyncronies. In fact, half a century later, one remains impressed with the astuteness of Kanner's early observations, which still hold up to current investigations.

Unfortunately, forces of contemporary thought in the 1950s and early 1960s transformed Kanner's early observations into a series of myths that have have been difficult to eradicate despite a lack of empirical support. The absence of a compatible theoretical framework is at least partially responsible for the controversies that have continued to surround the autistic syndrome. Because so little was known at mid-century about early social and communicative development, Kanner had to operate without a theoretical anchor for his observations.

Today our ever-expanding knowledge of early social, communicative, and cognitive development and its interlink with affective forces helps us understand the unusual developmental profiles associated with the syndrome of autism. While different sets of criteria have been used to define autism, the ways in which childhood autism and related pervasive developmental disorders are currently defined are remarkably congruent with the early decriptions of autism as formulated by Kanner. The current definition not only lists of a series of seemingly unrelated behavioral anomalies, but also portrays a cohesive constellation of behaviors that stem from a lack of reciprocal interaction and related imaginative activity (DSMIII-R, American Psychiatric Association, 1987).

COGNITION IN AUTISM

One ongoing source of controversy pertains to the cognitive status of individuals with autism. Based on his own clinical observations, Kanner referred to his first eleven cases as "cognitively well endowed." Nevertheless, approximately two-thirds of all individuals with autism have subsequently been described as intellectually impaired on the basis of large-scale intelligence testing (DeMyer, 1975). Yet views of people with autism as predominantly retarded continue to be challenged. For instance, Biklen (1990) has reported unprecedented literacy skills through assisted written communications, claiming that the behavioral peculiarites associated with the syndrome are a reflection of motor rather than of cognitive impairment. Moreover, differences of opinion continue to exist among those who claim cognitive impairments. While specific social cognitive impairments have been claimed in the context of research investigating the extent to which people with autism are able to entertain a so-called theory of mind (Baron-Cohen, Leslie & Frith, 1985), others (Prior, Dahlstrom & Squires, 1990) maintain that a more generalized cognitive deficit exists.

The controversies and debates are not merely academic. They resonate with sentiments commonly experienced by parents and teachers who feel at a loss in their attempts to access some type of smarts that they feel is locked inside their child or student. The often striking contradictions between apparent intellectual promise and immense deficiencies in adaptive skills are a source of great frustration for everyone closely involved with children with autism. Nevertheless, a rather cohesive picture emerges when available literature involving different lines of investigation, disciplines, and research methodologies is examined in conjunction with accumulated clinical experience. A cognitive profile appears that is rather consistent in the face of considerable variation across subtypes and overall functioning levels. In fact, much of the controversy and confusion could have been avoided if Kanner's differentiation between objects and people as a focus of thought had been taken more seriously. The following summary of pertinent research is presented to show how the specific profile of strengths and weaknesses may be explained as a discrepancy between the capacity to engage in people-referenced as opposed to object-referenced thought.

Evidence From Intelligence Testing

Despite the fact that it is difficult to administer standardized tests to individuals with autism, large-scale test data have been accumulated through careful testing and retesting. While the accumulated IQ scores are only marginally relevant to instruction and intervention, item-by-item analyses and accumulated test profiles have helped us to better understand the cognitive ramifications of the autistic syndrome. For instance, based on extensive comparisons, DeMyer (1975) concluded that the perceptual-motor skills of most autistic children were delayed, but that performance on visual-motor tasks was enhanced when the visual stimuli remained visible at all times. If the children were required to attend to a transient visual cue, their performance dropped. A similar drop was observed when the task became motorically more complex. When asked to imitate body movements or to engage in ball play, retarded children did better than matched autistic children. The performance of children with autism was enhanced when the tasks presented involved object matching or use of lower extremities. DeMyer went as far as to suggest that impaired visual-motor rather than poor verbal skills were linked to social withdrawal, and that both social withdrawal and nonfunctional object use were associated with lack of symbolic development. Interestingly, Rogers and Pennington (1991) recently argued that the primary deficit may lie in the area of imitation and related motor behaviors.

Based on analyses of accumulated intelligence test data, Prior (1979) has provided clear descriptions of the skill profiles typically associated with the autistic syndrome. She noted excellent rote memory for both auditory and visual information as well as proficiencies in tasks demanding visuo-spatial judgment and pattern recognition. Specific examples of such abilities include both recognition and production of melodic patterns; construction of visuo-spatial arrays from samples, such as in block construction; and the completion of jigsaw puzzles, formboards, block designs, and so forth. These skill profiles are consistent with common clinical experience and seem further validated by Temple Grandin's personal accounts of her thought processes in Chapter 2 of this volume, particularly her explanation of the differences between spatial vs. language-based thinking (Grandin, 1995).

Applied Learning Research

Peculiarites in learning have been reported in the context of data-based behavioral interventions incorporating mostly operant conditioning techniques. A phenomenon called *stimulus overselectivity* has been reported along with difficulties in the generalization of newly learned behaviors. Lovaas and co-workers first reported stimulus overselectivity in an experimental learning task where children were conditioned to press a bar when presented simultaneously with auditory, visual, and tactile stimuli (Lovaas, Schreibman, Koegel & Rehm, 1971). Subsequently, the three single stimulus components were presented separately in an attempt to determine which component had controlled the response. While typical children would maintain their responses to all components presented, the autistic children usually responded only to one component. This tendency to tune in to a single stimulus component was described as overselectivity.

Overselectivity was demonstrated repeatedly both across and within modalities. In other words, it did not vary as a function of sense modality or other stimulus attributes. Nevertheless, since overselectivity has subsequently been observed to vary as a function of task presentation, it could have been an experimental artifact. Moreover, it has been pointed out that the overselectivity may have been more a function of the developmental delay than of the autism. Overselective children may have performed similarly to normal children below the age of two (Ross, 1976). This possibility was confirmed by Schover and Newsom (1976) in a study that utilized proper developmental controls. Nevertheless, Grandin's account of her troubles with multiple input suggests that the concept of overselectivity may indeed have some validity. Observations by Schuler and Bormann (1983) suggest that overselectivity is likely to occur when the competing stimuli are of a transient, nonspatial nature. What is observed clinically may thus be a product of developmental delay and differences in processing style.

The construct of overselectivity does have some explanatory power. It could serve to explain some of the commonly encountered roadblocks in learning to relate to others and to use language. After all, learning about the meaning of words, facial expressions, and other affective signals depends on the integration of cross-modal stimulus input. Similarly, overselectivity would impede generalization because attention must be paid to a number of simultaneously occuring events or phenomena. For example, preoccupation with the ribbon around a teddy bear's neck or with other marginal features will make it unlikely that the word "bear" will be remembered in conjunction with its more pertinent features. However, given that younger children tend to be more selective in their attention, it is unclear whether these differences are the cause or the result of the autistic condition or both. Yet knowledge of these differences helps in interacting with people with autism. When we work with autistic children it's critical to ensure that they are indeed attending to what we think they are attending to, or want them to attend to.

**Information
Processing**

Information processing research, capitalizing on a by-now classic series of experiments conducted by Hermelin and O'Connor (1970), Hermelin (1976), and Frith (1971), has further helped to clarify the cognitive traits of individuals with autism. In this research the information processing capabilities of autistic children were compared with those of deaf, blind, and retarded children. The deaf and blind groups were included because of the often-noted behavioral similarities between children with autism and children with sensory impairments (Rimland, 1964; Wing, 1974). Autistic children were found to perform differently from blind children when visual information was presented in an accessible form—that is, when the information was coded in space. One of their best-known experiments examined how autistic children code positions in space when presented with a choice between an absolute visuo-spatial framework and a kinesthetic framework linked to the position of their fingers in space. Found to respond to spatial location rather than finger cues, the participating autistic children behaved more like normal and retarded children than like blind or blindfolded children.

Other often-quoted experiments dealt with the memorization of sequential information and the ability to detect patterns therein. It was reported that autistic children could recall series of unrelated words as well as words that were thematically related. Similarly, they were equally good at memorizing anomolous sentences and meaningful sentences. In other words, the autistic children did equally well recalling sense and nonsense both when visual stimulus input was presented and when auditory stimulus input was presented. Hermelin (1976) concluded that autistic children suffer from a central deficiency in the processing of incoming and outgoing information. She postulated that autistic children have trouble with the coding and categorization of information and that they employ an echo-boxlike memory store, a finding that is most pertinent to the prevalence of echolalic speech.

In another experiment, dealing with temporal vs. spatial digit recall, Hermelin observed autistic children perform like deaf children. Again, the autistic children recalled digits according to their spatial location and not according to the order in which they were presented. In doing so they acted like the deaf children. This experimental work has been interpreted to imply that central processing problems are at the core of the autistic syndrome. After all, both language and social interaction require that flexible rules are extracted. Literal rote forms of processing would be counterproductive. Again, it remains unclear whether the processing differences cause the social and linguistic delays or are the result of these delays. Frith (1989) interpretes the extremely literal ways in which individuals with autism process information as indicative of a limited appreciation of central coherence. She hypothesizes that this reflects a reduced awareness of one's own thoughts in relation to the thoughts of others. This ability to mentalize has recently become a major theme in the ever-expanding body of research dealing with so-called theory of mind, which is briefly summarized in the following passage.

Theory of Mind   A related series of experiments that has helped clarify our understanding of how individuals with autism differ in their thinking examines their ability to think of themselves and their intentions as similar to and different from others. The construct of "theory of mind" has been introduced to refer to our understanding of the feelings, beliefs, and desires of others. Differences between normal 3- and 4-year-old children were reported in research conducted by Wimmer and Perner (1983) in a now-classic experiment. Utilizing various dolls and props they presented the following scenario to the regular 3- and 4-year-olds:

"A girl named Sally enters the stage. She leaves after putting a marble into her basket. Next a different girl named Anne appears, who takes the marble out of Sally's basket to hide it in her own box."

Subsequently, the 3- and 4-year-olds are asked the following questions: "Where is the marble really?" "Where was the marble in the beginning?"

While these questions didn't present any troubles to either the 3-year-olds or 4-year-olds, the subsequent question: "Where will Sally look for her marble?" proved to be difficult for the 3-year-olds to answer. Somehow the younger ones found it difficult to apprehend that Sally's picture of the world doesn't match reality, but 4- and 5-year-olds showed better understanding of Sally's beliefs and intentions.

When this same scenario was presented to a group of autistic children who were compared to developmentally matched normal as well as children with Down syndrome, it was found that 80 percent of the autistic children predicted that Sally would look for the marble in its actual location rather than where she would be expected to look (Baron-Cohen, Leslie & Frith, 1985). These documented troubles in understanding the beliefs of others have been reported repeatedly and extended to include the desires of others. Similarly, when asked to sequence pictures that deal with people as opposed to object scenarios, children with autism did poorly when it was necessary to comprehend the beliefs of others (Baron-Cohen, Leslie & Frith, 1986). According to Hobson (1990a) this phenomenon may reflect the differences between our relations with others and our relations with the physical world. To account for these differences, Hobson introduced a differentiation between I–it and I–thou relations. Besides confirming the validity of Kanner's early differentiation between objects and people as a focus of reflection, such a theory also offers much explanatory power when differences in social interaction, communication, play, and language are examined.

COGNITION AND COMMUNICATION

Troubles within the domains of communication and language are so prevalent in individuals with autism that they have been used as the central descriptors of the syndrome. It has been estimated that about half of the children diagnosed as autistic never develop functional speech. With regard to the other half, their use of speech has been reported as largely echolalic or stereotypic at best. In other words, the bulk of the speech produced seems to consist of the immediate or delayed literal repetition of the speech of others, often without an appreciation of the conventional meaning of the utterances involved. Even when more creative utterances are produced, they tend to be used in a repetitive fashion. This dependence on memorized units of speech becomes very clear when samples of everyday conversations are transcribed. What should be pointed out here is that echolalic speech may nevertheless be meaningful and communicative (Prizant, 1983). Moreover, echolalia is not unique to autism (Schuler, 1979). Many children go through rather echolalic periods during the second year of life. The difference is again a matter of degree. Autistic children are merely better at it. They repeat longer units with greater precision and thereby draw attention to themselves. This is particularly so when they also manage to copy the intonation patterns involved in the most unsubtle ways.

Repetitive speech and an overall lack of differentiation of speech sounds are paralleled by a similar lack of differentiation of speech functions. Diversity is what is missing on all accounts. As noted by Kanner in his original case descriptions, it seems as if individuals with autism do not know how to put their vocalizations to work in an effort to communicate with others. Limitations in communicative intent and a restricted range of communicative functions have now been documented repeatedly through a number of studies (Curcio, 1978; Fay & Schuler, 1980; Wetherby & Prutting, 1984). What has been reported is that speech is used mostly for instrumental purposes, not for interactive purposes. Similarly, it has been pointed out that the semantic and the pragmatic dimensions of language are most affected in autism. The lack of differentiation of communicative functions is paralleled by a similarly limited repertoire of communicative means. Not only is speech underused as a means of communication, but nonverbal means that are normally used to augment communication are scarce. Those nonverbal means of communication that are used tend to be presymbolic. A common example of presymbolic communication is a child taking another person's hand and placing it on the doorknob of a door to be opened without acknowledgment of the person involved. What seems to be remembered is a series of actions associated with the opening of the door independent of the people involved in those actions. In this case communication is not outwardly directed but remains largely presymbolic. The child may be locked into a rigid routine that doesn't travel very well. Consequently, we need to be familiar with daily routines and contexts if we are to decipher the meaning of the behaviors involved. The behaviors involved may be unusual or even aberrant because more extreme behaviors trigger more consistent and predictable reactions of others. Biting one's own fingers or hitting one's own head may prove to be a very reliable means through which to get attention or escape from an unpleasant situation.

The communication patterns that have been described in cases of autism are congruent with the cognitive differences discussed previously. Attempts at communication seem more object oriented than people oriented. Because communicative intent is often only marginally established, the individuals involved may be unaware of their communicative behaviors. This may be evidenced by the fact that they are unlikely to notice communicative breakdowns, let alone repair them. The major problem is that the basic idea of comunication as a collaborative and reciprocal enterprise is not understood. Therefore the communicative potential of speech is often not capitalized on. When speech is lacking, alternative communicative means such as physical orientation, gesture, and gaze are not used in a compensatory fashion. Moreover, means of communication are often highly idiosyncratic because they fail to become conventionalized through reciprocal interactions. What we are facing is a limited communicative repertoire that seems mostly motivated by the desire to maintain the order of the surrounding physical world. Minimizing people-induced disruptions of an otherwise predictable physical world may become a major source of motivation.

A differerent style of language learning may also serve to illustrate the impact of cognitive differences on language development. The impact of a so-called gestalt vs. analytic language learning style was discussed by Prizant (1983) with particular relevance to echolalia and overall communicative behavior in autism. The term "gestalt language" refers to the use of memorized multiword utterances that are reproduced as single units without recognition of their constituent structure. By contrast, analytic language is produced when words are recombined in novel ways through application of linguistic rules, recognizing the meanings of the individual words. While these different language styles have been noted to normally co-occur in young children who are learning to talk (Peters, 1983), the gestalt style is most prominent in autism. Not only are whole phrases memorized as a single unit, they are also often associated with the contexts in which they occurred or with the associated physical state of the child involved.

A common frustrating example of such a learning style is when a particular phrase is taught in a specific setting and reproduced in that context only. It is as if the utterance is memorized together with the surrounding decorum, like Grandin's description in Chapter 2 of her image-based "video replay" mode of thinking (Grandin, 1995). When the complete image is not broken down into its component parts, generalization is unlikely to occur. While this processing style complicates language learning, it is not specific to autism: it merely presents a case of extreme variation along the normal continuum. Thus challenged, parents, teachers, and clinicians must stage communicative contexts that are most meaningful, incorporating immediate experiences, highlighting those words and gestures that carry the most relevant information. Once the routine of relevant events in a specific context is understood, larger chunks of memorized speech can be broken down into pertinent component pieces. By the same token, limited comprehension and a reliance on too-complex memorized phrases will invite more stereotypic speech.

COGNITION AND SOCIAL INTERACTION

Cognitive differences are also pertinent to idiosyncrasies in play and social interaction. What is becoming increasingly clear is that the differences in social behaviors cannot be attributed merely to a lack of interest. While

older literature has often portrayed people with autism as preferring aloneness and actively withdrawing from social contacts, extended contacts with
autistic people suggest otherwise. Affectionate exchanges and interactions
with caregivers as well as peers in predictable contexts are often enjoyed.
Such informal observations in the context of interactions over time are validated by research examining developmental differences. For instance, comparisons with other young developmentally delayed children indicated
that children with autism showed no significant differences when specific
attachment behaviors were compared in autistic, developmentally delayed,
and normally developing children (Sigman & Mundy, 1989). Both clinical
groups showed less separation distress and less involvement with their
caregivers, and did not differ much when they were reunited with their
caregivers after separation.

In an examination of interaction style, Clark and Rutter (1981) have
shown that children with autism are not less compliant or more negativis-
tic than other children matched for developmental level. Similar findings
were also reported by Volkmar, Hoden & Cohen (1985). Similarities as well
as differences were reported by Sigman and her co-workers (Sigman &
Mundy, 1989; Sigman, Mundy, Sherman & Ungerer, 1986). While the children with autism did not differ in the frequency of social behaviors such
as looking at, vocalizing to, and seeking the proximity of their caregivers,
they produced less speech and less often shared their focus of attention
with others.

Lack of joint attention is also reflected in the peculiarities of play
behaviors. If they play at all, children with autism tend to play in stereotypic ways with objects and they typically remain isolated from their peers.
They may play in proximity to others, but tend not to take turns sharing
toys or cooperating on play scripts. While their object manipulations may
be creative, they are nevertheless stereotypic and lack the imaginative qualities of pretend play. (For more detailed descriptions, see Wing, Gould,
Yeates & Brierly, 1977; Sigman & Ungerer, 1984; and Mundy, Sigman &
Sherman, 1987.) Their lack of understanding of people's intentions and scenarios of narrative thought in general keeps them stuck in the physical
exploration of objects. Children with autism seem to have too little understanding of the social world around them to act it out in play. Moreover,
their isolation from peers robs them of the opportunity to transform ritualized behavior patterns into more diverse forms of action. Normally, adults
as well as more competent playmates imitate and expand exhibited stereotypic behaviors into more conventional forms.

Despite the challenges encountered, some children with autism have
been noted to develop play over time. In addition, more advanced play
skills have been observed in more structured contexts (Lewis & Boucher,
1988; Rogers and Lewis, 1989). The findings with the integrated play
groups (Wolfberg & Schuler, 1993) also indicate that play can be pursued

successfully. When interactions with nonhandicapped peers were indirectly mediated by adults in supportive contexts, autistic school-age children showed surprising social and cognitive gains. Not only did the participating children learn to use objects in more functional and imaginative ways, they also learned to coordinate their play with others, demonstrating gains in joint attention. They became more communicative, producing more contextually relevant speech and seemed to enjoy the play sessions. It's possible that the common lack of play skills is more a reflection of the effects of social isolation than a fundamental representation and metarepresentational deficit.

It appears that the syndrome of autism presents us not with a specific deviance or pathology maintained throughout development, but rather with a distinct developmental imbalance that may take different forms as a function of ongoing development. The imbalance may be so extreme that it is perceived as deviance, a perception that in turn may negatively affect interaction patterns, accelerating the process of social isolation.

CASE STUDY: Developmental Imbalances

Since commonly used assessment tools are not specifically designed to be used with autistic children, a valid and comprehensive assessment is not easily obtained. Consequently, the magnitude of the developmental imbalances may be missed. This is particularly so when the children involved are considered "untestable." Yet all children can be assessed as long as assessments are individualized and tailored to the particular constellation of skills encountered. Completion of such a comprehensive series of assessments can be most enlightening in terms of our understanding of the magnitude of the discrepancies involved. Therefore the following is a brief synopsis of a most unusual cognitive profile observed in a child that was identified through a comprehensive series of individualized assessments. (For more detailed descriptions of such assessments, see Schuler & Bormann, 1983; Wetherby & Prizant, 1989; and Papy, Papy & Schuler, 1994.)

Initial Observations of a Child Named Tom

Tom was referred to us at age 10 because he made very little progress despite extensive teaching efforts. He puzzled, inspired, and disappointed teachers, caregivers, and other professionals because of the amazing speed with which he would learn some new behaviors in specific contexts, not learn others, and fail to generalize newly taught behaviors or use them in functional contexts. Despite his failures, Tom looked bright when concentrating on a task of his own choice, such as the completion of a jigsaw puzzle. In other contexts he demonstrated high rates of stereotypic or even aberrant behaviors such as finger biting, particularly when forced to complete tasks in which he showed little interest.

While Tom had been described as mute, he would vocalize occasionally, particularly when he was content and engaged in a favorite activity, such as paper tearing. Given that these vocalizations were not accompanied by other forms of nonverbal communication such as gaze, body orientation, and pointing and showing gestures, they were not indicative of communicative intent. Tom's most advanced communicative behavior involved the ritualistic reenactment of sequences of behavior in anticipation of specific consequences, but without evidence of communicative intent. For instance, Tom would indicate his desire to eat by setting the table in his own ritualized fashion and by pacing back and forth between the refrigerator and his place mat. Tom's limited understanding of the impact of his own actions may be best illustrated by the ritualistic behaviors he engaged in when thirsty. After Tom had been taught to pour himself a glass of water, he was observed to serve himself a second glass, a third one, and so on. Having no concept of the impact of his own action, he would restart the entire pouring routine by taking out another drinking glass when left thirsty after the first sips of water.

An extensive assessment of Tom's speech comprehension skills revealed that despite observed compliance with everyday spoken instructions, comprehension was minimal in the absence of visual and/or contextual cues. He could not discriminate one single word from another when presented without contextual support. Apparently, Tom's sensitivity to contextual cues and his memorization of everyday routines enabled him to compensate for limited speech comprehension. Tom exhibited some imitation skills when prompted, but he never used them spontaneously for social or cognitive purposes. He did not imitate gestures or vocalizations to initiate or maintain a social interaction, nor did he imitate the actions of others as a means to solve problems. When prompted to imitate, Tom was cued by the location of actions rather than by their progression over time. For instance, Tom was unable to discriminate between single and repeated pound-

ing motions despite extensive training. Discriminative responses were secured only when a particular location on the surface of the table top—that is, a spatial discrimination—was used to cue the temporal discrimination.

In marked contrast to Tom's severe communicative limitations, he demonstrated considerable skill in sorting, assembling, and matching tasks, evidencing a keen eye for visual detail. However, he failed to demonstrate such skills when spatial skills were assessed in a loosely structured, interactive context. It was as if Tom knew what to do as long as a reliable response mode was made available to him. In fact, Tom took on an alert and engaged appearance when adults structured learning tasks around objects and actions that fascinated him.

Tom's Knowledge of Objects Versus People

A series of highly structured nonverbal assessments were designed to supplement the information gathered by naturalistic or semi-structured observations. For this purpose an assessment format was adopted that incorporated discrimination teaching and subsequent generalization testing. This means that the true assessment trials were presented only after Tom had demonstrated to understand what he was supposed to do through training on practice items.

An examination of Tom's understanding of the world of objects surrounding him revealed that he could match not only identical objects but also similar ones. When asked to match objects because of their shared functions, he failed to do so, but would continue to match on the basis of single physical properties such as shape, color, size, symmetry, and so on. For instance, when asked to match a pen with a piece of scribbled paper, he selected another skinny long object, particularly if it was of a similar color or size. Shifting among a range of physical attributes, he demonstrated remarkably flexible problem-solving skills.

We wondered whether Tom's remarkable visual discrimination and memorization skills deserved any cognitive credit. Would he be able to categorize nonverbally? For instance, would Tom be able to figure out that the mirror-imaged versus parallel-imaged card was the one to be selected when presented with such contrasting pairs, and reinforcement was provided for the correct choice? To evaluate this, a series of nonverbal guessing games were designed that required Tom to figure out which card to select from a stack of paired cards, presenting all the same conceptual themes. Tom had no trouble figuring out any of the rules presented: big versus small, more versus less, same versus different, round versus sharp, centered versus off-centered, and rotated versus nonrotated. Moreover, Tom was extremely quick in doing so. The remarkable speed with which he operated suggested that he used a strategy different from the strategy most of us use when presented with such a task. Most likely he approached the task in a gestalt-like fashion, looking for analogies and regularities in spatial configurations.

Given Tom's demonstrated understanding of the physical attributes of objects and spatial images, his understanding of the numbers 1 through 5 was nonverbally assessed. Again, Tom could easily match all different configurations of the numbers 1 through 5, giving evidence of basic number conservation. Because these findings were congruent with Tom's overall performance on the nonverbal tasks summarized so far, it was felt that some cognitive credit was due. Apparently Tom was capable of some type of nonverbal reasoning that allowed him to make inferences and detect rules. Hence generalized cognitive failure was not a likely reason of his failure to communicate. Instead it could be a function of the stimulus properties of the communicative and linguistic signals involved and not of the linguistic operations as such. Tom might be able to express

communicative intentions and use principles of reference and grammar if the linguistic content would be presented through a nonspeech mode. For instance, it might be possible to teach Tom nonspeech labels for the numbers 1 through 5, mapping a referential operation onto demonstrated cognitive understanding. The next series of assessments were designed to determine whether nonspeech modes of communication would be preferable.

Tom's Acquisition of Spoken Versus Signed Versus Written Labels

To allow for a fair comparison of differential learning rates, Tom's prior knowledge was evaluated by taking baseline measures of his understanding of spoken versus signed versus written labels. For this purpose Tom was presented with ten common objects, which he was to manipulate physically when presented with either spoken, signed, or written word labels. When all extraneous cues were removed and percentages of correct responses to spoken, signed, and written word labels were compared, it was found that all of Tom's responses were at or below chance level. In other words Tom didn't comprehend any of the signed, spoken, or written word labels presented to him. Prior to the removal of those cues, Tom's performance had been considerably higher but completely inconsistent. It became evident that Tom's performance had been boosted by an amazing capacity to utilize inadvertent cues.

To ensure that a valid comparison of acquisition rates across modalities could be made, three sets of receptive labels were taught simultaneously through differential reinforcement and prompting. Three pairs of objects to be labeled were selected randomly from our collection of ten baseline objects. Written word labels were taught in reference to the presentation of either a block or a glass, signed labels to a book or a shoe, and spoken labels to a fork or a piece of soap.

Through use of differential reinforcement, Tom was trained to point to either the block or the glass when the corresponding written word label was placed in front of him. Similar procedures were used to teach the discriminations between the selected signed and spoken word pairs. At all times, equal numbers of differentially reinforced training trials were presented across all training modes so that fair comparisons could be made.

When no improvements in percent of correct scores were observed after extensive training (completion of 500 training trials) it was decided to discontinue signed and spoken word training. Tom would learn quickly to pick up one particular object in response to a particular spoken or signed word, but his responses would invariably drop to chance level when all extraneous cues were removed. In contrast, Tom would learn pairs of written word labels within the minimal number of trials possible (20) and without any errors, including the written word alternatives for the failed spoken and signed labels. In addition, the adults were unable to use the acquired written word labels as a prompt to teach him to discriminate between pairs of spoken and signed word labels. Tom's performance dropped back to chance level as soon as all extraneous written word cues were removed. It was as if he were incapable of making discriminations regarding the intrinsic features of the spoken and signed words themselves.

To further evaluate the quality of Tom's learning, more abstract forms of reference were introduced. The first question asked was whether Tom would be able to infer equivalence on the basis of second-order association. For this purpose, "cube" and "tumbler" were presented as synonyms of "block" and "glass" in the absence of the actual objects. Would Tom be able to associate the newly taught synonyms with the actual objects despite the fact that they had never been presented together?

The second question was whether Tom would be able to learn written word labels in reference to object attributes such as big versus little and same versus different as well as digital representations for the numbers 1 through 5. Tom was successful in all these endeavors. Despite initial hesitation, Tom scored 100 percent correct on the second order matching task. He made virtually no errors on any of the attribute labels and, more important, provided evidence of generalization. Apparently Tom was capable of more abstract levels of representation. The fact that Tom could handle an algorithm (if $a=b$ and $b=c$, then a=c) seemed quite an achievement given his overall developmental level.

Because the findings so far suggested that idiosyncracies of the mode of representation rather than the representative act as such may have been the major obstacle in language learning, the final assessment sought to determine if Tom could handle word combinations. The assessments examined whether Tom could comprehend and/or produce two- and three-word statements utilizing written word cards in reference to compound perceptual distinctions (for example, big cup versus little cup and three little cups versus two little cups). It was found that Tom could handle two-word combinations but no more than that. Expressing demonstrated conceptual understanding into serial order seemed a mind-boggling exercise.

Discussion

Tom's overall performance across domains, while highly discrepant, is nevertheless consistent across tasks and assessment contexts. His ability to think about spatial relations and objects and their physical attributes contrasts sharply with his limited understanding of the dynamics of communication. His lack of communicative intent and presymbolic levels of representation through memorized action sequences are remarkably out of line with his apparent ability to reason about the physical qualities of the world around him. The fact that the written-word mode of communication was much more accessible seems consistent with his facility for spatial forms of thinking. The specific cognitive profile and the associated learning style, while highly discrepant, are nevertheless remarkably consistent with the ways in which the relative strengths and weaknesses of autistic individuals have been described in the literature.

KANNER REVISITED

The symptomatology of the autistic syndrome may thus be best understood as the product of imbalances in evolving thought processes, not as a fixed collection of symptoms. Developmental processes transform the behaviors involved. For instance, a young child who shows a lack of eye contact may turn into an adolescent who demonstrates too much eye contact and positions himself or herself too close for comfort. The behaviors change, but what remains is discrepancy among dimensions of development. The syndrome of autism seems to specifically affect those aspects of cognition that were referred to as "dynamic" by Bates (1979) in her account of the symbolic development of our species. She includes imitation, symbolization, and tool use in this category as opposed to what she calls the "static" aspects of cognition, referring to object knowledge and the construction of objects in space. The most classic forms of autism may thus be conceptualized as resulting from the most severe limitations in social understanding contrasted by advanced or even precocious skills in those domains of development that are not dependent on social interaction, such as spatial, motor, and memory skills and object knowledge. By the same token, less pronounced discrepancies would be associated with less classic forms of autism and related disorders. Additional variation in symptomatology might stem from the heterogeneity in terms of causation, which seems to be generally acknowledged now.

Thinking About Objects Versus People

The cognitive profile exhibited by Tom and by so many others validates Kanner's speculation that thinking about objects and thinking about people are different enterprises. The finding that social use of communication is more affected than instrumental use in autism is consistent with Kanner's related observation that communication in autism may be motivated by the need to regulate one's physical environment rather than one's social environment. In Tom's case the most advanced forms of communication involved ritualized action sequences centered around daily eating ceremonies, the operation of mechanical devices, and the overall preservation of order in his everyday environment. While he would physically manipulate others to cooperate with his agenda, he didn't seem aware of them as communicative partners.

Current views of early communicative development that emphasize the importance of joint attention and action (Bruner, 1975) may explain why a lack of people-referenced thinking would compromise early communicative development. Normally, the integration of object- and people-referenced thinking sets the stage for the emergence of communicative intent. At around 9 months, typical children learn to combine their knowledge of objects and people by using objects to gain their caregivers' attention. And they learn to use those same caregivers to help them access desired objects.

Communicative intent is normally accompanied by the appearance of showing and pointing motions. Locked in their ritualistic behaviors, autistic children tend to remain object-oriented; hence pointing and showing motions generally fail to appear. It is as if sharing attention with others is a pursuit that they have not yet come to value. Their communicative efforts seem mostly prompted by more tangible pursuits such as the desire for particular foods or objects as well as the maintenance of routines and order. Lack of reciprocal action in autism may also serve to explain the prevalence of repetitive behavior. Normally, children learn to break down memorized routines through shared dialogue facilitated by joint action and attention. Because significant others had not been able to enter into Tom's world of strict schedules and ritualistic object manipulations, his behavior had not become diversified and normalized.

Limitations in people-oriented thinking interfere not only with learning how to intentionally impact on the behaviors of others, but also with the appreciation of other people's mental states. Clearly, the development of intentional communication and a "theory of mind" go hand in hand. To develop a theory of mind, we must expand our appreciation of intentionality. Moreover, the social functions of communication as well as pragmatic competence at large hinge on our understanding of the feelings, beliefs, desires, and perspectives of others. Therefore it's not surprising that more specific linguistic aspects of communication are often less impaired. In Tom's case it was most curious to see how quickly he learned to associate the written word label with its referent object. Nevertheless, learning to use such labels in a more pragmatic sense would be a different matter. The specific profile of communicative, social, and linguistic differences is thus consistent with the dissociation between object and people related thinking.

Behavior Differences and the Need for Sameness

Developmental imbalances have further-reaching consequences. They also account for much of the commonly associated behavioral excesses and deficiencies that make parenting and teaching such a challenge. A first point that needs to be appreciated is that many people with autism are more tuned in to the physical characteristics of their environments than other people are. They tend to perceive even the slightest changes—a misplaced chair, a new hairstyle, a different table setting—and are particularly sensitive to violations of routines. Their limited comprehension of both verbal and nonverbal communication leaves them unprepared for the continuous changes that are part of our species' lifestyle and culture. Consequently they rely on the predictability of routines and the preservation of physical order to deal with an otherwise too-unpredictable world.

Social intelligence is what enables people to cope with changes in scenarios and settings. An appreciation of the intentions and feelings of others and an understanding of the cause and effects of our own as well as their actions help us to interpret change. Anxieties associated with novelty and change are relieved by our ability to interpret the people cues, creating a coherent scenario. Confronted with covered-up furniture, paintbrushes, and ladders, we understand that someone must have been painting. When our social and object intelligences are balanced, we can explain perceived changes in our physical world. Given this need to understand the various scenarios that guide people's actions, people with autism could be helped if they could learn to generate interactive patterns as well as stories about themselves and others (see Chapters 7, 8, and 9).

The repercussions of the developmental imbalances we have discussed extend beyond the common need for sameness and literalness. They also affect the dynamics of personal interactions, particularly when observed in children who appear so competent in certain contexts and who look bright and appealing rather than handicapped. For instance, it is very easy to become frustrated with a child such as Tom, who might when we least expect it produce an approximation of the word "ball," yet fail to make any sound at times when we try hard to make him produce speech. It might be equally irritating that this messy eater is so meticulous when completing his own table setting. If we didn't recognize the developmental imbalances involved, we might attribute negative intentions to this child and be tempted to describe him as mischievous or uncooperative. Needless to say, these types of attributions can easily set the stage for power struggles. When our expectations about behavior are violated and our sense of control and predictability is undermined, we will look for ways to regain control and reduce the anxiety that comes from the unexpected.

Written Word Preferences

Tom's preference for written words did not come as a surprise given the accumulated literature and frequent case reports on unusual decoding skills. Their unusualness has prompted use of the term "hyperlexia" to refer to precocious reading skills that are perceived to be out of line with overall levels of intellectual and linguistic development. (For a recent detailed discussion of this phenomenon, see Welsh, Pennington & Rogers, 1987.) Nevertheless, the extent of the discrepancies is what was surprising. Since Tom's precociousness with written words was probably related to his superior spatial abilities, a careful consideration of how spoken words differ from written words is in order. With written words, the discriminations involved are of a spatial and not of a temporal nature. Consequently, integrity of temporal processing mechanisms is not required. The nontransient nature of the stimulus input involved eliminates sequential analysis and temporal processing requirements. When transient stimulus input is presented, information is coded in a time-dependent way; the information presented fades rapidly as a function of time.

Despite the fact that sign language involves the visual rather than the auditory modality, the same constraint applies, albeit to a lesser extent. Problems in the processing of transient stimulus input could thus account for the written-word preferences. Such a hypothesis seems further supported by Tom's inability to imitate repeated versus single hand motions and DeMyer's (1975) observations. These kinds of discrepancies invite etiological speculations such as those that might explain the possible contribution of perceptual dysfunctions or idiosyncracies.

Transient Versus Nontransient Stimulus Input

Tom's apparent preference for nontransient over transient stimulus input could be explained by a selective impairment in the processing of transient information. Both objects and their physical attributes as well as written words remain visible over time, whereas spoken words, gestures, and even signs are all transformed as a function of time. As discussed by Prizant and Schuler (1987), gestalt-like processing of nontransient information would suffice for the examination of objects and their physical surroundings.

Guided by factor-analytic research of standardized test performance, pertinent differences in information processing have been claimed by Das (1984). Commensurate with the processing of transient as opposed to nontransient information, Das made a differentiation between a so-called sequential as opposed to a simultaneous mode of processing. It is interesting that the differentiation made by Das resembles a similar distinction by Luria (1973) made within a larger developmental and neuropsychological framework. Thus the fact that we may truly be dealing with different modalities of mind is relevant to our theoretical understanding of the syndrome of autism as well as to our interactions with individuals affected by the syndrome.

The postulation of separate biological underpinnings and different evolutionary histories of these different modes of processing might explain the selective impairment in sequential analysis. Limitations in the perception of transient stimulus input would obviously thwart social development, as both the signals regulating social interactions and the interactions themselves are largely transient. Furthermore, such perceptual troubles would compromise the imitation of body movements, which, as Rogers and Pennington (1991) recently pointed out, would constitute a major impediment to social development.

Alternatively, the discrepancies in functioning demonstrated by Tom could be attributed to limited social experience. Normally, infants may be sensitized to transient signals by their active participation in social interactions with their caregivers. As claimed by Hobson (1990), more basic problems in affective relating might lead to a different cognitive style that operates in a gestalt fashion. Limited social responsiveness and the resulting lack of experience in processing social stimuli might result in atypical attention and processing patterns and ultimately differences in cognitive style. In addition, transactional effects could make perceptual troubles difficult to separate from problems in interpersonal relating.

While the presence and nature of perceptual problems and their interference with social functioning remains speculative, it is clearly helpful to present information in a visuo-spatial form. While the case study that was reported here would not predict major breakthroughs through this mode of communication, it would nevertheless not be surprising if Tom were to produce quite an array of written words given his excellent "gestalt" memory. In fact, with physical support he might be capable of producing an impressive collection of "echographic" utterances.

Multiple Intelligences

The cognitive discrepancies observed in autism are most pertinent to our understanding of nonverbal modes of thinking. What is suggested by the story of Tom is that considerable cognitive sophistication can be attained in the absence of language or related representational processes. Isolated areas of competence involving object knowledge and visuo-spatial skills challenge more traditional, unidimensional views of cognition and intelligence. While the notion of intelligence as a unitary entity has dominated the field of psychology, constructs of intelligence as one-dimensional have become increasingly subjected to criticism. Some of the fallacies surrounding the factor-analytic construct of -g- , referring to generalized capability, have been discussed by Gould (1981), and an alternative view of intelligence as composed of a number of multiple intelligences has been formulated by Gardner (1983). According to Gardner, linguistic intelligence is merely one of a number of intelligences that he believes to be distinct in terms of their neurophysiological makeup and relatively independent of one another. Such differentiations among types of intelligence have more explanatory power when we are confronted with striking developmental discrepancies and imbalances .

The prevalence of unidimensional views of intelligence may serve to explain the persistence of psychodynamic interpretations of autism as an emotional disorder favoring notions such as rejection and withdrawal. One is more likely to attribute developmental lags to some type of deviance when invested in unidimensional views of learning and intelligence. A limited appreciation of diversity along with a deficiency orientation may have limited opportunities for communicative growth for many individuals with autism. Portrayals of individuals as deviant or deficient easily leads to the construction of narrow deficiency-based categorical services as well as to coercion and aversive forms of behavior management. Such environments are also defined by externally imposed forms of learning, which fail to provide students with the opportunities to exert self-control and engage in reciprocal actions that constitute the core of communicative competence. The differences in cognition and learning style that were described here have profound implications for intervention and are reflected in the remaining chapters of this book. We hope they will inspire the type of changes in service delivery that are needed to promote social and communicative growth.

IMPLICATIONS FOR EDUCATION

The challenge of accessing a different form of intelligence with which we share neither a common symbol system nor even a mode of nonverbal exchange will color any educational intervention or clinical interaction. It seems that all such interventions and interactions should be designed to help reduce the confusion and uncertainty inherent to the autistic state of mind, and to generate a sense of efficacy, control, and predictability that comes from within and is not externally imposed. Externally imposed order and predictability is useful in reducing the anxiety of a world otherwise perceived as chaotic. Nevertheless, it presents the risk of mental submission. Such submission may surface as lack of spontaneity and initiative, may thwart generalization, and may ultimately lead to depression.

To enhance a sense of efficacy, we must establish an effective means of communication. The studies of Tom and the other accumulated evidence of more advanced written language skills suggest that the written word can provide a versatile alternative that can be supplemented by other means. Visuo-spatial modes of representation will always help to capture the order of daily schedules and events and to adopt modes of instruction that are not dependent on spoken language, capitalizing on areas of strength. Instruction should be built around the interests and initiatives of the individuals involved, even when most or even all of such initiatives take unconventional forms, including fascinations with objects and routines. Since autistic children may initially be incapable of establishing a joint focus of attention and action, reciprocity will fail to be established without such accommodations. Communication will remain a one-way enterprise if the child's initiations and fascinations are not acknowledged. Therefore close observation and ongoing evaluations of current levels of understanding and competence are critical. Such observations should be designed to determine the highest level of competence given the optimal amount of social assistance, allowing for scaffolded performance within the zone of proximal development, as defined by Vygotsky (1978).

In order to accomplish this, interventionists and clinicians need to examine their own levels of discomfort when common behavior expectations and norms are violated. It is conceivable that efforts to impose structure are more a reflection of the adults' anxiety, uneasiness, and need to reestablish control on their own terms. In order to provide children with a sense of control and a structure that serves them, adults need to become comfortable observers who can select motivating tasks and activity contexts that invite a sense of competence. They must be willing to scrutinize their own motivations, language use, and communicative style. Consequently, growth is pursued as a collaborative and increasingly reciprocal enterprise.

REFERENCES

American Psychiatric Association. (1987). *Diagnostic and statistical manual of mental disorders* (3rd ed., rev.). Washington, DC: Author.

Baron-Cohen, S., Leslie, A. M., & Frith, U. (1985). Does the autistic child have a theory of mind? *Cognition, 21,* 37–46.

Baron-Cohen, S., Leslie, A. M., & Frith, U. (1986). Mechanical, behavioural and intentional understanding of picture stories in autistic children. *British Journal of Developmental Psychology, 4,* 113–115.

Bates, E. (1979). *The emergence of symbols: Cognition and communication in infancy.* New York: Academic.

Biklen, D. (1990). Communication unbound: Autism and praxis. *Harvard Educational Review, 60,* 291–314.

Bruner, J. (1975). From communication to language: A psychological perspective. *Cognition, 3,* 255–289.

Clark, P., & Rutter, M. (1981). Autistic children's response to structure and interpersonal demands. *Journal of Autism and Developmental Disorders, 11,* 201–217.

Curcio, F. (1978). Sensorimotor functioning and communication in mute autistic children. *Journal of Autism and Childhood Schizophrenia, 8,* 181–189.

Das, J. P. (1984). Simultaneous and successive processing in children with reading disabilities. *Topics in Language Disorders, 4,* 34–48.

DeMyer, M. K. (1975). The nature of neuropsychological disability in autistic children. *Journal of Autism and Childhood Schizophrenia, 5,* 109–128.

Fay, W. H., & Schuler, A. L. (1980). Emerging language in autistic children. In R. L. Schiefelbusch (Ed.), *Language intervention series.* Baltimore: University Park Press.

Frith, U. (1971). Spontaneous patterns produced by autistic, normal and subnormal children. In M. Rutter (Ed.), *Infantile autism: Concepts, characteristics and treatment.* London: Churchill Livingstone.

Frith, U. (1989). *Autism: Explaining the enigma.* Oxford, England: Blackwell.

Gardner, H. (1983). *Frames of mind.* New York: Basic Books.

Gould, S. J. (1981). *The mismeasurement of man.* New York: Norton.

Grandin, T. (1995). The learning style of people with autism. IN K.A. Quill (Ed.), *Teaching children with autism: Strategies to enhance communication.* Albany, NY: Delmar.

Hermelin, B. (1976). Coding and the sense modalities. In L. Wing (Ed.), *Early childhood autism.* London: Pergamon.

Hermelin, B., & O'Connor, N. (1970). *Psychological experiments with autistic children.* London: Pergamon.

Hobson, R. P. (1990a). Beyond cognition: A theory of autism. In G. Dawson (Ed.), *Autism: New perspectives on diagnosis, nature and treatment.* New York: Guilford.

Hobson, R. P. (1990b). On the origins of self and the case of autism. *Development and Psychopathology, 2,* 163–182.

Kanner, L. (1943). Autistic disturbances of affective contact. *Nervous Child, 2,* 217–250.

Lewis, V., & Boucher, J. (1988). Spontaneous, instructed and elicited play in relatively able autistic children. *British Journal of Developmental Psychology, 6* (4), 325–339.

Lovaas, O. I., Schreibman, L., Koegel, R., & Rehm, R. (1971). Selective responding by autistic children to autistic children to multiple sensory input. *Journal of Applied Behavior Analysis, 6,* 131–166.

Luria, A. R. (1973). *The working brain.* Middlesex, England: Penguin Books.

Mundy, P., Sigman, M., J., U., & Sherman, T. (1987). Nonverbal communication and play correlates of language development in autistic children. *Journal of Child Psychology and Psychiatry, 27,* 657–669.

Papy, F., Papy, G., & Schuler, A. L. (1994). *Pensee Autiste sans language.* Paris: Centurion.

Peters, A. (1983). *The units of language acquisition.* London: Cambridge University Press.

Prior, M. (1979). Cognitive abilities and disabilities in autism: A review. *Journal of Abnormal Child Psychology, 2,* 357–380.

Prior, M., Dahlstrom, D., & Squires, T. L. (1990). Autistic children's knowledge of thinking and feeling states in other people. *Journal of Child Psychology & Psychiatry, 31,* 587–601.

Prizant, B. (1983). Language acquisition and communicative behavior in autism: Toward an understanding of the "whole" of it. *Journal of Speech and Hearing Disorders, 48,* 296–307.

Prizant, B., & Duchan, J. (1981). The functions of immediate echolalia in autistic children. *Journal of Speech and Hearing Disorders, 46,* 241–249.

Prizant, B., & Schuler, A. L. (1987). Facilitating communication: Theoretical foundations. In D. C. &. A. Donnellan (Ed.), *Handbook of autism and pervasive developmental disorders.* New York: Wiley.

Rimland, B. (1964). *Infantile autism.* New York: Appleton-Century-Crofts.

Rogers, S. J., & Lewis, H. (1989). An effective day treatment model for young children with pervasive developmental disorders. *Journal of the American Academy of Child and Adolescent Psychiatry, 28,* 207–214.

Rogers, S. J., & Pennington, B. F. (1991). A theoretical approach to the deficits in infantile autism. *Development and Psychopathology, 3,* 137–162.

Ross, A. O. (1976). *Psychological aspects of learning of learning disabilities and reading disorders.* New York: McGraw-Hill.

Schover, L. R., & Newsom, C. D. (1976). Overselectivity, developmental level and overtraining in autistic and normal children. *Journal of Abnormal Child Psychology, 4,* 289–297.

Schuler, A. L. (1979). Echolalia: Issues and clinical applications. *Journal of Speech and Hearing Disorders, 44,* 411–434.

Schuler, A. L., & Bormann, C. (1983). The interrelations between cognitive and communicative development; some implications of the study of a mute autistic adolescent. In C. L. Thew and C. E. Johnson (Eds.), *Proceedings of the Second International Congress on the Study of Child Language* (pp. 269–282). Washington, DC: University Press of America.

Sigman, M., & Mundy, P. (1989). Social attachments in autistic children. *Journal of the American Academy of Child and Adolescent Psychiatry, 28* (1), 74–81.

Sigman, M., Mundy, P., Sherman, T., & Ungerer, J. A. (1986). Social Interactions of autistic, mentally retarded, and normal children and their caregivers. *Journal of Child Psychology and Psychiatry, 27,* 647–656.

Sigman, M., & Ungerer, J. A. (1984). Cognitive and language skills in autistic, mentally retarded, and normal children. *Developmental Psychology, 20,* 293–302.

Volkmar, F. R., Hoden, E. L., & Cohen, D. J. (1985). Compliance, negativism and the effects of treatment structure in autism: A naturalistic behavior study. *Journal of Child Psychology and Psychiatry, 26,* 865–877.

Vygotsky, L. S. (1978). *Mind in society: The development of higher psychological processes.* Cambridge, MA: Harvard University Press.

Welsh, W., Pennington, B. F., & Rogers, S. (1987). Word recognition and comprehension skills in hyperlexic children. *Brain and Language, 32,* 76–96.

Wetherby, A., & Prutting, C. (1984). Profiles of communicative and cognitive-social abilities in autistic children. *Journal of Speech and Hearing Research, 27,* 364–377.

Wetherby, A. M., & Prizant, B. M. (1989). The expression of communicative intent: Assessment guidelines. *Seminars in Speech and Language, 10,* 77–91.

Wimmer, H., & Perner, J. (1983). Beliefs about beliefs: representation and constraining function of wrong beliefs in young children's understanding of deception. *Cognition, 13,* 103–128.

Wing, L. (1974). *Autistic children.* Secaucus, NJ: Citadel.

Wing, L., Gould, J., Yeates, S. R., & Brierly, L. M. (1977). Symbolic play in severely mentally retarded and autistic children. *Journal of Child Psychology and Psychiatry, 18,* 167–178.

Wolfberg, P., & Schuler, A. (1993). Integrated play groups: A model for promoting the social and cognitive dimensions of play. *Journal of Autism and Developmental Disorders, 23,* 467–490.

2

The Learning Style of People With Autism: An Autobiography

Temple Grandin

Some people are successful in teaching children with autism and others are not. Being successful requires an understanding of how people with autism think and feel. In this chapter, I will describe my experiences with autism and how my experiences relate to teaching methods. I will share my style of thinking and learning, perceptions of different sensory information, communication frustrations, and social and emotional issues. Scientific literature relevant to my experiences will be reviewed. I will also provide a model for thinking about general subtypes of autism that I recently developed (Grandin, 1993). This idea of general subtypes is based on my interviews with hundreds of parents and reviews of the scientific literature on autism. Finally, I will conclude the chapter with some teaching tips and suggestions for educators and parents.

COGNITIVE PROFILE

Observations by parents and testing by professionals both indicate that children with autism excel at tasks such as putting puzzles together and building things out of blocks. It is well known that children with autism perform well at spatial, perceptual, and matching tests and that they are most impaired at verbal tests that require comprehension and language expression (Prior, 1979). Autistic children and deaf children respond in a similar manner as stimuli are mapped in visual space (Hermelin, 1972). Normal children remember a series of numbers based on their order of presentation. Autistic children will recall the numbers based on their position on the page. The number on the far left is recalled first regardless of the sequence used to present the numbers.

Nine years ago I took some tests to determine my abilities and deficits. On the Hiskey-Nebraska Test of Learning Aptitude (Hiskey, 1955) Spatial Reasoning subtest, my score was at the top of the norms. On the Woodcock-Johnson Psycho-Educational Battery (Woodcock & Johnson, 1977) Spatial Relations Test, I got a middle-range score because it was a timed speed test. I am not a quick thinker, as it takes time for me to create the visual image. When I survey a site for equipment at a meat-packing plant, it takes twenty to thirty minutes of staring at the building to fully imprint the site in my memory. Once this is done, I have a "video" I can play back when I am working on the drawing. Research by Boucher and Lewis (1989) suggests that being able to look at a picture for a long period of time may aid an autistic child's memory.

When I was a child, I scored 120 and 137 on the Wechsler Intelligence Scale for Children. My adult scores on the Memory for Sentences, Picture Vocabulary, and Antonyms-Synonyms subtests of the Woodcock-Johnson were superior. On the Memory for Numbers subtest, I beat the test by repeating the numbers out loud. I have an extremely poor long-term memory for things such as phone numbers unless I can convert them to visual images. For example, the number 65 is retirement age and I imagine somebody in Sun City, Arizona. If I am unable to take notes, I cannot remember what people tell me unless I translate the verbal information to visual pictures.

At age 36, I got a second-grade score on the Woodcock-Johnson Blending subtest, for which I had to identify slowly sounded-out words. My performance on the Visual Auditory Learning subtest of the Woodcock-Johnson was very poor. I had to memorize the meaning of arbitrary symbols—for example, triangle means horse—and read sentences composed of symbols. I could learn only the ones where I was able to make a picture for each symbol: I imagined the triangle as a flag carried by a horse and rider. The Concept Formation subtest of the Woodcock-Johnson was another test with fourth-grade results. I am good at forming concepts of the real world. My ability to visualize broad unifying concepts from hundreds of journal articles has enabled me to outguess the "experts" on many livestock subjects. The Concept Formation subtest involved picking out a concept such as "large, yellow" and then finding it in another set of cards. The problem was, I could not hold the concept in my memory while I looked at the other cards. If I had been allowed to write the concept down, I would have done much better.

Visual Thinking

Most people in the so-called normal world think in words, but thinking in language and words is alien to me. I think totally in pictures. Visual thinking is like playing different tapes in a videocassette recorder in my imagination. I used to think that everybody thought in pictures until I conducted an informal thinking test on many people. The informal test consisted of asking people to "access their memory of cats" or some other object that was not in the person's immediate surroundings. Most "normal" people see an image of a cat that is a generalized generic cat image but they don't see a series of vivid cat "videos" unless they are an artist, an autistic child, or an engineer. They usually access their cat knowledge as auditory or written language. Some brilliant people have very little visual thought. One professor told me that facts just come to his mind instantly with no visual image. In contrast, I see in my imagination a series of "videos" of different cats. My cat concept consists of these series of "cat videos" that I have experienced. There is no generalized cat concept, and there is no language-based information in my memory. So to access spoken information about cats that I have heard in the past, I replay a "video" of the person talking to me. To retrieve facts about cats, I have to read them off a visualized page of a book or "replay the video" of some previous event. This method of thinking is slower than verbal thinking. It takes time to play the videotape in my imagination.

Visual thinking is a great asset in my career as a livestock equipment designer, and I have become internationally recognized in this field. Drafting elaborate drawings of steel and concrete livestock stockyards and equipment is easy. I can visualize a video of the finished equipment in my imagination and "test" to see if it will work. A brilliant autistic computer programmer told me that he visualized the entire program tree in his mind and then just filled in the code on each branch. A gifted autistic composer told me that he made "sound pictures." In all these cases, a hazy whole or gestalt is visualized and the details are added in a nonsequential manner. When I design equipment I often have a general outline of the system, and then each section of it becomes clear as I add details.

As a child and as a young adult, I was good at building things, but it took time to learn how the symbolic lines on a set of blueprints related to the "video" of a house or a piece of equipment that was in my imagination. After I learned to read plans, I could then instantly translate the symbols on the plans into a visualization of the finished structure. A similar problem was described by an articulate adult with autism. He was unable to associate diagrams of clock faces with telling time. He could have learned telling time more quickly if his teacher had used a real clock and turned the hands to different positions instead of using diagrams.

Visual thinking is also associated with intellectual giftedness. Albert Einstein was a visual thinker who failed his high school language requirement and relied on visual methods of study (Holton, 1971–72). His theory of relativity was based on visual imagery of moving boxcars and riding on light beams. Einstein's family history includes a high incidence of autism, dyslexia, food allergies, giftedness, and musical talent, and he himself had many autistic traits. An astute reader can find evidence of them in Einstein and Einstein (1987). Intellectual giftedness is common in the family histories of many persons with autism. In my own family history, my mother's grandfather was a maverick who started the largest corporate wheat farm in the world. One sister is dyslexic and is brilliant in the art of decorating houses.

When I think about abstract concepts such as relationships with people, I use visual images such as a sliding glass door. Relationships must be approached gently because barging forward too quickly may shatter the door. Thinking about the door was not enough; I had to actually walk through it. When I was in high school and college I had actual physical doors that symbolized major changes in my life, such as graduations. At night I climbed through a trap door on the roof of the dormitory to sit on the roof and think about life after college. The trap door symbolized graduation. The doors were a visual language for expressing ideas that are usually verbalized.

The use of visual symbols such as doors to describe abstract concepts is also reported by Park and Youderian (1974). Visualization enabled me to understand The Lord's Prayer. The power and the glory are high-tension electric towers and a blazing rainbow sun. The word "trespass" is visualized as a No Trespassing sign on the neighbor's tree.

I no longer use sliding doors to understand personal relationships, but I still have to relate a particular relationship with something I have read. For example, a fight between my neighbors was like the United States and Europe fighting over customs duties. All my memories are visual images of specific events. New thoughts and equipment designs are combinations and rearrangements of things I have previously experienced. I have a thirst to see and operate all types of livestock equipment because that programs the "visual computer."

Park (1967) explained that her daughter learned nouns first. Nouns are easy because they can be associated with pictures in one's mind. Inappropriate words are often used. For example, the name "Dick" was used to refer to painting. This happened because a picture of Dick painting furniture was seen in a book. Park also describes why her daughter had problems with pronoun reversal and won't say "I." She thinks her name is "you" because that's what people call her. Charlie Hart summed up autistic thinking with this statement about his autistic son Ted: "Ted's thought processes aren't logical, they are associational" (Hart, 1989).

Research findings indicate that verbal thinking and visual thinking work via different brain systems (Farah, 1989). The brain is compartmentalized by function (Damasio, 1991; Zeki, 1992). Studies of patients with brain damage indicate that one system can be damaged while another system may be normal. The brain has modular systems. These systems may work either together or singularly to perform different tasks. For example, people with certain types of brain damage can recognize objects with straight edges, but they cannot recognize objects with irregular edges. The brain module that recognizes irregular shapes has been damaged (Weiss, 1989). In autism, the systems that process visual-spatial problems are intact. There is a possibility that these systems may be expanded to compensate for deficits in language. The nervous system has remarkable plasticity; one part can take over and compensate for a damaged part (Huttenlocher, 1984).

Processing Problems

I have difficulty with long strings of verbal information. If directions from a gas station contain more that three steps, I have to write them down. Many people with autism have problems with remembering the sequence of a set of instructions. Children with autism perform best with written instructions that they can refer to, compared to verbal instructions or a demonstration of a task that requires remembering a sequence of steps (Boucher & Lewis, 1989).

Algebra is almost impossible, because I can't make a visual image and I mix up steps in the sequence. I have many dyslexic traits such as reversing numbers and mixing up similar-sounding words such as "over" and "other." Learning statistics was extremely difficult because I am unable to hold one piece of information in my mind while I do the next step. I had to sit down with a tutor and write down the directions for doing each test. Every time I do a t-test or a chi-square, I have to use notes. I have no problem understanding the principles of statistics, because I visualize the normal or skewed distributions. The problem is that I cannot remember the sequence for doing the calculations.

Donna Williams (1992), an autistic woman from Australia, describes similar difficulties. She was unable to learn math until she watched the teacher write out each step. Like me, she had to see every step written on paper. If the smallest step is left out, the autistic mind will be stumped. The visual image of all the written steps is essential. Donna also became very frustrated because her calculator did not have a button for finding percentages.

Words that have no concrete visual meaning such as "put" or "on" need to be seen in written form in order to be heard and remembered (Park, 1967). Written language is easier to understand than verbal language. Word processors should be introduced early to encourage writing, as typing is often easier than handwriting. Many people with autism have motor control problems that result in messy, illegible writing. Even highly verbal people with autism can often express themselves better using the written or typed word. When I want to describe how I really feel about something, I can express myself better in writing.

Difficulties in processing sequential information partly explain the problems some children with autism have understanding cause and effect. Hart (1989) describes an incident when his autistic son destroyed his favorite Mickey Mouse audio tape by pulling out the tape. He was trying to find Mickey inside the cassette. He finally understood that Mickey was not inside the cassette after the cassette was opened. Only then would he differentiate between the sound of Mickey and Mickey himself. Williams (1992) describes similar problems in that she always had difficulty with the concept of something being turned into something else; for example, flour being turned into cake or an animal being turned into a fur coat. To fully understand this concept she would need to actually see flour and other ingredients being converted into a cake.

Some autistic people who have severe cognitive impairments can be taught sequential activities such as cooking or doing the laundry but they do not have common sense when something goes wrong. Hart (1989) describes a mishap while his autistic brother was doing laundry. When the dryer broke, his brother just went on to the next step of the sequence he had learned and put the wet clothes in the dresser drawers. Children with autism have to be taught exactly what to do if something goes wrong. For example, if you miss the bus, you should call home or tell the teacher.

Learning to Read

Words are too abstract for me to remember. I would never have learned to read by the method that requires memorization of words. While children with autism vary in which method works best, old-fashioned phonics enabled me to learn to read. After I laboriously learned all the sounds, I was able to sound out words. Learning less than 100 sounds was easier for me than attempting to remember thousands of incomprehensible groups of symbols. One parent in Canada taught her autistic son to read in a similar manner, using Montessori methods. He eventually learned to communicate by typing.

Many nonverbal people with autism can understand speech, and some are capable of reading and writing. I learned how to write proper English because my parents spoke proper English with almost no slang. To determine correct grammar I "played a video" in my mind to see if the sentence sounded like Mom or Dad.

A visualized reading method developed by Miller and Miller (1989) has been reported to be beneficial for some children. In the Millers' method, each word has letters drawn to look like its respective meaning. For example, the word "fall" has the letters falling over, and the word "run" has letters that look like runners. A similar approach may also help some children learn speech sounds. For example, learning sounds would have been much easier if I had a picture of a choo-choo train for the "ch" sound and a cat for the hard "c" sound. Some children with autism might quickly memorize words that are associated with pictures. Williams (1992) explains that looking at the pictures in a book helped her to learn the meaning of the words. Words can be learned quickly if printed labels are placed on objects around the classroom. To recall the word, the child "replays a video" in his imagination of the object and its attached label. Reading books with clear pictures that realistically and accurately illustrate what the words are saying can also be very useful.

SENSORY SENSITIVITIES

For almost a decade, I have discussed sensory sensitivity problems in autism (Grandin, 1986, 1990, 1992a, 1992b). These problems are often overlooked in treatment programs for children with autism. Problems caused by noise sensitivity, oversensitivity to touch, and difficulties with rhythm all cause many behavior problems. These sensory sensitivities influence learning, communication, and social abilities.

Sound Sensitivity

Certain parts of the brain are underdeveloped and immature in people with autism. The areas of immature development are in the cerebellum, limbic system, and brain stem (Bauman, 1991; Courchesne, Yeung-Courchesne, Press, Hesselink & Jernigan, 1989; Hashimoto et al., 1992). They either overreact or underreact to sounds (Ornitz, 1985). Cerebellar abnormalities may play a role in sensory oversensitivity. The areas of the cerebellum that are abnormal in autism modulate sensory input (Crispino & Bullock, 1984). Stimulation of these areas with an electrode will make a cat hypersensitive to both sound and touch (Chambers, 1947).

Many behavior problems in the classroom are caused by noise sensitivity and fear of noises that hurt the children's ears. Bad behavior often occurs because the child is anticipating the onset of a hurtful sound. If a child screams when he sees a telephone, or tries to break it, he may be doing this because he wants to prevent it from ringing. Some children are afraid to go to the toilet because the toilet's flushing sound scares them. Other children with less severe sound-sensitivity problems may flush the toilet many times because they enjoy the sound. A child may scream when he is taken to gym because the loud echoes hurt his ears. Other sounds that can cause problems are high-pitched motor noises such as vacuum cleaners, air conditioning fans, and electric drills (Bemporad, 1979). Certain loud noises such as the school bell ringing hurt my ears like a dentist's drill hitting a nerve and it made my heart race.

All the behavior modification in the world is not going to stop a child from screaming if the sound of the bell hurts. Simple changes such as stuffing tissues in the school bell to soften the sound can really help.

Oversensitivity to sound is not uniform across the entire sound spectrum. A child is usually sensitive only to certain pitches or types of sound. High pitched sounds are usually more noxious than a low rumble. Other types of sounds that are often highly irritating and can cause fear reactions are rustling paper, electronic noises, or the sound of water flowing through a pipe (Stehli, 1991; Volkmar & Cohen, 1989). It has been reported that sound sensitivity may be reduced in some children after receiving auditory training (Stehli, 1991). Other methods that are helpful include using a Walkman and a favorite tape to mask noxious sounds, or having the child wear earplugs. Some children will hum or make odd noises to block out noxious sounds.

Repetitive stereotypic behavior is another way a child will screen out an overload of stimulation. I believe that children should not be allowed to spend over an hour a day engaging in rhythmic stereotypic rocking or flapping. There is a possibility that this may damage the developing nervous system by preventing the brain from receiving input. Experiments with animals indicate that certain areas of the brain become abnormal and hyperactive when sensory input is restricted (Melzack & Burns, 1965; Simons & Land, 1987).

Touch Sensitivity

Many people with autism, myself included, are hypersensitive to touch. When people hugged me at a young age, it sent an overwhelming tidal wave of stimulation through my system (Grandin, 1984, 1986, 1992a). Many children with autism seek deep pressure stimulation because it is calming to the nervous system, yet they show an aversion to other forms of touch. Touch sensitivity problems can sometimes be reduced by having the child work with an occupational therapist using sensory integration techniques (Ayres, 1979). Overarousal of the nervous system and hyperactivity can be reduced through the use of deep pressure and vestibular stimulation such as swinging or spinning (Grandin, 1992b; Bhatara, Clark, Arnold, Gunsett, & Smeltzer, 1981). Some simple methods for calming a child with deep pressure are rolling up in gym mats or getting under beanbag chairs. If parents report that a child has difficulty sleeping at night, suggest the use of a tight-fitting mummy sleeping bag (L. King, personal communication, July 1987). All of these activities should be conducted at a specific time each day as fun games. They must never be done immediately after bad behavior has occurred. This mistake would reward bad behavior. When the pressure stimulation is first introduced, the child may pull away from it. The therapist needs to be gently insistent to get the child to accept being touched. A firm touch is calming and a light touch will cause an alarm reaction in the child's overaroused nervous system. The stimulus should never be forced on the child (Grandin, 1989).

At the age of 18, I built a squeezing machine (Grandin, 1984, 1986, 1992). The machine consisted of two heavily padded boards that squeeze along the side of the body. The person using the machine has complete control over the duration of the pressure and the amount applied. It took a long time to relax in the machine and not try to pull away from it. This machine is now being used by several occupational therapists as part of a sensory integration program. Gradually, my overly sensitive nervous system became desensitized and I no longer flinched like a wild animal. My Siamese cat's reaction to me changed after I had used the squeeze machine. This cat used to run from me, but after using the machine I learned to pet the cat more gently and he decided to stay with me. I had to be comforted myself before I could give comfort to the cat.

Touch sensitivity can cause behavior problems. Both deep pressure stimulation and exercise can reduce self-stimulating behaviors. Deep pressure garments such as a Johst Vest used for pressure treatment of burns or bandages on the arms reduced self-injurious behavior, hand slaps, and self-stimulatory behaviors (Zisserman, 1992; McClure & Holtz, 1991). The beneficial effects of vigorous exercise on stereotypic behavior and disruptive behavior have been documented by Walters and Walters (1980) and McGimsey and Favell (1988). Opportunities for vigorous exercise each day can often improve classroom behavior.

Touch sensitivity problems may account for refusal to eat certain foods. Some children will limit their diet to three or four foods. I can't stand slimy foods because the feel of them in my mouth makes me gag. Other children may not like crunchy foods. One way to deal with the problem is to have an occupational therapist work on desensitizing the mouth. It is recommended to use a trained professional for the task and to make sure the child does not have a physical disorder that could cause choking. Another method is to mix small amounts of new foods with the child's favorite foods; for example, start with one pea in the middle of a pizza and gradually add vegetables and subtract pizza toppings.

Sometimes behavior may worsen when the seasons change. This may be due to touch sensitivity to clothes. After wearing shorts all summer, I could not tolerate the feeling of long pants against my skin. A normal person can adapt to the pants in several minutes, but my nervous system required over a week. New clothes also caused problems because scratchy seams and the label in the neck of a shirt scratched like sandpaper. Some simple changes in clothes can solve many of these behavior problems. I often wear a soft cotton T-shirt under blouses that would otherwise be intolerable. Even today I wear bras inside out because the scratchy feeling of the stitches is so intense I can't concentrate. Washing new clothes softens them and makes them easier to tolerate. Rough, scratchy fabrics should be avoided.

Rhythm Difficulties

Many people with autism, myself included, have problems with rhythm. I can generate a rhythm by myself, but I am unable to synchronize my rhythm with somebody else's rhythm. When people are clapping in time to the music at a concert, I am unable to synchronize my claps with theirs. The rhythm problems some children with autism display may also be related to speech problems. Research has shown that normal babies move in synchronization with adult speech (Condon & Sander, 1974). I think that autistic children fail to do this. They often have perfect pitch but have problems with the rhythm of music (O'Connell, 1974). Still, rhythmic activities with musical instruments can be very helpful. It is important to make sure that the music chosen does not hurt the child's ears. Female vocalists and high-pitched instruments such as the flute are most likely to cause problems.

As an adult, I find it difficult to determine exactly when I should break into a conversation. I cannot follow the rhythmic give and take of conversation. People have told me that I often interrupt, and I still have difficulty determining where the pauses are. Instead of breaking into the conversation when there is a pause, I break in a fraction of a second after the other speaker has started because there is a slight delay in my reaction. It is a physiological problem related to my difficulty in synchronizing my rhythmic clapping activity with somebody else. I still have difficulty with this problem and there is no easy way to deal with it because it seems to be an auditory processing deficit. The only thing I can do is wait for a really big gap in the conversation or interrupt at a time when it will seem least rude. I have learned from experience better times to interrupt.

Occupational therapists have found that speech can sometimes be induced in a nonverbal child if speech therapy is conducted while the child is swinging slowly on a swing (Ray, King, & Grandin,1988). Oscillating motion stimulates the vestibular system and the cerebellum. Swinging must be done as a fun game. If it ceases to be fun, stop immediately. Never force a child to swing, as forced vestibular stimulation can be dangerous.

Sensory Integration

A program that worked well for me may be painful and confusing to more severely impaired people with autism. For example, my speech therapist forced me to look at her. Some children with more severe sensory problems may withdraw further because the intrusion completely overloads their immature nervous systems. These children need a relaxed environment and receive input through only one sensory channel. Donna Williams, in her personal account of autism, explained that forced eye contact caused her brain to shut down. She said that people's words become a mumble jumble, and voices are often a pattern of sounds (Painter, 1992). She can use only one sensory channel at a time. She explained that if she listens to the intonation of speech, she can't hear the words. Only one aspect of incoming input can be attended to at a time. If she is distracted by the visual input of somebody looking in her face, she can't hear them. One man with autism explained that if somebody looked him in the eye, his mind went blank and thoughts stopped (Cesaroni & Garber, 1991). Another man with autism described confusing and mixing of sensory channels, as when sounds came through as color. He also said that touching the lower part of his face caused a sound-like sensation. Donna Willliams told me that she sometimes has difficulty determining her body's boundary. Sensory integration treatment, consisting of rubbing her skin with brushes, has helped. Even though she dislikes the tactile input from the brushes, she knows that it helps her different sensory systems to work together and become more integrated. Her sensory processing also becomes more normal when she is relaxed and is focusing on only one sensory channel.

COMMUNICATION FRUSTRATIONS

When I was a child, I usually could understand everything that adults said directly to me. When adults talked among themselves, it sounded like gibberish. I had the words I wanted to say in my mind, but I just could not get them out. It was like a big stutter. When my mother wanted me to do something, I often screamed. I screamed because it was the only way I could communicate. If something bothered me, I screamed. This was the only way I could express my displeasure. If I did not want to wear a hat, the only way I could communicate my desire not to wear the hat was to throw it on the floor and scream. Being unable to talk was utter frustration. I screamed every time my teacher pointed the pointer toward me. I was afraid because I had been taught at home never to point a sharp object at a person. I feared that the pointer would poke out my eye.

An observant teacher or parent can differentiate between screaming to communicate and screaming to avoid doing a task. If a child screams or spits during a lesson, the teacher must keep on teaching as if nothing has happened. If teaching is stopped, it reinforces bad behavior. If a child hits during teaching, just block the hit and keep on teaching. Sometimes I would have a tantrum just to see the adults get mad.

The speech therapist had to put me in a slight stress state so I could get the words out. She knew just how much to intrude. If she pushed too hard, I would have a tantrum; if she did not push enough, there was no progress. Often I would "space out" and the teacher would jerk me back to reality. Children with autism have also described buzzing or static in their ears that interferes with hearing. A man from Portugal wrote that carrying on a conversation was difficult because the sounds faded in and out like a distant radio station (White & White, 1987). Many children can learn to sing before they can speak. The brain circuits that control singing may be in a part of the brain with less impairment.

SOCIAL AND EMOTIONAL ISSUES

I was like a visitor from another planet who has to learn the strange ways of the aliens. I make social decisions based on intellect and logic. Memories of past experiences are used in the equation. I have learned from experience that certain behaviors make people mad. Sometimes my logical decisions are wrong because they are based on insufficient data. I compare experiences I have in my library of memories to a situation I am experiencing in the present. I then make a logical decision based on all the available data. For example, I often compare social relations with people with information I have read in the newspaper about international diplomacy; that is, a fight between Dick and Jane is like two countries fighting over trade rights. At the age of 45 I have a a vast data bank and am able to logically determine which people have good intentions and which people have bad intentions. When I was younger I was dismayed to discover that some people had bad intentions. This is something all people with autism have to learn. In business dealings I am now very good at figuring out a person's intentions.

Contact with normal children is essential to learn normal social behavior. I was mainstreamed into a normal kindergarten and first grade in small classes with experienced teachers. I needed to have normal examples of social behavior to emulate.

Social interactions are further complicated by physiological problems that autistic people have with attention shifting. People with autism require much more time to shift attention between auditory and visual stimuli (E. Courchesne, personal communication, July 1991). This would make it difficult to follow rapidly changing complex social interactions. Difficulties with remembering long strings of verbal information further hamper social interaction. These problems may be part of the reason adults with autism report that they become nervous and uncomfortable when they relate to people too much (Dewey, 1991).

Emotions

It is a mistake to assume that people with autism have no emotions. I definitely have emotions. When I was a child and other kids teased me, it really hurt and I became upset. I derive great emotional satisfaction from my career of designing livestock equipment. When a client is pleased with a facility that I designed, I am happy. Interviews conducted with other autistic adults indicate that it was important for them to please people (Dewey, 1991). If one of my projects fails to work or a client criticizes me unfairly, I become depressed and upset. Jack, a piano tuner interviewed by Dewey, reported similar sensitivities to criticism. I receive great emotional satisfaction by doing something that is of value to society. My work on livestock systems has resulted in improvements in animal treatment all over the United States. It also makes me feel good to help other people with autism and their parents. It is also very pleasurable for me to use my visualization skill to figure out a design problem. Exercising my cerebral cortex on an interesting design problem is fun. I have observed that my nonautistic engineering friends find intellectual use of the brain a very pleasurable activity. One major difference between me and many other people is that I use intellect and logic instead of emotions to guide my decision.

In a discussion about emotions in autism one must separate the variables of social interaction problems from emotions. People with autism desire emotional contact with other people but they are stymied by complex social interaction. Kanner (1971) states that an autistic person's obsessive and specialized interests are used to open the door of social contact. They become recognized for special knowledge of computers or trains. Asperger (1944) stated that normal children learn social skills instinctively, while people with autism learn everything by intellect. In people with autism, social adaptation has to proceed through the intellect. People with autism lack the basic instincts that make communication a natural process (Cesaroni & Garber, 1991).

Empathy is an emotion that is difficult for persons with autism to understand and express. I think that this is due to an overly sensitive, immature nervous system that prevents us from experiencing the comfort of being held. As a child, I wanted to feel the comfort of being held, but I would stiffen up, flinch, and jerk away for fear of losing control and being engulfed by a tidal wave of overstimulation. It was so intense that it was like the touch equivalent of finger nails scratching on a blackboard or screeching audio feedback from a public address system.

When I handle cattle in one of my handling systems at a feedlot or meat plant, and the animals remain calm and do not feel pain or discomfort, I have good emotional feelings. If the cattle become agitated or excited, I get upset. I often touch the animals as they walk up the chute because it helps me to be gentle with them. Recently I designed a new restraining chute for holding cattle during slaughter. It is operated with hydraulics. After some practice I learned to manipulate the controls so that the device would hold the cattle gently. When the cattle remained calm, I felt peaceful. Operating the device gently is an act of kindness, and a person has to really love the cattle in order to operate it humanely. Most people who love animals have such a negative emotional reaction to being in a slaughter plant that their emotions interfere with really empathizing with the cattle. As I operated the chute, I concentrated on holding the animal gently and was very careful not to squeeze him too hard. I wanted to make him as comfortable as possible during the last moments of his life. It was like being a hospice worker. When I think about this experience by replaying it on the "video" in my imagination, I feel good.

Directing Fixations

A review of the literature indicates that some successful high-functioning autistics have directed their childhood fixations into careers (Simons, 1974). Bemporad (1979) reported a case in which a childhood fixation for arithmetic formed the basis of a career of preparing fiscal efficiency reports. Kanner identified autism in 1943, and he followed up his original eleven cases in 1971 to see what had happened to them. There were six failures, two unknowns, one partial recovery, and two successes. The most successful individual, who had a childhood fixation with counting, works as a bank teller. In the fourth grade my fixation was election posters, buttons, and bumper stickers. At that time, I thoroughly disliked social studies and had little comprehension of how government worked. My fixation should have been drawn on to motivate study in history, social studies, and math.

A tour of the legislature would have stimulated my interest if I had seen the people I had previously learned to recognize on posters. Math could have been used in an assignment calculating Electoral College points. I could have been given reading assignments in newspapers and magazines throughout the course of an election. If a child is interested in vacuum cleaners, reading could be motivated by using a vacuum cleaner instruction book as a reading text. Principles of science and physics could be taught by learning how the vacuum cleaner motor works.

Another of my fixations was automatic sliding doors in supermarkets and airports. A teacher might wonder, "How can I use math, science, and English in a door fixation?" At the elementary level, tasks could be simple, such as requesting the door company to send its catalog. Adults might think such a catalog boring, but the autistic child with door fixation would find it fascinating. Math and geography could be involved by asking the child to find the door company on a map and measure the miles to it from the school.

I have made a successful career based on my fixation with cattle squeeze chutes. I have designed livestock handling systems for major ranches and meat companies all over the world. When I was in high school, many of my teachers and psychologists wanted to get rid of my fixation on cattle chutes. I am indebted to Mr. Carlock, my high school science teacher, who suggested that I read more about my interests in scientific journals.

More limited compulsions such as playing in water, twiddling coins, and looking at and jiggling keys can be broadened out and expanded into useful activities. Simons and Oishi (1987) describe a little boy whose compulsion was grabbing keys from strangers. The boy was told that he would be allowed to play with keys at two specific times each day and the rest of the day he had to leave them alone. The teacher then taught him concepts such as shapes and counting by playing games with keys. Fixations are powerful motivators. It is a mistake to try to stamp out fixations. They will be replaced by another fixation.

During my travels to many autism conferences I have observed many sad cases of autistic people who have successfully completed high school or college but have not been able to make the transition into the world of work. Some have become perpetual students because they thrive on the structured environment, and intellectual stimulation of college. For many able people with autism, college years were their happiest (Szatmari, Bartolucci, Bremner, Bond, & Rich,1989).

I would like to stress the importance of a gradual transition from an educational setting into a career. My present career of designing livestock facilities is based on an old childhood fixation. I used that fixation to motivate me to become an expert on cattle handling. Equipment I have designed is in all the major meat plants. I have also stimulated the meat industry to recognize the importance of humane treatment of livestock. I started visiting local feedlots and meatpacking plants while I was in college. Mentors in the business community helped me learn the livestock and meat industry and allowed me to visit their operations every week. They recognized my talents and tolerated my eccentricities. My mentors bluntly told me that I had to improve my clothing and grooming habits. In one of Kanner's papers about autistic people who that make a successful adaptation, he indicated that they made a conscious effort to do something about their peculiarities (Kanner, 1971).

The freelance route has enabled some people with autism to be successful and exploit their talent area. To get the business started, the person with autism needs someone to help secure some initial jobs. A freelance business also helps avoid some of the social problems with a job in one place. I can go in, do the design job, and then get out before I get involved in a social situation where I could get into trouble. I just spend my time excelling in my area of expertise and my clients appreciate my specialized knowledge. Other freelance businesses that can work well for people with autism are computers, piano tuning, motor repair, and graphic arts. These jobs all make use of skills that many people with autism have, such as perfect pitch, mechanical ability, and artistic talent.

AUTISM SUBTYPES

My interviews with hundreds of parents and reading in the scientific literature indicate that autism may be conceptualized as divided into two broad categories. I have termed these subgroups the Kanner/Asperger types, named after the doctors who discovered autism (Kanner, 1943; Asperger, 1944) and the Regressive/Epileptic type. This is my own hypothesis about the subgroups of autism. It is based on my personal experiences, interviews with hundreds of parents and people with autism, and my interpretation of the scientific literature. It is presented in the hopes of clarifying some of the confusion that exists about autism, its etiology, and its expression.

First, I believe that both types probably have a strong genetic basis. Talks with parents indicate that they both have the same family history profile (Grandin, 1991a, 1992a). An interview with Margaret Bauman indicated that both types have the same pattern of brain abnormalities (Bauman, 1991). The very different clinical symptoms between the two types might possibly be explained by subtle variations of brain abnormality within the larger framework of a basic abnormality in the limbic system, hippocampus, amygdala, and cerebellum.

**Kanner/
Asperger Type**

Kanner/Asperger types can range from individuals with very rigid thinking patterns and a relatively calm temperament to people with more normal thinking patterns with lots of anxiety and sensory sensitivity problems. They tend to be good at visual thinking. Hart (1989) described his son as rigid and calm, while my book (Grandin & Scariano, 1986) and Stehli's (1991) description of her son included normal thinking patterns with anxiety. I had very severe problems with anxiety, nervousness, and sensitivity to touch and sound. The anxiety felt like a constant state of stage fright, and caused me to resist changes in routine because changes made me more anxious. I was in a constant state of stress and my nervous system was running 100 miles per hour. Proper use of the right antidepressant medication changed my life. My speech became more modulated and I became more social when the anxiety eased. The individuals with anxiety and nervousness are likely to respond well to small doses of antidepressant drugs. I required very low doses of the drug to prevent problems with agitation and irritability (Grandin, 1984, 1991b, 1992). After I had been on medication for three months, the anxiety and nervousness returned. I stayed on the same low dose and the "nerve" relapse subsided. It is a big mistake to raise the dose of a drug every time there is a return of anxiety or bad behavior. I have had five or six major anxiety relapses but the same drug dose has been effective for eleven years.

Regressive/ Epileptic Type

Unlike the Kanner/Asperger type, the regressive type has a period of normal development for 18 to 24 months. The child starts to talk in either single words or sentences and then loses speech. Many children with this type of autism have signs of subtle seizure activity such as staring and spacing out. Some may have sensory jumbling and mixing that is severe. Whereas children with the Kanner/Asperger type of autism have good receptive speech and can usually understand what people are saying, the regressive child with autism may just hear a jumble of noise. Allen and Rapin (1993) state that children with autistic behavior who are totally mute and uncomprehending have to be introduced to language through the visual modality. Some of these children may learn to speak when they are taught to read. Interviews with many parents also indicate that this group is most likely to have a favorable response to vitamin supplements (Rimland, 1990), seizure medications, and/or beta-blocker drugs (Ratey et al., 1987). Children in the Regressive subgroup also appear more likely to have seizures and sudden temper tantrums that come "out of the blue." These tantrums may be a frontal or temporal lobe epilepsy that is very difficult to detect on a simple EEG test (Gedye, 1989).

Fred Volkmar and Donald Cohen (1989) at Yale University were the first researchers to recognize the Regressive or "late onset" autism. Some of the children with late onset autism may have good cognitive skills hidden by their problems with sensory jumbling and mixing, while others are probably retarded. The anecdotal reports of individuals successful with facilitated communication (Biklen, 1990) appear to be in the Regressive subgroup with no speech and obvious movement problems. There has been much controversy about facilitated communication, and in many cases the facilitator has pushed the child's hand. However, some low-functioning nonverbal individuals may be able to read and write, so facilitated communication or some other augmentative communication system should be tried.

IMPLICATIONS FOR EDUCATION

Based on my experiences with autism, and my interviews with hundreds of parents and other people with autism, I would like to offer the following suggestions for educators and parents. Many of these suggestions are discussed in great detail in the remainder of this book.

1. Use visual methods of teaching and avoid long strings of verbal information. People with autism often communicate better with the written word. Introduce typewriters and word processors at an early age. Due to motor control problems, typing may be easier than handwriting.

2. Direct and broaden fixations into useful activities. For example, a fixation on trains can be used to motivate interest in reading or math. Use a train book to teach reading. Compulsions and repetitive behaviors with coins and keys can be broadened into games to teach counting and sharing. Try to broaden and redirect a fixation instead of eliminating it.

3. Develop talent areas such as drawing, music, and computer programming. People with autism who have a successful career often have a career that is based on a talent area. There needs to be more emphasis in developing areas of ability.

4. Treatment and awareness of sensory problems is often overlooked in many education programs. Sensory integration therapy from an occupational therapist should be made available to children with autism. Teachers should be made aware of sensory problems and how many bad behaviors are the result of fear and stimuli that cause pain and confusion.

5. Mainstreaming and meaningful contact with children who have normal social behavior is essential if a child with autism is to learn social skills. It is not always practical to mainstream a severely impaired individual in all classes but it is essential that he interacts with normal children.

6. Early intervention improves the prognosis. Ideally, children should be in a structured nursery school program by age three.

7. A structured, predictable classroom environment helps children with autism learn. Due to high levels of anxiety and nervous system overarousal, changes in routine will often cause temper tantrums and other behavior problems. The routine should be structured but not

absolutely rigid. Meal times and the basic schedule of the day should remain constant, but the child should be given limited choices such as making a snowman or building a fort during playtime.

8. Exercise can help reduce disruptive behavior. Periods of vigorous exercise each day have a calming effect on the nervous system.

9. Sensible use of behavior management techniques is part of a good treatment program. An observant teacher or parent can differentiate between bad behavior caused by biological problems and outbursts that have a behavioral basis. Behavior management methods work well on behavioral problems and poorly on biological problems. Examples of biological problems are sound sensitivity, touch sensitivity, visual sensitivity, pain from an undiagnosed medical condition, frontal/temporal lobe epilepsy, and anxiety or panic attacks. Behavioral methods work well when a child uses disruptive behavior to avoid a task, is frustrated because of an inability to communicate, or uses tantrums to get attention.

10. The correct medications used properly can improve both behavior and the quality of life. A common mistake with many medications is to keep increasing the dose every time there is a deterioration in behavior. I have been on the same low dose of an antidepressant drug for the last eleven years. During this time I have had relapses when the anxiety and panic returned, but I stayed on the same dose and each anxiety relapse subsided after a few weeks. An effective medication should have a fairly dramatic effect on behavior and not just cause sedation. Consult with a physician who is knowledgeable about autism.

REFERENCES

Allen, D. A. & Rapin, I. (1993). Autistic children are also dysphasic. In H. Naruse and E.M. Ornitz (Eds.), *Neurobiology of autism*. Amsterdam, Netherlands: Elsevier Science Publishers.

Asperger, H. (1944). Dic Autistischen Psychopathen 1m Kindersaltr, *Archive fur Psychiatier Und Neruenkrankhieten*, 117, 76–136.

Ayres, J. A. (1979). *Sensory integration and the child*. Western Psychology Service, Los Angeles, California.

Bauman, M. L. (1991). Microscopic neuroanatomic abnormalities in autism. *Pediatrics*, 78, 791–796 (supplement).

Bemporad, M. L. (1979). Adult recollections of a formerly autistic child. *Journal of Autism and Developmental Disorders*, 9, 179–197.

Berger, C. L. (1992). *Facilitated communication guide*. Eugene, OR: New Breakthroughs.

Bhatara, V., Clark, D. L., Arnold, L. E., Gunsettt, R., & Smeltzer, D. J. (1981). Hyperkinesis treated with vestibular stimulation: An exploratory study. *Biological Psychiatry*, 61, 269–279.

Biklen, D. (1990). Communication unbound: Autism and praxis. *Harvard Educational Review*, 60, 291–314.

Boucher, J., & Lewis, V. (1989). Memory impairments and communication in relatively able autistic children. *Journal of Child Psychology and Psychiatry*, 30, 99–122.

Bowler, D. M. (1992). "Theory of Mind" in Asperger's Syndrome. *Journal of Child Psychology and Psychiatry*, 33, 877–893.

Cesaroni, L., & Garber, M. (1991). Exploring the experience of autism through firsthand accounts. *Journal of Autism and Development Disorders*, 21, 303–313.

Chambers, W. W. (1947). Electrical stimulation of the interior cerebellum of the cat. *American Journal of Anatomy*, 80, 55–93.

Condon, W., & Sander, L. (1974). Neonate movement

is synchronized with adult speech. *Science, 183,* 99–101.

Courchesne, E., Yeung-Courchesne, R., Press, G. A., Hesselink, J. R., & Jernigan, T. L. (1989). Hypoplasia of cerebellar vernal lobules VI and VII in autism. *New England Journal of Medicine, 318,* 1349–1354.

Crispino, L., & Bullock, T. M. (1984). Cerebellum mediates modality specific modulation of sensory responses of midbrain and forebrain of rats. *Proceedings of the National Academy of Science (USA), 81,* 2917–2929.

Delaccato, C. H. (1974). *The ultimate stranger.* Novato, CA: Arena Press.

Damasio, A. (1991). Category-related recognition defects as a clue to the neural substrates of knowledge. *Trends in Neuroscience, 13,* 95–98.

Dewey, M. (1991). Living with Asperger's Syndrome. In U. Frith (Ed.), *Autism and Asperger Syndrome* (pp. 184–206). Cambridge, England: Cambridge University Press.

Einstein, A., & Einstein, M. W. (1987). *The collected papers of Albert Einstein* (A. Beck & P. Havens, Trans). Princeton, NJ: Princeton University Press.

Farah, M. J. (1989). The neural basis of mental imagery. *Trends in Neuroscience, 12,* 395–399.

Gedye, A. (1989). Episodic rage and aggression attributed to frontal lobe seizures. *Journal of Mental Deficiency Research, 33,* 369–379.

Grandin, T. (1984). My experiences as an autistic child. *Journal of Ortho Molecular Psychiatry, 13,* 144–174.

Grandin, T. (1989). An autistic person's view of holding therapy. *Communication, 23,* 75–76.

Grandin, T. (1990). Needs of high functioning teenagers and adults with autism. *Focus on Autistic Behavior, 5,* 1–16.

Grandin, T. (1991a). Autistic perceptions of the world. *Proceedings of the Autism Society of America Conference* (pp. 85–94) Indianapolis, IN: ASA.

Grandin, T. (1991b). New drug treatments for autistic adults and adolescents. *The Advocate* (newsletter of the Autism Society of America) (Fall), pp. 6–7.

Grandin, T. (1992a). An inside view of autism. In E. Schopler & G. B. Mesibov (Eds.), *High functioning individuals with autism.* New York: Plenum.

Grandin, T. (1992b). Calming effects of deep touch pressure in patients with autistic disorders, college students and animals. *Journal of Child and Adolescent Psychopharmacology, 2,* 63–70.

Grandin, T., Dodman, T. N., & Shuster, L. (1989). Effect of naltretone on relaxation induced by lateral flank pressure in pigs. *Pharmacology, Biochemistry & Behavior, 33,* 839–842.

Grandin, T., & Scariano, M. (1986). *Emergence: Labelled autistic.* Novato, CA: Arena.

Hart, C. (1989). *Without reason.* New York: Harper and Row.

Hashimoto, T., Tayama, M., Miyazaki, M., Sakurama, N., Yoshimoto, T., Murakawa, K., & Kurodo, Y. (1992). Reduced brain stem size in children with autism. *Brain & Development, 14,* 94–97.

Hermelin, B. (1972). Locating events in space and time: Experiments with autistic, deaf and blind children. *Journal of Autism and Childhood Schizophrenia, 3,* 288–298.

Hiskey, M. S. (1955). *Hiskey-Nebraska test of learning aptitude.* Lincoln, NE: College View.

Holton, G. (1971–72). On trying to understand scientific genius. *American Scholar, 41,* 102.

Huttenlocher, P. R. (1984). Synapse elimination in the cerebral cortex. *American Journal of Mental Deficiency, 88,* 488–496.

Kanner, L. (1943). Autistic disturbances of affective contact. *Nervous Child, 2,* 217–250.

Kanner, L. (1971). Follow-up study of eleven autistic children originally reported in 1943. *Journal of Autism and Childhood Schizophrenia, 1,* 112–145.

McClelland, D. G., Eyre, D., Watson, G. J., Sherrard, C., & Sherrard, E. (1992). Central conduction time in autism. *British Journal of Psychiatry, 160,* 659–663.

McClure, M. K., & Holtz, Y. M. (1991). The effects of sensory stimulatory treatment on an autistic child. *American Journal of Occupational Therapy, 45,* 1138–1142.

McGimsey, J. F., & Favell, J. E. (1988). The effects of increased physical exercise on disruptive behavior in retarded persons. *Journal of Autism and Developmental Disorders, 18,* 167–179.

Melzack, R., & Burns, S. K. (1965). Neurophysiological effects of early sensory restriction. *Experimental Neurology, 13,* 163–175.

Melzack, R., Konrad, K. W., & Dubrobsky, B. (1969). Prolonged changes in the central nervous system produced by somatic and reticular stimulation. *Experimental Neurology, 25,* 416–428.

Miller, A., & Miller, E. E. (1971). Symbol accentuation, single-track functioning and early reading. *American Journal of Mental Deficiency, 76,* 110–117.

Newson, E., Dawson, M., & Everard, P. (1982). *The natural history of able autistic people: Their management and functioning in a social context.* Nottingham, England: University of Nottingham, Child Development Research Unit.

O'Connell, T. (1974). The musical life of an autistic boy. *Journal of Autism and Childhood Schizophrenia, 4,* 223–229.

Ornitz, E. (1985). Neurophysiology of infantile autism.

Journal of the American Academy of Child Psychiatry, 24, 251–262.

Ozonoff, S., Roger, S .J., & Pennington, B. F. (1991). Asperger's syndrome: Evidence of empirical distinction from high functioning autism. *Journal of Child Psychology and Psychiatry, 32,* 1107–1122.

Painter, K. (1992, November 11). Autistic and writing close the gulf. *USA Today,* p. D1.

Park, C. C. (1967). *The siege.* Boston, MA: Little, Brown.

Park, D., & Youderian, P. (1974). Light and number: Ordering principles in the world of an autistic child. *Journal of Autism and Childhood Schizophrenia, 4,* 313–323.

Prior, M. (1979). Cognitive abilities and disabilities in autism: A review. *Journal of Abnormal Child Psychology, 2,* 357–380.

Ratey, J. J., Mikkelsen, E., Sorgi, P., Zuckerman, S., Polakoff, S., Bemporad, J., Bick, P., & Kadish, W. (1987). Autism: The treatment of aggressive behaviors. *Journal of Clinical Pharmacology, 7,* 35–41.

Ray, T. C., King, L. J., and Grandin, T. (1988). The effectiveness of self initiated vestibular stimulation in producing speech sounds. *Journal of Occupation Therapy Research, 8,* 186–190.

Rimland, B. (1990). Dimethylglycine (DMG) a non-toxic metabolite and autism. *Autism Research Review, 4,* (2), 3.

Simons, D., & Land, P. (1987). Early tactile stimulation influences organization of somatic sensory cortex. *Nature, 326,* 694–697.

Simons, J., and Oishi, S. (1987). *The hidden child.* Kensington, MD: Woodbine House.

Simons, J. M. (1974). Observations of compulsive behavior in autism. *Journal of Autism and Childhood Schizophrenia, 4,* 1–10.

Stehli, A. (1991). *Sound of a miracle.* New York: Doubleday.

Szatmari, P., Bartolucci, G., Bremner, R., Bond, S., & Rich, S. (1989). A follow up study of high functioning autistic children. *Journal of Autism and Developmental Disorders, 19,* 213–225.

Volkmar, F. R., & Cohen, D. J. (1989). Disintegrative disorder or "Late Onset" autism. *Journal of Child Psychiatry, 30,* 717–724.

Walters, R. G., & Walters, W. E. (1980). Decreasing self-stimulatory behavior with physical exercise in a group of autistic boys. *Journal of Autism and Developmental Disorders, 10,* 379–387.

Wechsler, D. (1967). *Wechsler intelligence scale for children.* New York: Psychological Corp.

Weiss, R. (1989, November 11). Why a man may mistake his wife for a cat. *Science News,* p. 309.

White, G. B., & White, M. S. (1987). Autism from the inside. *Medical Hypothesis, 24,* 223–229.

Williams, D. (1992). *Nobody nowhere.* New York: Times Book.

Woodcock, R. W., & Johnson, M. B. (1977). *Woodcock-Johnson psycho-educational battery.* Allen, TX: DLM Teaching Resources.

Zeki, S. (1992, September). The visual image in the mind and brain. *Scientific American,* pp. 69–76.

Zisserman, L. (1992). The effects of deep pressure on self stimulating behaviors in a child with autism and other disabilities. *American Journal of Occupational Therapy, 46,* 547–551.

CHAPTER 3

Teaching Children with Autism: What Parents Want

Charles Hart

I'll never forget my first walk down the hallway of Bagley Elementary School. It was 1976, and my wife and I had known about our son's disability for only two years. Like so many children diagnosed with autism, Ted didn't fit into the neighborhood school program. From age 4, he attended a "communication classroom" operated by the University of Washington, but, as his sixth birthday approached, he needed to transfer into the public school system.

Ted's pediatrician visited many classrooms, looking for the best possible fit. He suggested that I observe a combination kindergarten and first-grade program for the neurologically impaired. Accordingly, I called the school to schedule a visit.

My visit took place in March. Plum trees were blooming in the school-yard and ivy covered the entire building, except for the windows and the wide double doors. As I stood on the front steps, everything seemed fresh and green. Indoors, I could smell pine oil cleaner and wax on the dark oak floors. That odor carried me back to my own childhood. Suddenly I sensed the similarities—and the differences—between my son's educational opportunities and my own.

Thirty years earlier, I had walked down a similar hallway. It, too, had seemed ancient and awesome to a 6-year-old's eyes. So much was the same, yet so much was different. When I was six, my parents simply enrolled me in the neighborhood school, expecting me to flourish until I turned eighteen and was ready for college or a career. A generation later, I faced a challenge my parents had never known. I couldn't take my child's success for granted as they had. They expected the teachers to know what would be best for their child. I wasn't so sure. My son wouldn't coast through school or make the honor roll. Perhaps he wouldn't even graduate. In that hallway of Daniel Bagley Elementary School, I faced the fear of the unknown.

MOVING THROUGH THE SPECIAL EDUCATION MAZE

I didn't know what to expect from this thing called special education! Through the Autism Society we had met other parents who told us about PL94-142, the law that would guarantee a free appropriate education for Ted. They said the law also gave us "parental rights." We were supposed to sign an IEP (Individualized Education Program) every year, indicating we agreed with the school's educational goals for our son, but we didn't know how to judge the school's goals or the teacher's competence. We were in a quandary, knowing neither what to accept nor what to challenge. How could we be partners in a system we didn't understand?

Like so many other parents whose child is a focus of concern, we had a double challenge to deal with. We were still struggling to understand our child's diagnosis, but we were already given the responsibility of helping plan his education. Most parents are not asked to evaluate their child's curriculum or the teacher's methodology, but we had to be partners in the educational system while still grieving over our son's newly identified handicap.

Our pediatrician had spared us an ordeal that confuses many parents, the search for a placement. We didn't have to subject ourselves to the whims of the bureaucracy or deal with the ideological conflicts of segregation versus full inclusion. That wasn't an issue in 1976 as it is today. Neither is placement a concern in this book, for this is a manual about methods that can work in virtually every type of educational placement.

As I walked down the stairwell of the Bagley school to the classroom in the basement, I had only two questions: "What is the teacher like?" and "Will my son fit in with the other kids?"

The Early Years   Ted's first teacher, Mrs. Habeggar, passed my test with flying colors. She obviously liked the children and they liked her. The school day began with group greetings, the pledge of allegiance, and a sing-along to a recording of the national anthem. The teacher easily won my confidence.

I didn't think in terms of "behavioral objectives" and "task analysis," but I could tell this was an environment for achievement. Regardless of competence each child participated in everything. The bulletin board announced the leader of the day. Children's names were rotated so that each child would have a regular turn, perhaps the first or only chance that child had ever had to lead others to recess, lunch, and other group activities. Through trial and error, the teacher had learned each child's strengths and weaknesses. She knew each child was unique, but she wanted all of them to practice the same social skills: turn taking, waiting in line, and sharing. Since there were only twelve children in her class, Mrs. Habeggar was able to keep track of social interactions. She knew which children to seat together and which to separate, keeping behavior problems and sensory distractions to a minimum. Simply put, she created an environment for learning.

Even though I didn't know much about educational theory and the learning disorders connected with autism, I knew Ted would do well in this classroom. We enrolled him in the Bagley school and looked forward to the next September.

For the first three years, everything went well. When Ted completed the combined kindergarten and first-grade class, Mrs. Habeggar transfered to the second grade with him. As long as the same caring teacher tracked Ted's progress through introductory academic skills, he flourished. However, as he and his classmates aged, their neurological differences became more obvious.

By the time Ted and his classmates advanced to the third grade, a new teacher had to cope with different learning styles and emerging behavior problems. Several of the children had dyslexia, so the teacher conducted daily drills with rhymes and games to practice recognition of the letters of the alphabet. In the meantime our son, who could read upside down, backwards, sideways and mirror image, lost interest in the class activities. He drifted more and more into his own daydreams, totally bored with a redundant academic exercise. Unfortunately, this meant he also missed out on the social aspects of the school lesson—the turn taking, sharing of attention, and focus.

My wife and I finally realized that we had to take a more active role in our son's education plan. We couldn't simply assume that the general curriculum, even in a special education class, would match our son's needs. Fortunately, the teacher agreed and requested help from a communication disorder specialist. Unfortunately, the head of the district's speech and hearing services disagreed. She insisted that our child didn't need communication therapy because he neither lisped nor stuttered during his irrelevant babbling. Her professional training had not included pragmatics, the use of language, so we had to go outside the district for our son's language assessment.

One Person Makes a Difference

We really didn't know what to expect from a communication assessment. We knew that our son's language development was "atypical." In fact the other third graders had begun teasing him for his irrelevant and often nonsensical speech. As parents, however, we had no training in the field. We didn't even have a descriptive vocabulary to explain the language we heard from our son.

We were intrigued when a communication specialist at the University of Washington described our son's receptive and expressive language abilities. After only a few hours of testing and observation, she identified language problems and learning disorders, explaining how one could impact the other. She noted that our child had problems with sequencing. He couldn't follow more than two instructions in a row, or identify which of two pictures represented "before" or "after."

The communication specialist won our confidence for two reasons. First, her language assessment described our son's speech better than we could ourselves. We didn't think she'd missed anything we'd seen. Her observations went beyond ours, connecting the various language problems into a larger pattern that enabled us to understand him better than ever before. Second, she knew what to *do* about it! She prescribed play activities that would involve an ever-increasing number of steps. She showed us strategies for teaching pronouns, those mysterious words that change reference, depending on the speaker: "When *I* am talking to *you*, *you* are *you* and *I* am *me*, but when *you* are talking to *me*, *you* are *me* and *I* am *you!*"

The communication disorder specialist gave us our first formal training in autism. Sadly, most teachers don't get enough training in this subject. Every year we had to break in a new teacher, reciting the communication problems that had been diagnosed at the University of Washington. Eventually, people started calling my wife and me "the autism experts." However, we found that role hard to fill. We weren't trained in the field, so the various education theories baffled us. Hearing stories from other parents only confused us more. We met families that were committed to every treatment known to science and the *National Enquirer*!

TREATMENT OPTIONS: IN THE NAME OF HOPE

Most parents don't even question the scientific validity of treatments. They take ideas from *Reader's Digest*, "St. Elsewhere," or overheard in the supermarket. They're a true cross section of the American public. No one taught them the principles of scientific investigation when they were students in regular education, so they can't apply it to special education! Our education system has failed us twice: first as students, then as parents.

One of our friends joked that parents who try every treatment for autism belong to the "cure-of-the-month club." But, there's nothing funny about parents chasing every report of a miracle. They're misled by fads, often with unrealistic and unsupported claims. The rumors of miracles and recoveries never subside, even after professional journals have disproven a treatment. Every year another group of children will be diagnosed with autism, their parents will recoil with shock, and then they will pursue every discredited treatment a friend or relative discovers in a magazine article.

While you read this chapter, another woman is giving birth to a child with autism. He won't be diagnosed for a few years, but when he is, his mother will probably want the same thing for him that Barbara Christopher wanted for her son with autism. In a written account of living with her son, she recalls listening to Glenn Doman, founder of the controversial Doman-Delacato physical patterning program at the Institute for the Development of Human Potential , and shares her feelings:

> He [Doman] said the words that made us know we were in the right place. "I know what you want. You want your child to be well." . . . We understood exactly what he meant . . . until the day came that [our son] Ned could be called normal, we would not be satisfied. We kept listening. (Christopher & Christopher, 1989, p. 106)

They listened and followed his program not because they had seen any research or another form of evidence, but because a master salesman had read their minds and made the siren call: *"I know what you want. You want your child to be well."*

Berneen Bratt (1989), another parent who has shared her personal story, offers a more cynical view of her experience with the Doman-Delacato program:

> After only a few minutes of listening to Glenn Doman, I realized that he continually focused on the mothers' attachment to their children . . . "You have a deep emotional problem and you get up every morning with a heavy heart because your child is not well." It was apparent that this man . . . was a gifted and dynamic speaker and a master psychologist. (p. 63)

Like the Christophers and the Bratts, thousands of families have wasted time and money to follow Doman's methods. Yet the American Academy of Pediatrics censured the Doman-Delacato program as far back as 1982. The Academy concluded its policy statement with this warning:

> Based on past and current analysis, studies and reports, we must conclude that the patterning treatment offers no special merit, that the claims of its advocates are unproven, and that the demands on families are so great that in some cases there may be harm in its use. (p. 810)

Professionals have nothing to learn from Doman's pseudoscientific treatments, but they have plenty to learn from his marketing strategy. He bases his charisma on a formula that recognizes what the consumers (parents) want and then markets to their hopes and fantasies. Responsible professionals find Doman hard to accept and consider it unprofessional to let their clients, patients, or students cling to unrealistic hopes. But while professionals need not nurture false hopes, neither should they ignore the power of hope and the parents' emotional needs. Parents need to feel positive about their children and about their own role raising a child with a disability. Parents need to feel useful; they need to believe that they can make things better for their child.

In 1988, *The Advocate,* a quarterly newsletter of the Autism Society of America, published interviews with prominent mothers of children with autism. The interviewer asked, "Is there a time to accept professional opinion and, if so, how can a parent decide when to accept and when to fight?" Parent and author Mary Callahan replied:

> I always noticed that I felt a lot better when I was working on a new idea and that idea offered hope. On the other hand, it seemed to me that many professionals think it's their job to make parents accept the worst and give up hope. It's as if they think giving up hope is a necessary step for parents to accept their child's prognosis, and that often makes the professionals discourage the parent's search for a solution. (ASA, *The Advocate,* 1988, p. 7)

In the name of hope, some parents will draw a child out of school to give him ten or twelve hours of one-on-one therapy a day. Doman encouraged this, and so does Kaufman (1976, 1981). Ivar Lovaas, respected for innovations in behavior modification, raises high expectations for home programs based on his methods. He claims that fifty percent of his students "recover" from autism (1987). One parent, writing under a pseudonym, recently recorded her experiences with the Lovaas program, crediting him with her 6-year-old daughter's and 4-year-old son's "recoveries" (Maurice, 1993). Sadly, this young mother doesn't seem to understand the meaning of developmental disability and the many challenges that lie ahead for her children.

THE PROFESSIONAL'S RESPONSIBILITY

As a professional, how would you respond on behalf of your district if a parent brought a book of miracles or a reprint from *Reader's Digest* to an IEP meeting? If a mother demanded an intensive program based on the theories of Kaufman, Doman, or Lovaas, would you be able to convince her that your district offers something just as appropriate?

Professionals shouldn't be surprised if parents ask for a treatment they've learned about on a television show. Commercial TV and trade magazines are the oracles of our society and they'll publicize anything that boosts audiences. They rarely interview skeptics who would raise the troublesome questions: Does this really work? Will every student benefit? Will the alleged benefits last or transfer to another setting?

When a parent asks for services that a district can't—or won't—provide, it is the responsibility of the professional to investigate it. Families should be encouraged to discuss what they've heard. To understand the concept, professionals should watch the program or read the article that inspired the parents. They should admit it if they find value in the program, for they have to appear as credible as talk show hosts! If professionals believe the "miracle" reported on TV isn't valid or that the strategy won't work for a specific student, they need to explain why. Professionals are dealing with a fragile entity, parental hope. They want to direct the parents' energy away from an unreasonable program and toward something constructive they can do for their child.

Assessment

The best defense against unreasonable demands is a good assessment. This can reassure the parents that someone understands their child as well, or better, than the family. Once a professional has observed the child's language and motor development, the information must be explained in terms the parents understand. My wife and I will always be grateful to the occupational therapist who explained our son's motor development to us. In thirty minutes she identified signs of developmental delay we hadn't noticed in eight years! Then she told us what he could do in the present, what was reasonable to expect in the near future, and how we could enhance his progress.

Realistically speaking, many schools don't have occupational therapists and communication specialists with training in autism. Sometimes the teacher hasn't taught a student with this disability before. Perhaps the school's psychologist has no experience with nonverbal IQ tests. What should be done?

It is important that professionals don't try to bluff the parents. It's better to go into the IEP meeting with questions than with pat answers. If school staff have incomplete information, they need to be honest about it. Most parents will respect professionals who say they need more time to evaluate the child or want the parents' opinion on issues.

The best investment is an outside assessment of the child by someone with expertise in autism. A smart administrator will order one before the parents are driven to request it. A thorough assessment shows a school district's good faith, it reassures the parents that the school has the child's interests at heart, and it helps the staff identify the starting point for the education plan.

An assessment should give as much information as possible about the child's receptive and expressive language, gross and fine motor coordination and academic, personal, and social skills. How does this child express his needs? How does he behave in class, on the playground, and at home? A good evaluation considers the youngster's performance in different settings. Assessment will probably reveal wide variations in his abilities.

Some findings may even surprise the parents. They may have no idea how their child responds to the school bell or the line in the cafeteria. Remember, autism is a "social and communication disorder," and these children are notoriously unreliable as communicators. The child won't go home and tell you that he learned to tie his shoes and doesn't need help anymore. Nor will he tell you when the teacher sends him to the hall after he bites someone, which explains why he is biting his brother in order to get away from him too!

The child has probably acquired behaviors at school that he doesn't use at home or vice versa. Parents and teachers need a system of ongoing communication to share their vision of the student's performance. Some schools use a journal that travels from school to home and back on a daily basis. If something unusual occurs at school, the teacher records it for the parents to read that night. When a new skill or behavior surfaces at home, the parent notes it in the journal so the teacher reads about it the next morning.

When professionals request an outside assessment, they need to tell the parents the type of information they're looking for. Don't let them assume it's going to be a medical report prescribing paramedical treatment, drugs, or diets. The evaluation doesn't point toward a cure, but it does show what the child can do now, what he is ready to learn, and the best pathways for teaching him. If a child watches better than he listens, the evaluation should show that. It should also indicate if the child understands more than he can express.

The consultant/evaluator should write the report in understandable, everyday terms, not psychological jargon. After all, this assessment is going to be discussed not only with the parents, but also with the educational team, including the teachers' aides and the bus drivers. They don't want to hear test scores, numbers, or percentiles. They want specific details about the child's achievements and delays.

When a written assessment is completed, parents should be allowed to read it before the IEP meeting so they can compare their own observations with the specialist's. After all, they've lived with this child for a long time and seen him in different situations, twenty-four hours a day, year in and year out. A good assessment may help the parents understand behaviors they've seen before but have never known how to interpret. For example, it might explain why the child ignores his mother's requests, or why he walks on his toes.

Sometimes the family will challenge the assessment or contribute more details. Since the parents have probably seen responses at home that the specialist couldn't observe during an evaluation, this anecdotal information should be encouraged. Find out what the family has seen at the dinner table, in the bathroom, or at the park. Remember, these children probably behave differently from one setting to another.

Children with autism have trouble transferring skills from one setting to another. This simply means that learning a task under one set of conditions (in the classroom, after lunch) may not prepare the child to repeat the task in a different location or time (at home, before lunch). Changing the environment or the sequence of events might cause a change in behavior. Accordingly, the family and staff would observe different skills. It's important that these observations are shared to reach agreement on the child's current abilities and a starting point for the education plan.

**Developing
a Plan**

Once everyone agrees on the child's starting point, they must decide where they want him to go, and how he'll get there. They should choose the destination (goals and objectives) before selecting the path (methods and activities). As Mager (1968) warns in his manual about preparing instructional objectives, "People who don't know where they are going are bound to end up somewhere else!" (p. vii).

Setting appropriate goals is very hard for professionals and parents alike. Our society hasn't done a very good job of articulating the goals of regular education, let alone special education. Parents generally have a fuzzy recollection of their own school experience, recalling nine months a year with time divided between academics and recreation; classrooms and playgrounds; tests and proms. Perhaps they think the only educational objective was graduation and preparation for college or a work program.

Parents assume special education will be different from regular education, but they don't know what to expect. The uncertainty can add to their uneasiness. They already have a child they can't fully understand; now they have to deal with an educational service that hasn't been defined! Some parents hope special education will help their child catch up with other students. They may hope for a total recovery by graduation. But most parents recognize that their child's disability won't fade with age. Rather, the child with a disability will become an adult with a disability. Eventually, even the most hopeful parents face their compromise with destiny.

When parents recognize their child can't be cured or perfect, they at least want him to get *better*. However, it's harder to define *better* than it is to define *perfect*. Better is a relative term. It can't be seen as an icon, the ideal that parents envisioned before the reality. The word "better" requires comparisons: Better than who? Better than what? Better *at* what?

Better Than Who?   This shouldn't be an issue for any child, especially one with a disability such as autism. We hope no parents think their youngster has to compete with others, learning faster or more than classmates and siblings. Compare the child's performance with his own potential, not the standards that others set. This applies to all children, whether in special education or regular education.

Better Than What?   Usually this can be defined as better than he is now. The assessment helps here. If the professionals and the parents have pooled their observations, they will have a comprehensive portrait of the child, including his academic, language, social, and self-help skills. It will be easy to see many needs for improvement. In fact, everyone will want to see him improve in so many areas, the next question may overwhelm them.

Better At What?   Set priorities. The parents probably want to see many changes, bad behaviors dropped and new skills learned. They may not know where to start or which goals to include in the IEP. Teachers also have a hard time choosing a focus when the child presents many challenges. The following list outlines the kinds of problems a child may have.

1. Behaviors may include poor eye contact, toe walking, and other gestures that make the child conspicuous in public. Some behaviors such as hand-flapping, rocking, or spinning may interfere with school work and bother other students.
2. Social delays may prevent the child from playing with other children, being accepted on the playground, or accompanying the family to malls and restaurants. He may be unwilling to share toys or space, take turns, or wait in lines. Perhaps he hits other children and attempts to escape from the classroom or run away from adults.
3. Uneven academic skills may concern parents and teachers. Perhaps the child reads and spells but doesn't appear to comprehend. He may do math assignments by memory, but can't comprehend premath terms such as more, less, enough, and many.
4. The communication problems keep teachers and parents from knowing how much the child understands. This makes it hard to negotiate with the child and to teach appropriate requesting behavior, how to express needs, or say "no."
5. Sensory problems may trigger bizarre or unpredictable behaviors and fears. The child may scream, place hands over his eyes or ears, and even flee from certain sounds, movements, or odors. He may avoid touch, seek isolation, or engage in excessive repetitive movement.
6. Problems with disorganization make the child seem irrational and confused. He appears confused by the order of events, loses track of time, or shows extreme impatience. He may resist transitions, or changing from one activity to another. Perhaps he doesn't understand cause and effect.

For this child, how would *better* be defined? Parents will want to see improvement in all the problem areas. They can list dozens of behaviors they'd like to see less of, and others they'd like to see more often. They want their child to outgrow maladaptive habits and learn socially acceptable ones. Parents have no problem identifying goals. Their challenge is deciding which are the most important. They want their child to be better, but the definition evades them.

Some parents and teachers think better means less disruptive. An adult in charge of several children wants them to cooperate, sit quietly, and take turns. In the name of compliance, children have been tied in chairs, slapped, and locked in time-out boxes. Believers in these strategies defend their methods by claiming that children must sit still and face the blackboard before any real learning can advance. So they're willing to constrain and punish the youngster, thinking it will prepare him to learn something when he's ready. This definition of learning needs examination. If a task is so alien, so foreign to a student's interests that the teacher uses punishment as a learning tool, the student won't practice that task out of class.

It may be tempting to target the student's eccentricities such as self-stimulation and echolalia and change those behaviors to make him seem more like other children. However, a superficial or cosmetic approach to behavioral differences doesn't take the child's needs into consideration. You can't motivate someone to change a behavior he needs or enjoys. In Chapter 9, Carol Gray reminds us that the teacher and the child are working from two "equally valid but different perspectives." If adults want the child to cooperate, they'd better take into account his perspective. A learning plan should offer the student something he can value, not something only the teacher values. If the child can't see a payoff, he won't cooperate for long. Learners with autism need immediate personal reinforcement or they won't practice a new skill. They have a hard time comprehending cause and effect, so long-term benefits don't impress them as much as short-term ones.

Some people think better means more normal in appearance. They'll use *abnormal* methods to make children with autism act "normal." In *A Child Called Noah*, Greenfield (1971) recalls hearing Lovaas explain his theory of education:

> The trouble with most of these kids, according to Lovaas, is that they don't have any fear at all. And to begin to make them function, you must forget all etiology, and implant fear in them. (p. 158)

Today the philosophy remains essentially the same: "forget all etiology" and pay little attention to the neurological problems. Make the child look you in the eye, stop the odd gestures, hide every tell-tale symptom! Lovaas (1987) says his best children "recover." I believe that he calls them normal because they're normal in appearance. Upon meeting one of the children, you might be fooled by the appearance until the conversation drifts away from the tightly rehearsed script. Years of one-on-one training can teach a child to perfect social rituals such as greetings and a handshake. These gestures seem flawless, but there is often little behind the appearance: no communicative intent, no personal expression, no functional value. The child may have mastered the style or *form* of communication but hasn't learned the *function*, the natural choice of gesture and words for self-expression to communicate personal interests and desires.

FAMILY PRIORITIES

When teachers and parents meet to plan educational goals, they have to choose from among many possible values, each defining progress in a different way. For example, they may select one of the following:

1. The student will be less disruptive. He will kick, scream, hit, yell, run, cry, or bite less often, for a shorter length of time, or with less intensity.

2. The student will act more normal. He will do less toe walking, hand flapping, finger flicking, head banging, spinning, or rocking, and he will do more eye contacting, handshaking, quiet sitting , turn taking, or waiting in line.

3. The student will be more verbal. He will imitate more words, use complete sentences, say "please" and "thank you" routinely, and identify objects when asked "What is this?"

4. The student will learn more functional communication. He will point at objects he wants, signal to the teacher when he needs help, shake his head or nod to indicate "yes" or "no."

5. The student will make academic progress. He will increase his reading level, complete one mathematics workbook, learn programs in computer class.

For one child, teachers and parents might want to see progress in all of these areas. Each issue could become the focus for an entire year, perhaps longer. It's hard to choose between academic goals, language skills, and social development. However, someone has to decide which problems need immediate attention and which can wait. Most parents want help setting these priorities. They need the teacher's cooperation to choose reasonable, achievable goals. All of the adults want to see the child "better," but sometimes it's hard to define that term.

It helps to remember that a child spends 30 hours a week or less at school, whereas he spends another 138 hours with his family! Parents should be encouraged to discuss home life and their child's behavior in the neighborhood and general community. A family's concerns will be influenced by myriad social and economic factors, ethnic heritage, religion, and various lifestyle choices. The teacher should get to know the child's home environment. One family may want to take their son into a restaurant for a formal dinner, whereas another may want their daughter to join them on a camping trip. People who live on busy streets want their children to learn traffic safety, whereas families on farms or cul de sacs are less concerned with it. If there is a helpless infant at home, parents probably worry about the aggressive behavior of the child with autism, whereas tantrums and violence may be better tolerated in a family with older children. If the child with autism happens to be an only child, the parents may teach many skills at home, but they'll need the school's help to arrange social contact with other children.

It is important to find out which behaviors and self-help skills will enhance individual children's lives and help them become more independent in their homes. Children need to be taught the community's standards of behavior so that they can use the rest room, browse the mall, and maybe even hop aboard a bus. These skills make the children look "better" not only to the parents, but also to the rest of society.

Communication should be a primary concern when setting priorities. However, adults should be careful not to confuse form with function. Many parents think better means more verbal. If their son doesn't speak, they want him to talk. If their son talks, they want him to make sense. Problems with language are not the only symptoms associated with autism, but they are the most noticeable, the most dramatic. The popularized image of autism is a nonverbal child. If this disability had a poster child, he would be a handsome little boy whose abilities were locked behind a wall of silence.

It's easy to understand why so many parents emphasize speech therapy in the IEP. Some evaluate their child's program according to hours of therapy provided each week, assuming that more means better. They may focus on spoken language to the exclusion of other communication styles. Some will ask teachers to drill children in speech exercises, believing that if they can talk, everything will be all right. Unfortunately, these parents need to have their concern redirected. Making a nonverbal child practice sounds is like fixing the turn signals when the car has a broken steering wheel! The language and communication specialist should help parents understand the problems behind their child's speech failure. Some children have a hearing distortion that makes it hard to recognize language, so they can't decode our spoken words. Others may not understand our language rules and parts of speech, so they can't create original sentences.

The language program should help clarify the child's communication abilities. When a language strategy (such as picture boards) works in one environment, it should be tried in another. If communication boards are used at school, the parents need to be offered training so they can reinforce the system at home. If wall charts and calendars help the child organize information at home, they should be used in the classroom too. Remember, the children need to communicate their needs and desires more than they need to build a repertoire of sentences. The educational goal should be "more communicative," not "more verbal."

Perhaps the youngster will never become as fluent with speech as with augmentative communication. For many parents, facilitated communication has become the last and most irresistible hope. They've heard that nonverbal people may reveal normal or even superior intelligence with facilitation. However, this may prove to be another avenue of false hope, as Layton and Watson suggest in Chapter 4.

Children with autism vary tremendously in the nature and extent of their neurological differences. Many have distorted sensory perceptions. They have trouble processing sounds or shifting attention from one stimulus to another. Even the highest-functioning adults with autism admit, as Temple Grandin does in Chapter 2, that problems with comprehension and recognition remain.

When children do show an ability to read and write, adults often change the focus of their education plans from social and self-help skills to academic ones. Does everyone who reads belong in history and geography classes? Are illiterate, nonverbal students the only ones who need to learn self-care and community orientation? Reading and writing enable some students to cope with academic challenges, but that doesn't mean they've outgrown their special needs. Individuals may still have problems with socialization and self-control. They may have sensory disturbances and problems with concentration. We should try to keep bigotry and status out of the education plan. Don't assume better means more capable of learning academic subjects.

After teachers and parents set learning objectives, they should have consistent standards for communication and behavior, so the child faces the same expectations at home and at school. The child won't make progress if problem behaviors are ignored in one environment and rewarded in another. The child can't be expected to ask the teacher for help, if Mom always anticipates his needs and never waits for him to ask at home. The parents can't eliminate a behavior by ignoring it at home, if that same behavior gets attention at school. The rules should be the same in every classroom as they are at home.

RESPECT THE CHILD

Parental love operates on dynamic tension between the opposing goals of protection and freedom. On the one hand, we want to shelter our children from pain, humiliation, and corruption. On the other hand, we want to give them as many choices as possible. We want them to have every opportunity we've had, and then some! We want them to be as happy as they can, to go places and do things.

Occasionally, the protective instinct gets out of hand. A parent may confuse love with control. Some will request a controlling environment for their child, perhaps a residential school or a self-contained classroom. Some people try to control their child's behavior with drugs. Children have even been bound and locked in windowless time-out rooms because a parent or a teacher thought they needed to be controlled. Odd as it may seem, these strategies have even been written into education plans because adults feared what a child might do without restraints.

If teachers and parents must err, err on the side of freedom, not on the side of control. Public education is supposed to prepare youngsters for citizenship. Children with autism may not all choose to vote, but they'll have that right. They'll be legal citizens in a freedom-loving society. They shouldn't waste their formative years, imprisoned in classrooms that don't offer training that interests them. We should pay more attention to what their behavior means, rather than changing them for the sake of an ideal we call "normal."

The child who constantly tries to escape from the classroom or bolt from the schoolyard has an agenda. He may be curious about his community, want to explore the other end of the playfield, *investigate the road not taken*. Maybe it would be better to hire an aide to accompany the youngster as he explores the community than to pay that same aide to restrain the child.

Instead of fighting to extinguish stereotypic behaviors, try thinking of them as forms of recreation or entertainment. Some creative teachers use those behaviors as rewards. Try saying, "You can flap your hands for five minutes after you finish your math sheet." Maybe the emphasis needs to be to negotiate around these behaviors. Include them in a menu of rewards, so the student has to choose: "Since you finished your project, you can twirl your keychain or you can have a snack with us."

It shouldn't be surprising to find that these students act a lot like other people! The more we give them *choices*, the less stubborn they seem. Forbidding something only makes them want it more. When we relax our rules, their anxiety seems to subside. We should pay more attention to these common human qualities rather than their differences. We should remember that each child with autism is a human being first. He has needs, interests, and fears that deserve our attention, not our impulsive reaction, our desire to control what we can't understand.

Consider teaching the child something he wants to learn rather than what others have decreed is relevant. You'll be amazed how much faster he'll learn, for it is always easier to teach children what they want to know. They pay more attention, and they find opportunities to practice the skills they've chosen themselves. Temple Grandin (1986) emphasizes this when she credits a science teacher for helping her follow her own interests. Ideas that others considered "odd," perhaps even "autistic" in their intensity, led Grandin to a career and an international reputation.

In the preceding chapter of this book, Grandin described how it feels to have autism; how hard it is to sit still and behave when clothing hurts, sounds annoy, and instructions don't make sense. She tells us that occupational therapists can explain a child's sensory differences and the way those differences affect learning style. Grandin also pleads on behalf of these children: help them set their own learning goals instead of just imposing yours.

How would you like school if you had no interest and no comprehension of the teacher's agenda? You'd wonder why you were in school at all, why your parents made you go there five days a week. The day might seem interminable if you had no clue what you were supposed to do or when one irrelevant ordeal would end and the next pointless one begin! The authors of this book urge you to give the children a chance. We need to try to figure out the children's perceptions—how they view our rules, our agenda, and our authority. The better they understand their home or classroom, the more competent and independent they become. Since we can't make them adopt our perspective, we have to discover theirs. It's easier for us to change our customs than it is for them to change for our convenience.

SUMMARY

The annual IEP meeting is a caucus where adults plan changes for the child. But parents and teachers have learning needs too. Often they lack the information or skills they need in order to serve a child with autism. In the spring of 1978, I was as ignorant about my son's perceptions as any other neophyte parent. Fortunately, I had the cooperation of an expert teacher, but this is not always the case. Many times the teacher has less understanding than the parents.

In 1990, the director of OSERS (Office of Special Education and Rehabilitation) reported that 40 percent of the special education teachers were "conditionally certified" because they didn't meet their individual state's mininimal training standards (Schrag, 1991). Furthermore, 25 percent of the personnel left the field every year to be replaced by new—and probably "conditionally certified"—replacements. Accordingly, most students with autism have to break in four or five teachers, as well as train their parents, before they graduate!

These statistics inspired me to consider the teachers' and the parents' learning needs. Perhaps they too should have annual education plans, so that they'll be able to recognize their children's learning styles, their needs, and the best routes for reaching them. Children's IEPs project the learner's progress over the school year. However, we can't offer teachers and parents the luxury of nine full months to identify the child's needs and learning style. Their responsibility begins with the first day of school even though it takes adults a few weeks to fully recognize a child's individuality. Let's give the parents and the teachers thirty days to meet the following objectives from their own individual plan. The teacher's goals should be to recognize how the child responds to different sensory stimuli, identify the child's best channels for learning, identify activities and interests that motivate the child, develop a reward system based on the child's interests, evaluate the child's current skills, set educational objectives for the year, and design a home-school communication system. The parents' goals would be to meet the teachers and/or therapists, discuss the family's long- and short-term goals, share information about any earlier assessments, request an outside assessment if the school personnel seem to lack the expertise, agree on a system for exchanging information between school and home, find out how to reinforce educational objectives at home, and request written permission before any changes are made to the child's curriculum or disciplinary procedure.

We never know what to expect for our children's future, even if they're typical or gifted. It seems harder to foretell the future when our child has a disability. The uncertainty can be frightening, as I found on my first visit to the Bagley school nearly twenty years ago. The difference between my school career and my son's overwhelmed me. My senses were jumbled by contrasts, the familiar and the unknown, the expected and the unexpected. The nearly forgotten smells of pine oil and floor wax caught me off guard, but later I'd recall them as a premonition, my first scent of a truth that would take years to register. My instincts carried a powerful but simple message: my child needed the same thing that I—and every other child— needed from education: opportunities to grow and to become as capable, as independent, and as happy as it was within his nature to become!

REFERENCES

Autism Society of America. (1988). Pioneering mothers make a difference. *The Advocate, 20* (2), 6–8.

American Academy of Pediatrics. (1982). Policy statement: The Doman-Delacato treatment of neurologically handicapped children. *Pediatrics, 70* (5), 810–812.

Bratt, B. (1989) *No time for Jell-O: One family's experiences with the Doman-Delacato patterning program.* Cambridge, MA: Brookline Books.

Christopher, B., & Christopher, W. (1989). *Mixed blessings*: Nashville: Abingdon Press.

Grandin, T., & Scariano, M. (1986). *Emergence: Labeled autistic.* Novato, CA: Arena.

Grandin, T. (1995). The learning style of people with autism. In K.A. Quill (Ed.), *Teaching children with autism: Strategies to enhance communication.* Albany, NY: Delmar.

Gray, C. (1995). Teaching children with autism to "read" social situations. In K.A. Quill (Ed.), *Teaching children with autism: Strategies to enhance communication.* Albany, NY: Delmar.

Greenfield, J. (1971). *A child called Noah.* New York, N.Y.: Holt, Rinehart & Winston.

Hart, C. (1989). *Without reason: A family copes with two generations of Autism.* New York: Harper & Row.

Kaufman, B. (1976). *Son rise.* New York: Harper & Row.

Kaufman, B. (1981). *A miracle to believe in.* New York: Doubleday.

Layton, T., and Watson, L. (1995). Enhancing nonverbal communication in children with autism. In K.A. Quill (Ed.), *Teaching children with autism: Strategies to enhance communication.* Albany, NY: Delmar.

Lovaas, O.I. (1987). Behavioral treatment and normal educational and intellectual functioning in young autistic children. *Journal of Consulting and Clinical Psychology, 55,* 3–9.

Mager, R. (1968). *Preparing instructional objectives* (2nd ed.). Belmont, CA: Fearon-Pitman.

Maurice, C. (1993). *Let me hear your voice.* New York: Knopf.

Schrag, J. (1991). *The reauthorization of PL94-142: How this will impact the states.* Presentation given during a panel discussion at the Autism Society of America National Conference, Indianapolis, IN.

Communication Enhancement

CHAPTER 4

Enhancing Communication in Nonverbal Children With Autism

Thomas L. Layton
Linda R. Watson

To the best of our knowledge, there is no known common single physical factor linked to the cause of autism. At best, it has been associated with a cluster of behaviors that differs from one individual to another and, when viewed as a collective, provides the distinction of autism. It is the severity of the problem, along with the number of associated symptoms, that forms each child's level of disability. Some children with autism are highly verbal, while some say only a few words (Frith, 1989); more than half seem to be unable to speak at all (Rutter, 1978); some exhibit unique behaviors, such as hand flapping or unmitigated squealing, while others do this less often; and some of the children love to be hugged and cuddled, while others prefer not to be touched (Frith, 1989).

It is not the intent of this chapter to describe the common behaviors associated with autism or to describe the uniqueness of the behaviors found in each child, but it is important to have a good understanding of the individual differences found in these children. With this understanding comes a more effective communication intervention program tailored to each child's individual needs. All too often, children with autism are viewed as members of a group, with little interest or concern shown toward each child as an individual. This is clearly not the intent of this chapter. The goal here is to strengthen the perceptions toward the unique qualities of each child. The recommended intervention strategies should be considered for each child individually and should be modified or adapted when the particular needs of the child demand it.

This chapter is written for those children who are considered functioning at a lower level or who are nonverbal. Within this subgroup there are, however, many differences in how the children attempt to interact with people in their environment. It is helpful to begin by determining how these children interact and how they develop social, cognitive, and language behaviors.

DEVELOPMENTAL BEHAVIORS

Social Behavior   Social behaviors enable one to relate to the environment and to interact with others in a social setting. If a child ignores the people around him or her, there is no reason or need to communicate or to learn to deal with problems he or she might encounter in the community.

Several reviews on social deficits in children with autism have appeared recently (Howlin, 1986). To restate what is already known about the topic is not the purpose of this section; it will merely summarize some of the evidence. Nonverbal children with autism have been known to withdraw, to ignore people, and to demonstrate a general problem in getting along with others socially. Their social expressions have been limited to extreme displays of emotion, such as screaming, crying, or laughing profusely, with infrequent signs of subtle expressions such as smiling or frowning.

They are often resistant to social change or disruption in daily routines and prefer to keep their world the same. They can become easily upset if minor changes occur, such as moving the furniture around in their classroom, taking a different route to school, or even eating at a different time during the day. These changes upset them to the extent that they can become more withdrawn or increase their inappropriate behavior.

The children frequently display self-stimulating behaviors: hand flapping, rocking back and forth, producing constant noises, or self-inflicting injuries such as biting, scratching, or picking at a spot on the arm. These behaviors have often been considered noncommunicative by professionals, but actually have been documented in several controlled research studies to be attempts at interacting in different social situations (Donnellan, Mirenda, Mesaros, & Fassbender, 1984; Iwata, Dorsey, Slifer, Bauman, & Richman, 1982; Mundy, Sigman, Ungerer, & Sherman, 1986).

Although these unusual behaviors can be common among nonverbal children, they do not occur to the same degree in each child. One child may have only one or two of these behaviors, while another may demonstrate several. Furthermore, research has found that adults' interactive style can help to improve their social awareness. For example, Dawson and Galpert (1990) reported that mothers' use of imitative play behavior facilitated social responsiveness and toy play in their young children with autism. Compared to a free play session, the children increased their gaze toward the mother and decreased the amount of time looking at the mother's interactions with the toy. Dawson and Galpert (1990) concluded the children did not simply find their mother's contingent interactions with toys more interesting, but rather found social interaction more interesting.

Self-stimulating behaviors occur more frequently at different times of the child's life or during different social situations (Iwata et al., 1982). These behaviors occur more often when the child is left alone than when he is busy working on a task, and less frequently after the child has learned to communicate (Carr & Durand, 1985). The following vignette will help to explain this point.

VIGNETTE Allen was a 5-year-old autistic boy who had little use of language and was being taught to communicate by sign. When Allen was signing and using his language in a structured setting, he attended quite well and enjoyed learning. He rarely displayed atypical behaviors. Part of the language lesson, however, was to have Allen use his newly acquired signs in a free play situation or in an unstructured environment. Allen would pace back and forth across the room and continually vocalize unintelligible utterances. He would stop suddenly, begin to squeal loudly, and then repeat the sequence over again. This behavior would continue until the clinician drew him back to the more structured language lessons or would intervene by attempting to communicate with him. Allen certainly understood the differences between social-communicative situations and those times when he was left alone.

Kara was a 6-year-old autistic girl who had fairly poor communication skills and had also been taught to communicate by sign. She differed from Allen in that when she was given free time, she would seek out her favorite telephone book (a large metropolitan book) and fan through the pages endlessly. This fanning would continue until someone would approach her or would interact with her. She would then put the book down and attend to her communicative partner.

These children are different in obvious ways, but both were able to reduce their atypical behaviors in communicative-social situations or under more organized and controlled conditions. Eventually Allen and Kara were able to learn to reduce their behaviors during unstructured situations. This occurred after they learned to increase communicative skills and began to request things from others. Allen and Kara's atypical behaviors occurred less and less the more they learned to communicate.

Cognitive Behavior

Cognition is reflected in how the child solves problems or achieves tasks that require thinking (Frith, 1988; Leslie & Frith, 1988). It is axiomatic to think that children with higher intelligence solve harder problems with greater ease than do less intelligent children. Even children with normal intelligence can find it difficult to solve various types of problems.

There are nonverbal children who can problem solve in one area but not in another. They can, for example, arrange beads in a complex manner to match a picture but cannot sort colored socks; or they can add and subtract numbers but cannot count money. Nonverbal children may be able to put simple puzzles together or dress themselves if they do these things in a different way. One younger autistic boy could put any puzzle together if it was turned upside down and over. He was not able to put the puzzle together when he looked at the picture because it confused or distracted him, but when it was turned over he could focus on the shapes and put the puzzle together quickly. In fact, he could do it faster than the clinicians could when they were using the picture to help them. This unique ability in problem solving seems related to the basic inability of these children to think abstractly. They may, for instance, be able to see a glass of milk and understand that you drink it, but may not be able to understand that the spoken word "milk" refers to a glass of milk.

Playing with toys and handling objects can also be a unique experience with many nonverbal children with autism (Doherty & Rosenfeld, 1984). Whereas most children learn that a car makes a noise, runs on its four wheels, sometimes crashes into other cars, and can go either fast or slow, the child with autism may not play with cars in this manner. He might notice the wheels move on the car, so he will spin them until someone tells him to stop; or he might notice the car door opens and closes, so he will open and close it until the door falls off. These children have idiopathic play behaviors that often lack normal cause-effect relationships. One primary goal of intervention with these children, therefore, should be to teach them appropriate problem-solving strategies and to help them learn how to play. For more on this topic, see Pamela Wolfberg's discussion in Chapter 8.

Communication Behavior

Language includes forming words, learning the rules for putting the words together, and knowing the purpose or reason for using language (i.e., pragmatics). Pragmatics is the interpreting and use of language in social, physical, cognitive, and linguistic contexts. Pragmatics and communication are closely related. To be a successful communicator, a child must have knowledge of the language he or she is using, as well as the understanding of the human and nonhuman dimensions of the world.

Communication is more than being able to speak or being able to put words together in proper order (Wilson, 1987). It is the ability to let someone else know that you want something, to tell someone about an event, to describe an action, and to acknowledge another person's presence. This can be done either verbally or nonverbally. It can be accomplished through gestures, through the use of signs, or by pointing to a picture or word.

Communication also implies a social situation between two or more individuals. The person who is sending the message is the initiator, while the listener is the receiver. In communication exchanges, the role of the initiator and the receiver switches back and forth. To be fully competent in pragmatic skills, the child must know and understand both roles—that of initiating and that of receiving information (Watson, 1987).

Many children with autism have an especially difficult time in the area of pragmatics (Baron-Cohen, 1988). Kanner (1946), for instance, described the children as not being able to initiate conversation despite being able to talk. When they converse, they tend to request objects, a toy or food, or request the adult to complete an action, but they rarely convey communicative acts such as acknowledging others, commenting on something (a dog outside, a unique picture drawn by the child), or expressing feelings or social etiquette (like saying thank you or good-bye).

Nonverbal children with autism are often receivers of information and frequently respond to their parent's or teacher's requests with a good deal of consistency. For instance, an adult might say to the child, "What do you want to eat?" And the child might respond by giving a picture of a cookie, or pointing to the object, or even saying the word. This is a communicative exchange because the child acknowledged the adult as a partner in the communication exchange and understood what the teacher was asking him to do. The child was both the receiver and the responder in this request.

Helping the child learn to respond in such communicative exchanges is a relatively new intervention approach. It is a great improvement over earlier intervention techniques. The earlier strategies required the child to imitate a word being produced in association with an object (Lovaas, 1977). There was little communication going on in this type of language exchange. At best the child was a receiver of the information but was taught only to label specific items. The usefulness of this information outside the language training environment has been highly questioned. In this approach the child never had the opportunity to learn the necessary communicative exchange to ask someone else to get the car so he could play with it, nor did he or she learn to address someone else socially as a communicative partner. This approach has had little utilitarian value; it never allowed the child to learn that language was about communication with others.

In the role of initiators of communication, children with autism have a good deal of difficulty starting conversations (Feldstein, Konstantareas, Oxman, & Webster, 1982). Therefore any intervention approach should be geared toward helping these children become foremost communicators by learning to be both initiators and receivers of information. A related goal should be to help them become social partners in a world where interaction is of prime importance.

BEHAVIORS NECESSARY TO BE A COMMUNICATOR

There are a number of important elements nonverbal children should have in order to be more successful communicators. They need an understanding of cause-effect, the desire to communicate, someone with whom to communicate, something to communicate about, and a means of communication.

Understanding Cause and Effect

Understanding cause and effect relationships relates to whether the child recognizes that his or her behavior can have a clear outcome. Is the child aware, for instance, that turning the switch on makes the light come on, or opening the cabinet door gives him access to the cookie jar? In communication, if the child does not understand cause-effect, he or she will have difficulty asking someone else to help open the cabinet door or to assist in reaching for an item on the top shelf. Without cause-effect reasoning, the child can not request actions or objects from others, which is one of the earliest communicative acts acquired by typical children.

It is important to look for evidence of understanding cause-effect in informal or observational assessment conditions. The child with autism may not pass specific cause-effect items on a test but may demonstrate understanding of cause-effect relative to his or her own area of interest.

It is important to surround the child with daily activities that will expose him or her to cause-effect events. While being exposed to these activities, the child is also exposed to various forms of symbolic communication associated with the experience; examples are the use of a manual sign for representing the experience (Layton, 1987) or a picture for use in a communication exchange (Bondy & Frost, in press). If the child likes to be tickled, teach the child the sign for tickle or present a picture of "tickling" as a means for the child to request the continuation of the tickle game. While the child is being allowed to explore his environment and learn social exchanges, the environment needs to be structured so that cause-effect happenings occur. When these happenings occur, they then should be paired with some form of communication exchange.

Desire to Communicate

Having the desire to communicate with another person is often a tough task for nonverbal children, since one of their primary challenges is the inability to relate to others in expected ways. They often do not acknowledge or show a particular interest in others. A major reason for this stems from the poor cause-effect relationship discussed earlier. That is, if the child does not have an understanding that someone can help him, or if the child does not understand that his actions will result in getting something, there is little need to relate to others. Often parents and teachers anticipate and respond to the needs of these children too quickly. They just provide the child with everything he needs without expecting the child to communicate with them.

Daily routines and communicative exchanges should be planned where the child is required to interact with others. During these situations, the structure should be planned so that the child learns the value of communicating with others. If the child is never expected to interact with others, he will be deprived of the opportunity to learn the benefits of communicating. The more frequently the child is required to interact with teachers and peers, the more willing he is to do so.

Someone With Whom to Communicate

Frequently teachers and clinicians take the position of initiators in the communicative exchange while the child is allowed merely to be a responder. When the child's needs are interpreted and provided for without him having to ask for anything, then the child is deprived of a communicative partner. Children often use an augmentative communication system or speak a word only on request; for instance, a cookie and a cracker may be displayed on the table and the teacher might ask the child which one he wants. The child gives a picture card to request the cookie after being cued by the teacher. This scenario, however, has two problems with it. First, teachers and parents all too often do not progress beyond this level. Since they do not expect the child to initiate a communicative exchange, they do not wait for it to occur. After a few requested exchanges, the child learns to merely wait patiently for the teacher to direct him and he will receive what is wanted. The child needs opportunities to ask for the cookie independently or initiate the conversation. Otherwise, the child becomes a passive participant in the social and linguistic communicative exchanges.

Something to Communicate About

If the child with autism does not have something to communicate about, he or she will remain noncommunicative. What should the child be asked to communicate about? Some professionals recommend that learning the names of objects is important, because nouns and tangible objects are concrete. Others recommend selecting only functional nouns, as these are the words that typical children learn first (Nelson, 1973). Functional nouns are objects that serve a useful purpose to the individual, such as a key for opening a door, a bat for hitting a ball. They are not merely the names of objects that serve no useful function, such as the floor, a window, a tree. Other clinicians recommend teaching initially the names for foods because specific foods seem to be a reward for many of these children and are self-reinforcing to the child.

Watson, Lord, Schaffer, and Schopler's (1989) recommendation is to let the child be the one to determine what to communicate about. The child should take the lead and direct the conversational interaction. If the child is interested in an action like hugging or swinging, then that is where the conversation should begin. If the child shows a real interest in an object such as a toy car or running water, start with it. To know the child's likes and dislikes can hasten the beginning of early communication. After communication has begun, the teacher or parent can then work on extended vocabulary such as food items and functional nouns.

A Means of Communication

For the nonverbal child, learning to speak may not be the best or preferred system to communicate. In order to communicate with speech, the child must be able and motivated to speak, but this may not be the case initially with many children with autism. The clinician has few options in terms of shaping speech in a nonverbal child. Several research investigations have demonstrated that although nonverbal autistic individuals have a decidedly difficult time learning to speak, they do communicate when using alternative systems such as signing, picture/pictograph exchange, whole word communication boards, and computerized devices. This topic will be discussed in detail in the following section.

ALTERNATIVE COMMUNICATION SYSTEMS

Table 4.1 presents several strategy steps that the authors have found useful in selection of alternative communication systems for children with autism.

Sign Language

The use of signs as a communication system has several strengths but also some weaknesses. One of its major strengths is the fact that during the initial stages of communication signs can be shaped by the parent/teacher and paired with the appropriate reinforcer. One may find an unwillingness to communicate during the initial communicative exchanges with nonverbal children. These children do not have the basic understanding of what communication means or the importance of interacting with someone else, and the use of signs can assist them in learning the importance of communicating. Pairing the sign with the object or the action teaches the child this first important step to communication; it tells the child, "If I make this sign, then I will receive this object or action."

Signs are also quite flexible and can be used anywhere at any time. Signs can express what the child wants quite rapidly and can be easily chained together to make a sentence. Signs frequently are made in such a manner that they closely resemble the object or action associated with them. This is termed iconicity. The sign for drink, for example, is made by shaping the hand as if it is holding a cup and tipping it up to the lips. Thus the sign is readily associated with the object or action the child desires. This iconicity of signs seems to help the child in the learning process (Konstantareas, Webster, & Oxman, 1980).

One concern often expressed by parents and teachers regarding the use of signs and other augmentative systems is whether their child will learn to talk if he or she signs. Using augmentative communication does not seem to inhibit the development of speech. In fact, research (Carr & Dores, 1981; Konstantareas et al., 1980; Layton, 1988; Layton & Baker, 1981; Yoder & Layton, 1989) has clearly demonstrated that learning to communicate initially by sign transfers to the spoken word after the child learns approximately 200 signs and starts to chain two or more signs together. It should be pointed out, however, that even after intensive training with signs, a significant number of nonverbal children continue to be mute and acquire only a few useful signs (Layton, 1983, 1988).

There are some concerns about using sign with nonverbal children (Prizant & Wetherby, 1985). If the child is to become an effective signer, he needs a good model as a communicator. His parents and teacher must know how to sign and preferably be skilled enough to sign in conversational situations. Being able to merely label an object with a sign, as typically occurs with unsophisticated signers, does not help the child become a good communicator. The child should be able to sign sentences, request objects, ask questions during a dialogue with his teacher or parent.

Signing can also be a problem in that only a few people know sign language. Frequently, the child's teacher is the only other person who knows sign language. The child's parent, the bus driver, the music teacher, the occupational therapist, the typical peers, the local sales clerk are not typically signers. Therefore the child does not have an opportunity to communicate in many situations outside the classroom. This is a problem if the child is to become an effective communicator. Essentially the more people who are willing to learn to sign, the more effective the child will become as a communicator, and the sooner he or she will be code switching from a sign system to the spoken system.

Another concern is that some children with autism appear to need static visual cues to aid their communication. Although it is possible to "hold" a sign in place to give the child a longer time to process input, signing systems do not allow a child to visually scan an array of choices to choose the appropriate output. In order to initiate communication with signs, he or she must retrieve the appropriate sign from memory.

Objects for Communicative Exchange

Selecting a set of objects that the child shows interest in can enhance the early stages of communication. If the child wants something, then the child must go and get the object representing what he or she wants. It is important that the object the child seeks does not completely fulfill his or her desire. The child must give the object to someone in order to use it communicatively. At snack time, for instance, giving a cup can serve as a request for juice, giving a plate as a request for a cracker, and giving a knife as a request for peanut butter. In other situations a child might learn such things as bringing a key to someone to ask to go for a ride, giving a bubble wand in order to ask to blow bubbles, or bringing a page from a telephone book to ask for the whole book. Children with autism often use objects spontaneously to communicate, but instead of giving the object to another person, they put the object near the thing that is desired. For instance, the child might put a cup next to a pitcher of juice without acknowledging the person who will pour the juice into the cup. It is important for the child to learn to give the object to a person to help him understand that another person can be the means to a desired end.

Pictures/ Pictographs for Communicative Exchange

Bondy and Frost (in press) have used a similar strategy to establish communication with pictures. They have detailed a program entitled Picture Exchange Communication System (PECS). According to these authors, the use of pictures can provide an immediate functional communication system. The teacher initially observes and determines what items or objects are needed for communication in the child's environment. The child is then taught to associate a picture with the appropriate item. The child is required to pick up a picture and hand it to the teacher, who then exchanges the picture for the item and gives the item to the child. The pictures have been placed on a Velcro communication board where the child must peel off the word before giving it to the teacher. According to Bondy and Frost, the exchange or handing the picture to the teacher has made their approach more successful than simply having the child point to the picture.

Mirenda and Schuler (1986) advocate a somewhat different strategy, which involves prompt-free training to establish pictorial communication in children with autism. Their position is based on work by Mirenda and Santogrossi (1985) with a nonspeaking 9-year-old girl. In this approach, the child is seated at a table, and a high-preference item is within view but out of reach. A picture of the item is placed in front of the child. No verbal cue or physical prompts are given. Rather, the child is engaged in an activity that makes it highly likely the child will touch the picture accidentally. As soon as the child touches the picture, the high-preference item is provided for a brief period of time. Over time the actual item is faded from view. Next, the child learns to choose the picture of the high-preference item when picture cards are also provided. Throughout the entire training, no prompts are employed. This strategy avoids a problem often observed in working with people with autism, that they become readily prompt-dependent.

deVilliers and Naughton (1974) reported on the use of magnets, each with a written label attached, to teach two nonverbal autistic children a communication system. Both children were relatively successful with the system. LaVigna (1977) similarly used word cards to teach the expressive and receptive use of three words by nonverbal autistic adolescents. LaVigna's results indicated that this was an effective procedure for establishing functional use of first words.

▶**TABLE 4.1** Steps for Assisting in Selection of Alternative Communication Systems

	Signing	Pictures/Pictographs	Written Words
Easily Shaped:	Yes	Yes	Yes
	Signs are easy to teach because the teacher can take child's hands, shape them to form appropriate sign, and reinforce the child with the object, action, or concept.	It is easy to physically prompt a child to touch or give a picture card, then reinforce with the action, object, or concept represented by the picture.	Same as pictures.
Active Participation:	Not initially	Not initially	Not initially
	Initially, the child does not have to be a willing participant in the communicative act.	The child does not have to be a willing participant in the communicative exchange for pictures to work.	To use written words for communication, the child does not have to be a willing participant.
Portable:	Yes	Somewhat	Somewhat
	Signs are flexible and portable. They can be used in any entironment—in the classroom, on the playground, at home, in the community.	Pictures are not as easy to carry around for purposes of communication. They can be mounted on a board, strung together and carried around, or put into a wallet-size picture book.	Written words, like picutres, are not as portable for general communication. Child could have a series of words on index cards to carry them around and readily display a word or series of words in discourse situations.
Transient:	Yes	No	No
	In typical input, sign is transient. However, to facilitate processing, an individual sign can be "frozen" in space.	Picture and pictograph systems are nontransient visual spatial systems that allow a child to scan options and select appropriate picture(s) to communicate.	Same as pictures.
Speed:	Yes	Less	Less
	Speed of communication is quite fast, although slower than speech.	Process of communication is slower than for speech, signs, or written words, but faster than using pictures.	Process of communication is slower than speech or signs.
Sentences:	Yes	Limited	Yes
	It is relatively easy and quick to chain more than one sign together during communication.	Pictures are awkward to string together to make a connected sentence.	Written words can be easily chained together, but not as quickly as signs.

TABLE 4.1   (cont.)

	Signing	*Pictures/Pictographs*	*Written Words*
Iconicity:	Yes	Yes	No
	Some signs are iconic, while others are arbitrary. Exact concepts can be represented by signs.	Pictures provide concrete images, but it may be difficult for a child to determine what concept is represented by an image, especially when the concept is not concrete.	Written words represent concepts more exactly than do pictures, but in almost all cases they are related arbitrarily to the concepts.
Other factors:	For signs to be understood, someone else must be able to interpret and use them.	Pictures can be used to represent things in the child's immediate environment. Pictures are easy for the child to use in initial communication because they picture the actual thing the child is attempting to request.	More people can read words than can interpret signs or pictures.
	To be effective, a sign partner needs to be skilled enough to sign in discourse, not simply able to label items.		Written words can be used for expressing ideas and can lead to reading comprehension.
	If the child has a motoric problem (especially in hand coordination), signs may be difficult to form. Often two different signs are formed essentially the same way. This can be confusing to the child as well as to the interpreter.	People can understand what a child wants if the picture is of an object, but it is harder to understand a picture of an action, or other related concepts. However, using written words below pictures can help make communication clear to partners who read.	Reading can enhance one's overall language skills; that is, reading can help to improve sentence structure, increase vocabulary concepts, and define multiple meanings.
		Parents and teachers don't usually use pictures for conservation. Child gets oral input but is expected to express himself by showing or pointing to the picture.	Parents and teachers do not usually use written words for conversation. Child gets oral input and is expected to respond by pointing to written words.

Reading and Computers for Communication

Hyperlexia, or an ability to read beyond what would be predicted based on a person's cognitive abilities, is a phenomenon that has been frequently reported among individuals with autism (Goldberg, 1987). Hyperlexia is not restricted to higher-functioning children. It is sometimes apparent in children functioning cognitively in the severely impaired range and/or in children who have very limited verbal communication abilities. Although comprehension of material being read is at a lower level than the ability to recognize or decode the words, the work of Frith and Snowling (1983) indicated that children with hyperlexia and autism do process meaning at the word level.

It is of interest to utilize these hyperlexic abilities in order to promote functional communication. As with children developing normally, the first print symbols that children with autism recognize are often those from product labels or familiar logos (e.g., McDonald's, Cheerios). Communication with print might involve utilizing such logos on communication cards. For instance, a child named Andrew began to read "Teddy Grahams" from the graham cracker box. The cutout box label was added to his communication cards, which had previously included a generic picture of a cracker that was used to facilitate his requesting of all types of crackers. Andrew learned quickly to read his "Teddy Grahams" card in order to request these particular snacks. Andrew also learned to play a stop-and-go game with his clinicians when they used replicas of traffic signs first to give him directions and then to have him give them directions for "stop" and "go."

The important role of literacy artifacts, or various print materials in the environment, has been stressed in the literature describing the development of emergent literacy in children following a typical course of development (Sulzby & Teale, 1991). Watson, Layton, Pierce, and Abraham (1993) believe that it is important to maximize the exposure of children with autism to print in the environment. For a child who is using a picture communication system, printing words underneath the pictures will not only provide greater cues for the person with whom the child is communicating,

---

VIGNETTE Andrew, the child described earlier, loved to look at books and magazines from an early age. He did not seem to care whether there were pictures accompanying the print or not. At age 4 there was no evidence that he was recognizing any words. He enjoyed, however, having a clinician read a sing-song repetitive book about a teddy bear doing different things in his daily routine (washing his hands, brushing his teeth, etc.) and was soon able to recite the lines corresponding to the page in each book. (Andrew's articulation was not very distinct, but he used the correct prosodic patterns, and some words were intelligible.) It was important to know if Andrew could understand the meaning of the book, so he was taught to act out the different actions using a stuffed teddy bear and other appropriate props. He was able to do this after only a few sessions and could carry out the appropriate actions even if the clinician had him skip around in the book. It was not determined, however, if he was successful because of the pictures or the printed words or some combination of the two. Andrew, along with other children with autism in his program, are now regularly involved in "story time." Attention is given to choosing books that allow very concrete role-playing of this type in order to promote language and literacy skills. By age five, Andrew was demonstrating hyperlexia, and a written word system became central to his communication.

but also expose the child to the words that he or she may then begin to recognize because of the consistency of this exposure. Using picture and word schedules, or printed instructions that include familiar product labels (for example, in a "recipe" for making a peanut butter sandwich) can also help the child with autism begin to understand that print can be used to communicate whether you are an initiator or a receiver of information.

There are several programmable devices with speech output available for children who are able to use visual symbols, whether pictures or printed words, to communicate. Some of these are the Wolf, available through the Wayne County Regional Education Service Agency in Wayne, Michigan; the IntroTalker; and the McCaw. A potential advantage of a speech output device is that it gives the child a "voice" and possibly makes the power of communication clearer to him or her in this way. A potential problem, at least initially, is that the children are so interested in the cause-effect relationship between pushing the panel and having the device speak, that they would rather explore the device itself than use it to communicate with someone. This can be dealt with by programming into the device communication related to the child's favorite routines.

VIGNETTE   Nathan loved to take a bin of crayons, blocks, or other multiple items and "sift" the objects repetitively through his fingers, picking them up and letting them fall back into the bin. For this routine, a computer device was programmed with four squares: "Nathan's turn," "Karen's [the clinician's] turn," "Drop blocks," and "Finished." This activity was sufficiently interesting to Nathan that it was at least in even competition with the device itself. Then the clinician responded to Nathan based on what he made the device say. For example, when he pushed "Finished" (which was the first square he activated when beginning this session), Karen put the top on the bin and said, "Finished? Okay." Nathan protested vocally when he saw her starting to put the blocks up, so Karen responded, "No? Nathan's turn?" and she prompted Nathan to activate the appropriate panel on the device. She then traded the bin of blocks for the device, and let him play with them for a while. During this time, she modeled "Nathan's turn" and "Drop blocks" both with her own comments and by activating the device.

Karen next made a request for "Karen's turn" with the device, and traded Nathan the device for the bin of blocks. It was interesting that Nathan never again, during that session, pushed "Finished" on the device. He seemed to settle on using "Drop blocks" as a request to get the blocks back, rather than using it as a comment on his or Karen's action, and Karen responded to it as a request. Other routines have since been programmed into the device and used with Nathan, and he now clearly understands that the clinician will act in ways that are contingent on which panel he activates on the device.

As is true with speech, sign language, picture-card communication, and so forth, the nonverbal child will lack an initial understanding of using a high-tech device for communication. Getting the child to use any augmentative communication system with a communicative intent is probably the biggest hurdle a clinician or parent will face, and the sophistication of the technology does not matter when one is trying to get over this hurdle. However, because computers and other electronic devices hold so much intrinsic interest for children with autism, a computer will often be something about which a child is motivated to communicate. Thus, the authors have used different computer software programs with children, not because of an expectation the children will learn how to communicate by interacting with the computer, but because they learn to communicate with people in order to get to interact with the computer.

There are only a few studies reporting the use of computers with nonverbal children with autism. Waite and McAloon (undated) reported on a case study using the Wolf with a young nonverbal child. They reported the subject progressed from using one-inch pictures for requesting food, toys, activities, and songs, to the use of the Wolf during story time, and later used it for an entire two-and-a-half-hour classroom morning. Colby (1973) also reported using microcomputers with nonverbal children and found an increase in voluntary use of speech for social communication after interaction with games and symbols on the computer. Frost (1984) described using a computer as an instructional tool with a nonverbal girl with autism. He found that the child's social communication away from the computer expanded in that she began to communicate with a peer rather than only to her teacher when she was asked to talk about the computer. Ratusnik and Ratusnik (1974) reported using an alphabet communication board with a nonverbal child. The child showed an increase in the number of items used in nine syntactic categories, consistent formulation of basic sentences, the ability to express simple wants, needs, and feelings, as well as to relate to past experiences. It was noted, however, that the boy

---

VIGNETTE Two 3-year-old boys with autism were enrolled in a toddler language group along with two nonautistic children. The IBM Speechviewer was used for a group activity with them. The Speechviewer puts up pictures as well as words to show the different programs available, and the clinicians showed the children how to use these pictures on the screen to choose the desired activity. They would take turns using the microphone to activate the animation on the screen. They would have to ask the other child for a turn using words or a gesture, depending on what each was capable of doing. The clinician would terminate the program after a brief period of interaction, so that comments such as "bye-bye" and "all gone," and requests for "more" or another program could be facilitated.

rarely initiated conversation with his augmentative communication system. Although there are only a few studies where computers have been used with nonverbal children, taken together they do suggest that with some children computers can aid in the language learning process and may even facilitate some additional social-communicative interactions.

Facilitated Communication

The strategy for enhancing communication in nonverbal individuals with autism that has received the most attention during the past several years is facilitated communication (FC). The authors of this chapter have followed the literature on FC closely, but have not had personal experience with this approach. As articulated by Biklen (1990), the underlying assumption for FC is that people diagnosed with autism suffer from an expressive communication disorder rooted in a neuromotor disturbance of praxis. In other words, the brain is not able to effectively tell the body how to move in the intended way to produce speech, gestures, written forms, and so forth. Using FC involves providing physical support to the individual at the hand, wrist, elbow, or shoulder. The individual being facilitated typically communicates by pointing to letters or striking keys to spell out a message, although facilitated pointing to words or pictures has also been reported (Biklen, 1990; Calculator & Singer, 1992). The purpose of the physical support is to provide stability, assistance in isolating the index finger, and prevention of impulsive or repetitive responses by pulling the hand back from the communication board or keyboard after each point. The facilitator's role is not to physically prompt a correct response. The eventual goal is to fade physical support so that independent communication is occurring. Facilitators are instructed to provide emotional support by assuming the person is competent, and by being positive and encouraging in their interaction (Biklen, 1990).

Facilitated communication was developed by Rosemary Crossley in Australia, initially in working with individuals with cerebral palsy. Later she began to use this method with individuals with other developmental disabilities, including autism. Crossley and Remington-Gurney (1992) described 430 subjects served by the Dignity through Education and Language Communication Centre (DEAL) in Melbourne, Australia. Of these, 117 had been primarily diagnosed with autism. The authors reported that although only 12 of the individuals with autism were known to have some literacy skills before attending DEAL, 91 of them showed spelling skills adequate for communication during initial FC assessment. They concluded that FC revealed previously existing skills that were obscured by the expressive language impairments of these individuals.

Biklen, Morton, Gold, Berrigan, and Swaminathan (1992) reported on forty-three subjects with autism who had received seven to fifteen months of FC training. The authors noted that the time required to move an individual from the highly structured "set work" that characterizes early stages of FC training to open-ended conversation varied widely among subjects and ranged from one hour to months. Proficiency achieved with one facilitator did not consistently carry over to a new facilitator. The authors claim validation of FC based on the following observations made in this qualitative investigation:

1. Patterns of fine motor movements were consistent for an individual across different facilitators.
2. Typographical errors were consistent across different facilitators.
3. Unique phonetic or invented spellings were used across facilitators.
4. Some unique phrases were typed that would not have been expected from facilitators, such as swearing at the facilitator.
5. Information was communicated that was not known to the facilitator.
6. Personalities were revealed through sarcasm, humor, and so forth.

None of the subjects in this study had moved to communicating without physical support at the time of the report, although some reportedly were being supported lightly at the elbow rather than at the hand.

Adherents of FC proscribe the use of confrontational testing and advocate the use of qualitative research to validate FC. The Biklen et al. (1992) study was a beginning in this regard. As Silliman (1992) pointed out, however, stricter adherence to accepted qualitative research methodology and a more complete report of findings will be needed to advance the claims made based on qualitative approaches.

A number of controlled experimental investigations of FC have been completed to date, resulting in almost uniformly negative findings. One exception is a pilot investigation by Calculator & Singer (1992) in which controlled methodology was applied to the testing of five school-age students, three of whom had autism or "autistic-like" characteristics. In this case each student was facilitated in pointing to pictures while being tested with the Peabody Picture Vocabulary Test-Revised (PPVT-R). Facilitators were prevented from hearing test stimuli by playing masking noise through the headphones they wore. In addition, they were not permitted to look at the examiner, in order to prevent lipreading. The three students with autism all improved their performance on the PPVT-R markedly with facilitation compared with the nonfacilitated administration. With facilitation, they attained scores in the normal to advanced range.

In all other experimental studies of FC involving individuals with autism, there has been a failure to confirm that messages were originating with the person with autism rather than the facilitator, or a failure to reveal previously unknown literacy skills. These include studies by Wheeler, Jacobson, Paglieri and Schwartz (1993) of twelve subjects with autism; Eberlin, McConnachie, Ibel and Volpe (1993) of twenty subjects with autism and one with pervasive developmental disorder; Bligh and Kupperman (1993) of one child with autistic characteristics involved in a court case pursuant to the child alleging sexual abuse through FC; and Smith and Belcher (1993) of eight individuals with autism. While all of these investigations have involved what FC advocates would consider confrontational testing, the investigators were consistently attentive to issues such as making subjects comfortable and familiar with the testing situation, and obtaining informed consent through FC for participation in the studies.

Facilitated communication is a topic currently characterized by controversy and often emotional exchanges between its adherents and skeptics. It is being used on a widespread basis in some parts of the country, and parents and professionals alike often feel compelled to "give it a chance." Unfortunately there are no agreed-on guidelines to suggest which individuals would be good candidates for FC, how its validity can be evaluated for each individual in the absence of independently produced communication, and how long FC should be continued in pursuing the goal of independent production. The decisions are not easy ones. The hope of unlocking an individual's previously untapped potential is set against the expenditure of large amounts of resources in both time and money, and the concurrent lack of implementation of other approaches that might be more appropriate than FC for the individual. Another issue is that accusations of abuse via FC are becoming increasingly common, with far-reaching implications for the importance of validating the source of the communication, protecting the individual with a disability, and also protecting family members, teachers, and other caregivers from false accusations that wreak emotional and financial havoc (Rimland, 1993).

COMMUNICATION INTERVENTION

Intervention Goals

The first goal in working with nonverbal children with autism is to increase their expression of communicative intent, or to help them communicate intent in interpretable rather than idiosyncratic ways. Bates, Benigni, Bretherton, Camaioni and Volterra (1979) have defined intentional communication as "signaling behavior in which the sender is aware *'a priori'* of the effect that a signal will have on his listener, and he persists in that behavior until the effect is obtained or failure is clearly indicated" (p. 36). Foster (1990) suggests the following behaviors might occur during a child's intent:

1. Continuing with a behavior (i.e., reaching or vocalizing until responded to)
2. Showing distress at an object or a person, but ceasing when the person responds
3. Reaching toward something that is clearly out of reach
4. Gazing at an object
5. Proximation, standing beside or in front of

6. Using consistent or "ritualized" facial expressions, gestures, or vocalization to indicate

7. Combining gaze at a person with some other behavior such as a vocalization or gesture

Research has indicated there seems to be a stage development to these intents through which children advance. According to Bates, Camaioni, and Volterra (1976), children begin their intent by reaching for something. The mother observes the reaching and assists by providing the item. The child then learns that reaching "means" the child can obtain an item. The next stage is the child reaching and looking at the parent. This, according to Bates et al. (1979), is the first evidence of intentionality in the child. The last stage occurs when the child vocalizes and uses words to request (Bates et al., 1979).

Wetherby and Prutting (1984) studied the intentional communicative acts among children with autism and found the children used as many intentional communicative acts as did typically developing children. The children with autism, however, used a higher proportion of communicative acts for regulating adults' behavior, and a lower proportion for attracting and directing adults' attention.

In another study, Layton and Stutts (1985) investigated the communicative intent in sixty children with autism. These were children involved in a research project looking at the use of signing as an alternative communication system. As part of that investigation, the researchers analyzed all of the communicative acts that occurred spontaneously throughout the sessions. The results indicated that the children who were high verbal imitators used communicative acts differently from those who were low verbal imitators. The high verbal imitators used more descriptions and performatives and fewer requests. The low verbal imitators, on the other hand, used more requests and descriptions. The low verbal imitators were also limited to regulating or controlling the teacher's behavior or communicated for purposes of describing their immediate environmental conditions. These findings suggest that children with autism do demonstrate the ability to communicate intentionality, albeit this may be at a less advanced level. Second, the children are not a homogeneous group and performance across various communicative tasks is needed.

Once a base level of interpretable communicative intent is established, parents and clinicians are ready to help the child with autism *expand his or her communicative abilities*. There are a number of paths to pursue. Watson et al. (1989) have described a procedure for observing the communicative intent of children with autism and developing goals and objectives based on these observations along with parent and teacher information about what is important for the child to learn in order to be a more effective communicator in his or her environment. In this approach the child's communicative intent as expressed in natural, everyday situations is recorded. An observer records fifty spontaneous communicative acts, or records for a total of two hours of observation time during a variety of typical daily activities in classroom or home. The acts recorded can be either verbal or nonverbal communication, as long as the observer judges the act to have communicative intent.

These communicative acts are then categorized according to several different dimensions, including the purpose or function of communication; the mode or form of communication; the vocabulary used; the types of meaning or semantic categories represented; and the context in which the communication occurred. Table 4.2 shows the taxonomies used for this

▶**TABLE** 4.2
Dimensions of
Communication

I. SEMANTIC CATEGORIES
Most Frequently Observed

Object:	wanted, being acted on, labeled, or described
Action:	own action, other person's action, object's action
Person:	person doing, person desiring
Location:	own location, other person's location, object's location

Less Frequently Observed

Additional Person Words: addressed, acted on, feeling, possessing
                                             of an object, of a person

Observable Qualities:	
Affirmatives	Desire or Need
Internal States	Negatives
Quality of an Event	Social or Routinely Used Words

II. COMMUNICATIVE FUNCTIONS

Request	Give Information
Get Attention	Seek Information
Reject or Refuse	Express Feelings
Comment	Social Routine

III. FORMS OF COMMUNICATION

Motoric	Written
Gestural	Sign
Vocal	Verbal
Pictorial	

IV. CONTEXTS

People	*Places, Activities*
Teachers/Parents	Group Session
Classmates/Siblings	Individual Session
Familiar Adults	Independent Activity
Other Adults	Meals
Other Peers	Leisure Time

Adapted from Watson, Lord, Schaffer, & Schopler, 1989.

categorization process. When the process is completed, it provides a picture of what the child is able to communicate and why, how, where, and with whom he or she is communicating. This type of assessment can be applied to children with autism who have no verbal skills as well as to children who are communicating using spoken words put into simple sentences. This information is then combined with information from parents, teachers, and other significant people in the child's life regarding what communicative needs the child has. In other words, what are the perceptions of these people regarding what will make the child a more effective communicator? These needs can also be categorized according to the preceding dimensions. The child may need to learn to communicate for still other purposes. He or she may need to learn a new form of communication in order to communicate more effectively and may need to expand vocabulary, or learn to express some different types of meaning. For instance, the child's existing vocabulary may be restricted to a set of objects, and the child may need to learn to communicate in some way about actions. Last, the child with autism may need to learn to communicate with more or different people and/or in a broader range of situations.

While using this approach, the child is more likely to achieve a goal if the steps toward that goal do not require the child to learn many new things at once. For example, if the goal is for the child to learn a new form of communication, then the first step should be to teach that new form as a means of communicating for an "old" purpose, using "old" vocabulary, in an "old" context. "Old" skills are those that the child has already exhibited with some consistency in his or her spontaneous communicative behavior. Once the new form of communication has been taught in conjunction with these other established skills, then the child is ready to learn to expand on his or her communicative behavior in other dimensions that have been given high priority in the needs assessment.

One question often asked by parents and clinicians is where to begin with children who are nonverbal. In the current approach, it is strongly recommended that each parent/clinician develop an individual vocabulary list for each child. To help determine this, Layton (1983) has developed a child information sheet that either the teacher or the parent can fill out. The information sheet provides a listing for each child's skills and interests (see Appendix 4.1) and lists the words the child uses spontaneously (either orally, in sign, or through gestures). The data from the information sheet is an excellent place to begin an intervention program. This information, along with the research provided by Nelson (1973) and Bloom, Lightbown, and Hood (1975) based on their research with normal developing children, provides a guide for what vocabulary should be introduced initially—that is, start with what the child knows and build from there.

Introducing early vocabulary items means more than just teaching the names for a few objects. Layton (1983), for example, found that the first words acquired by nonverbal children expressed a variety of concepts, including action words, recurrence, locatives, and attributes as well as general and specific nominals. Nonverbal children have similar needs and desires similar to those of normally developing children and therefore should be exposed to a variety of early vocabulary concepts.

CASE STUDY

Ralph was a middle school age student diagnosed with severe autism. He had learned some signs for communication, but acquired new signs very slowly. His predominant mode of communication was motoric in that he would go to locations or objects associated with his needs, and if he was not able to independently meet those needs, he would intermittently look toward a teacher. He would also move the teacher's hand toward objects that he wanted. The three signs he used most consistently were "ball," "drink," (semantic category of *object wanted*) and "shoe" (to get help in tying his shoe-semantic category of *object acted on*). All of his communication appeared to serve the function of *requesting*. A high priority goal for Ralph was to learn a different form of communication that would be more readily acquired than signs and could be an effective means of communication in a sheltered workshop, which was his next probable placement.

The decision was made to attempt a picture communication system. The "new" element in this case was the form of communication—that is, pictures. In order to begin teaching the new form, the teachers looked at Ralph's "old" skills and determined that they should begin by teaching him to use pictures to communicate a *request* for an *object wanted* or *object (to be) acted on*. In addition, they examined his communication sample to determine what objects he had requested through signs or motoric communication and determined several "old"

vocabulary items, including "ball," "shoe," "key," "toothbrush," "screwdriver," and "drink."

The teachers then removed the objects represented in Ralph's vocabulary from their usual locations and put a picture of each respective object in the location instead. When Ralph went to get the objects during the course of his daily routine, a teacher would prompt him to hand her the picture, and then she would respond by giving him the object. Once Ralph was exchanging the pictures for objects without prompts, the teachers added one or two distracter pictures to the appropriate picture in each location. The teachers found that Ralph had no difficulty selecting the appropriate picture from among the choices; apparently he did have the concept that a picture represented a specific object.

Once Ralph was consistently using a picture to request each of five objects, the pictures were put on a picture board. At least twice a day one of these objects was removed from its usual location. When Ralph went to get the object and could not find it, one of the teachers prompted him to get the appropriate picture from his picture board and give it to a teacher. The prompts were faded as Ralph learned to get and exchange the cards independently. Then, to expand Ralph's skills, the teachers began to add new vocabulary to the picture communication system, focusing largely on vocabulary that Ralph would be able to use in his home, school and vocational setting.

Intervention Strategies

Rutter and Bartak (1973) found when teaching methods were structured (i.e., consistency in daily routines, consequences of inappropriate behavior, and task organization), children with autism obtained the most benefits. In addition, the benefits were greater for the nonverbal than for the more able children. Schopler, Brehm, Kinsbourne, and Reichler (1971) observed children with autism playing in structured and unstructured conditions. The results indicated that the structured condition yielded better performance of attending, appropriate effect, relating to others, and minimized atypical behaviors.

Svavarsdottir (1992) recently completed an ethnographic investigation in three structured classrooms for children with autism looking at how structure enhanced communication. The most frequent interactions that occurred were routine bound. They were either a teacher-child-teacher or child-teacher sequence where the child failed to respond back to the teacher. The teacher, in other words, was mostly controlling the communicative interactions, while the child's communicative purpose was frequently responding back to the teacher's initiations.

MacDonald (1985) and Mahoney and Powell (1988) have demonstrated that a controlling style can limit the options for a child's participation. Nonverbal children can be limited in their communicative style in a highly structured classroom unless the teacher learns to nurture child initiations. Svavarsdottir (1992) observed several naturally occurring incidents throughout the day where the teachers could have followed the child's lead and encouraged a communication initiation. The teachers, however, usually responded to a child's eye gaze or vocalizations by providing the child what he or she wanted. Instead, they could have explanded the child's communication efforts by asking what he or she wanted, clarified the communication attempt, modeled a word, or helped the child use a more effective means of communication. Svavarsdottir presented a number of useful examples of how children related to early communicative attempts in the three classrooms:

1. Gestures involving the hands (e.g., putting another person's hand on a desired item, reaching, pointing, dropping, refusing to take items, taking someone to a desired object)
2. Signals involving eye gaze (e.g., looking at the teacher, looking at a location where a desired object is kept, looking at the desired object, refusing to look at an item)
3. Proximity (e.g., putting himself or herself where somthing happens, moving toward a communicative partner, moving away from an undesired item, standing up from the table)

These signals need to be responded to consistently by teachers, clinicians, and parents. If adults respond to these child attempts, many opportunities for functional communicative intents will occur.

One of the benefits of a highly structured environment is the subsequent establishment of routines. Structure begets routines. One intervention strategy that incorporates the elements of structure is the use of routines or unexpected events. Routines are a powerful means of promoting communication.

Snyder-McLean, Solomonson, McLean, and Sack (1984) are given most of the credit for establishing joint action routines (JAR) with severely impaired individuals. The basic tenet of this approach is to arrange the environment so as to increase the probability that the child will initiate

VIGNETTE A snack-time routine was established for a boy named Troy who liked to eat peanut butter on crackers. Following the suggestion by Snyder-McLean et al. (1984), his clinician wanted to make sure the snack time was a social interactive routine. Troy was taught over several days to ask for peanut butter so he could spread it on some crackers. It was important for Troy to understand that he was expected to ask for it and he was going to do the spreading by himself. In order to do this, he learned to request the peanut butter, the crackers, and a knife to spread it. After he became comfortable with this routine, the next step was to change the environment (or routine). The crackers were no longer made available for him to see; the peanut butter was there and so was the knife, but there were no crackers. His clinician waited for Troy to ask for the crackers. Waiting has been found to be an important facilitator of initiation (Halle, 1982; Snyder-McLean et al., 1984). Halle (1983), for example, recommends waiting by counting silently to oneself for approximately ten seconds. If the child has not initiated a request or a communication, then the adult should make a general statement such as, "I am waiting!" and again wait for the child to communicate, but this time do so with an inquisitive look. If still no initiation comes from the child, then the adult should ask, "What do you want?"

Troy soon learned to ask for the crackers. He then learned that he had to go and find the crackers behind the cabinet door. Following this, the crackers were still moved to another location. When Troy went to the cabinet to look for the crackers, they were gone. His clinician waited for him to request. He said, "Crackers." The clinician said, "That's right, crackers, bring them here." Nothing happened. He then commented, "No crackers." This was the first time he had used a negative word in conjunction with another word. Later on, the routine was again altered by making the knife unavailable to him. Troy had to ask for it. His clinician provided him with a cracked knife so when he tried to scoop out the peanut butter, it broke. The clinician waited to see what he would do or say. This is an unexpected event (Constable, 1983). Finally, she switched the peanut butter with frosting in the jar, so when he opened it up he was surprised to find frosting instead of peanut butter. When he did this, he commented "No peanut butter."

communication. For children with autism, this becomes most effective if initially the environment has been established as a routine. Constable (1983) describes four ways of modifying routines:

1. Violation of routine events (e.g., putting on a coat and hat, and lying down for a nap)
2. Withholding objects or turns (e.g., passing out juice at snack time, but no cups)
3. Violation of object function (e.g., attempting to scoop out peanut butter with a broken knife)
4. Hiding objects or making objects inaccessible (e.g. placing a desirable toy on a high shelf)

Recently, McClenny, Roberts, and Layton (1992) evaluated the use of routine events with ten developmentally delayed children. In their investigation, they included several types of routines, including mislabeling objects or actions (e.g., calling a cup an elephant), making objects inaccessible (e.g., placing a desired object in a closed plastic bag), and violating object function (e.g., trying to pour from a closed bottle). In general, they found that children communicated more frequently during the session that used the unexpected events compared to a simple play session. In addition, the unexpected event of withholding objects was associated with more communication attempts than were the other two events. Violation of object function, however, was more effective than mislabeling objects. Some examples of unexpected events, joint action routines, and alternative choice activities may be found in Table 4.3.

▶**TABLE 4.3**

Sample Unexpected Events, Joint Action Routines, and Choice Activities

I. UNEXPECTED EVENTS
- Spoon too large for jar of applesauce
- Batteries too large for flashlight
- Two opaque juicers—one empty, and one full
- Container with lid sealed
- Spoon with holes to serve liquid

II. JOINT ACTION ROUTINES
- Snack: place small amount in juice container for child to pour.
- Meals: have child set table; eventually have spoons misplaced.
- Cooking: use hand mixer to stir water.
- Play: let child learn how to do a windup toy, then switch to a broken one.

III. ALTERNATIVE CHOICE ACTIVITIES
- Use Pringles and Cheetos containers, child chooses—later switch contents.
- Cans of chocolate and vanilla frosting, child chooses—later switch labels.
- Crackers with peanut butter or cheese spread—later switch labels.
- Two flavors of juice drink, child chooses—later switch contents.

There is one modification to Snyder-McLean et al.'s (1984) JAR that benefits children with autism. It is useful to provide the child with alternative choices. Following the suggestions made by Crystal, Fletcher, and Garman (1976), the adult might ask, "Do you want juice or an apple?" remembering that one of the items is what the child really wants. This approach is used when, no matter what is tried, the normal routine does not elicit initiations from the child. It may be that the child does not yet know the label for the object or he has not learned how to request things. Providing the alternative choice makes the situation more of a recognition task than a recall task. Recognition tasks are easier to process because the child merely needs to decide which one he or she wants. The recall task requires the child to pull from his or her memory the appropriate lexical items. Should the alternative choice technique be used, it is important to remember not to always make the desired choice the last item because children frequently select last items. The adult should also be prepared to provide the child with the wrong choice if one is made by the child. This helps the child to understand the connection between his or her communication and its consequences. It also allows for the child to say "no" or to correct his or her request by asking for the correct item. Recognition tasks seem to occur at a higher level of communication than just asking a child to imitate a word.

SUMMARY

Over the past two decades we have been fortunate in the expanded knowledge about autism. There now is a clearer understanding of the problems associated with autism, especially in the area of communication. Through the use of augmentative and alternative communication systems—signs, picture exchange, written symbols, and computer programs—many of these children have been helped to express their needs and desires. Understandably, parents and teachers are usually concerned about whether the child will speak. In the authors' estimation, it is more important that these children learn to communicate by any means, at least initially. The challenge is to determine what communicative system is best for each child and how to effectively implement it. In this chapter several ideas and strategies were discussed that have been found useful with these children. It needs to be recognized that each child with autism is a unique individual who differs from all other children. With such an understanding, it is hoped that a more productive and communicative individual will emerge.

REFERENCES

Baron-Cohen, S. (1988). Social and pragmatic deficits in autism: Cognitive or affective? *Journal of Autism and Developmental Disorders, 18*, 379–402.

Baron-Cohen, S., Leslie, A., & Frith, U. (1985). Does the autistic child have "a theory of mind"? *Cognition, 21*, 37–46.

Bates, E., Benigni, L., Bretherton, I., Camaioni, L., & Volterra, V. (1979). *The emergence of symbols: Communication and cognition in infancy.* New York: Academic.

Bates, E., Camaioni, L., & Volterra, V. (1976). Sensorimotor performatives. In E. Bates (Ed.), *Language and context.* New York: Academic.

Biklen, D. (1990). Communication unbound: Autism and praxis. *Harvard Educational Review, 60*, 291–314.

Biklen, D., Morton, M.W., Gold, D., Berrigan, C., & Swaminathan, S. (1992). Facilitated communication: Implications for individuals with autism. *Topics in Language Disorders, 12*, 1–28.

Bligh, S., & Kupperman, P. (1993). Brief report: Facilitated communication evaluation procedure accepted in a court case. *Journal of Autism and Developmental Disorders, 23*, 553–558.

Bloom, L., Lightbown, P., & Hood, L. (1975). Structure and variation in child language. *Monographs of the Society for Research in Child Development, 40*.

Bondy, A., & Frost, L. (in press). Educational approaches in preschool: Behavior techniques in a public school setting. In E. Schopler & G. Mesibov (Eds.), *Learning and cognition in autism.* New York: Plenum.

Calculator, S.N., & Singer, K.N. (1992). Preliminary validation of facilitated communication [Letter to the editor]. *Topics in Language Disorders, 12*(5), ix–xvi.

Carr, E., & Dores, P. (1981). Pattern of language acquisition following simultaneous communication with autistic children. *Analysis and Intervention in Developmental Disabilities, 1*, 25–38.

Carr, E., & Durand, V. (1985). Reducing behavior problems through functional communication training. *Journal of Applied Behavior Analysis, 18*, 111–126.

Colby, K. (1973). The rationale for computer-based treatment of language difficulties in nonspeaking autistic children. *Journal of Autism and Childhood Schizophrenia, 3*, 254–260.

Constable, C. (1983). Creating communicative context. In H. Winitz (Ed.), *Treating language disorders: For clinicians by clinicians.* Baltimore: University Park.

Crossley, R., & Remington-Gurney, J. (1992). Getting the words out: Facilitated communication training. *Topics in Language Disorders, 12*(4), 46–59.

Crystal, D., Fletcher, P., & Garman, M. (1976). *The grammatical analysis of language disability: A procedure for assessment and remediation.* London: Edward Arnold/Whurr.

Dawson, G., & Galpert, L. (1990). Mother's use of imitative play for facilitating social responsiveness and toy play in young autistic children. *Development and Psychopathology, 2*, 151–162.

Deich, F., & Hodges, P. (1977). *Language without speech.* London: Souvenir.

deVilliers, J., & Naughton, J. (1974). Teaching a symbol language to autistic children. *Journal of Consultation in Clinical Psychology, 42*, 111–117.

Doherty, M., & Rosenfeld, A. (1984). Play assessment and the differential diagnoses of autism and other causes of severe language disorders. *Developmental and Behavioral Pediatrics, 5*, 26–29.

Donnellan, A., Mirenda, P., Mesaros, R., & Fassbender, L., (1984). Analyzing the communicative functions of aberrant behavior. *Journal of the Association for Persons with Severe Handicaps, 9*, 201–212.

Eberlin, M., McConnachie, G., Ibel, S., & Volpe, L. (1993). Facilitated communication: A failure to replicate the phenomenon. *Journal of Autism and Developmental Disorders, 23*(3), 507–530.

Feldstein, S., Konstantareas, M., Oxman, J., & Webster, C. (1982). The chronography of interaction with autistic speakers: An initial report. *Journal of Communication Disorders, 15*, 451–460.

Foster, S. (1990). *The communicative competence of young children.* New York: Longman.

Frith, U. (1988). Autism: Possible clues to the underlying pathology: Psychological facts. In L. Wing (Ed.), *Aspects of autism: Biological research.* London: Gashill, Royal College of Psychiatrists.

Frith, U. (1989). *Autsim: Explaining the enigma.* Oxford: Blackwell.

Frith, U., & Snowling, M. (1983). Reading for meaning and reading for sound in autistic and dyslexic children. *British Journal of Developmental Psychology, 1*, 329–342.

Frost, R. (1984). Computers and the autistic child. In D. Peterson (Ed.), *Intelligent schoolhouse: Readings on computers and learning.* Reston, VA: Reston.

Garfin, D., & Lord, C. (1986). Communication as a social problem in autism. In E. Schopler & G. Mesibov (Eds.), *Social behavior in autism.* New York: Plenum.

Goldberg, T. (1987). On hermetic reading abilities. *Journal of Autism and Developmental Disorders, 17*, 29–34.

Halle, J. (1982). Teaching functional language to the handicapped: An integrative model of natural environment teaching techniques. *Journal of the Association for the Severely Handicapped, 7,* 29–37.

Helmer, S., Layton, T., & Wolfe, A. (November 1982). *Patterns of language behavior in autistic children.* Paper presented at the ASHA Annual Convention, Toronto.

Howlin, P. (1986). An overview of social behavior in autism. In E. Schopler & G. Mesibov (Eds.), *Social behavior in autism.* New York: Plenum.

Iwata, B., Dorsey, N., Slifer, K., Bauman, K., & Richman, G. (1982). Toward a functional analysis of self-injury. *Analysis and Intervention in Developmental Disabilities, 2,* 3–20.

Kanner, L. (1946). Irrelevant and metaphorical language in early infantile autism. *American Journal of Psychiatry, 103,* 242–246.

Konstantareas, M., Webster, C., & Oxman, J. (1980). An alternative to speech training: Simultaneous communication. In C. Webster, M. Konstantareas, J. Oxman & J. Mack (Eds.), *Autism: New directions in research and education.* New York: Pergamon.

LaVigna, G. (1977). Communication training in mute autistic adolescents using the written word. *Journal of Autism and Childhood Schizophrenia, 7,* 135–149.

Layton, T. (1983). *The acquisition of language and communicative skills by speech and by sign in infantile autism.* Final report, National Institute of Neurological and Communicative Disorders and Stroke, University of North Carolina at Chapel Hill.

Layton, T. (1987). Manual communication. In T. Layton (Ed.), *Language and treatment of autistic and developmentally disordered children.* Springfield, IL: Charles C. Thomas.

Layton, T. (1988). Language training with autistic children using four different modes of presentations. *Journal of Communication Disorders, 21,* 333–350.

Layton, T., & Baker, P. (1981). Description of semantic-syntactic relations in an autistic child. *Journal of Autism and Developmental Disorders, 11,* 385–399.

Layton, T., & Stutts, N. (1985). Pragmatic usage by autistic children under different treatment modes. *Australian Journal of Human Communication Disorders, 13,* 127–152.

Leslie, A., & Frith, U. (1988). Autistic children's understanding of seeing, knowing, and believing. *British Journal of Developmental Psychology, 6,* 315–324.

Lovaas, O. (1977). *The autistic child: Language development through behavior modification.* New York: Irvington.

MacDonald, J. (1985). Language through conversation: A model for intervention with language-delayed per-

sons. In S. Warren & A. Rogers-Warren (Eds.), *Teaching functional language: Generalization and maintenance of language skills.* Baltimore: University Park.

Mahoney, G., & Powell, A. (1988). Modifying parent-child interaction: Enhancing the development of handicapped children. *Journal of Special Education, 22,* 82–96.

McClenny, C., Roberts, J., & Layton, T. (1992). Unexpected events and their effect on children's language. *Child Language Teaching and Therapy, 8,* 229–264.

Mirenda, P., & Santogrossi, J. (1985). A prompt-free strategy to teach pictorial communication system use. *Augmentative and Alternative Communication, 1,* 143–150.

Mirenda, P., & Schuler, A. L. (1986). Teaching individuals with autism and related disorders to use visual symbols to communicate. In S. Blackstone (Ed.), *Augmentative communication: An introduction.* Rockville, MD: American Speech-Language-Hearing Association.

Mundy, P., Sigman, M., Ungerer, J., & Sherman, T. (1986). Defining the social deficits of autism: The contribution of nonverbal communication measures. *Journal of Child Psychology and Psychiatry, 27,* 657–669.

Nelson, K. (1973). Structure and strategy in learning to talk. *Monograph Society for Research in Child Development, 38* (1-2, Serial No. 149).

Prizant, B., & Wetherby, A. (1985). Intentional communicative behavior of children with autism: Theoretical and practical issues. *Australian Journal of Human Communication Disorders, 13,* 21–59.

Ratusnik, C., & Ratusnik, D. (1974). A comprehensive communication approach for a ten-year-old nonverbal autistic child. *American Journal of Orthopsychiatry, 43,* 396–403.

Rimland, B. (1993). F/C under siege. *Autism Research Review International, 7*(1), 2.

Rutter, M. (1978). Language disorders in infantile autism. In M. Rutter & E. Schopler (Eds.), *Autism: A reappraisal of concepts and treatment.* New York: Plenum.

Rutter, M., & Bartak, L. (1973). Special educational treatment of autistic children: A comparative study. II. Follow-up findings and implications for services. *Journal of Child Psychology and Psychiatry, 14,* 241–270.

Schopler, E., Brehm, S., Kinsbourne, M., & Reichler, R. (1971). Effect of treatment structure on development in autistic children. *Archives of General Psychiatry, 24,* 415–421.

Silliman, E. R. (1992). Three perspectives of facilitated communication: Unexpected literacy, Clever Hans, or enigma. *Topics in Language Disorders, 12*(4), 60–68.

Smith, M., & Belcher, R. G. (1993). Evaluating the facilitated communications of people with developmental disabilities. *Journal of Autism and Developmental Disorders, 23*, 175–183.

Snyder-McLean, L., Solomonson, B., McLean, J., & Sack, S. (1984). Structuring joint action routines: A strategy for facilitating communication and language development in the classroom. *Seminars in Speech and Language, 5*, 213–228.

Sulzby, E., & Teale, W. (1991). Emergent literacy. In R. Barr, M. Kammil, P. Mosenthal, & D. Pearsons (Eds.), *Handbook of reading research* (Vol. II) . White Plains, NY: Longman.

Svavarsdottir, S. (1992). *Spontaneous communication in structured classrooms.* Unpublished master's thesis, University of North Carolina at Chapel Hill.

Waite, B., & McAloon, M. (undated). *Integrating the Wolf into the augmentative communication strategies of a verbally limited preschooler with autism.* Crossroads Rehabilitation Center, 4740 Kingsway Drive, Indianapolis, IN.

Watson, L. (1987). Pragmatic abilities and disabilities of autistic children. In T. Layton (Ed.), *Language and treatment of autistic and developmentally disordered children.* Springfield, IL: Charles C. Thomas.

Watson, L., Layton, T., Pierce, P., & Abraham, L. (1993). Facilitating emerging literacy in a language preschool. *Language, Speech and Hearing Services in Schools.* Under review.

Watson, L., Lord, C., Schaffer, B., & Schopler, E. (1989). *Teaching spontaneous communication to autistic developmentally handicapped children.* Austin, TX: Pro-Ed.

Wetherby, A., & Prutting, C. (1984). Profiles of communicative and cognitive-social abilities in autistic children. *Journal of Speech and Hearing Research, 27*, 364–377.

Wheeler, D. L., Jacobson, J.W., Paglieri, R. A., & Schwartz, A. A. (1993). An experimental assessment of facilitated communication. *Mental Retardation, 31*(1), 49–60.

Wilson, M. (1987). Aspects of language. In T. Layton (Ed.), *Language and treatment of autistic and developmentally disordered children.* Springfield, IL: Charles C. Thomas.

Wolfberg, P. (1995). Enhancing children's play. In K.A. Quill (Ed.), *Teaching children with autism: Strategies to enhance communication and socialization.* Albany, NY: Delmar.

Yoder, P., & Layton, T. (1989). Speech following sign language training in autistic children with minimal verbal language. *Journal of Autism and Developmental Disorders, 18*, 217–229.

APPENDIX 4.1   **Child Information Sheet (Nonverbal)**

Child's name_____ Date of birth_____

School or center_____ Address_____

Parents_____ Home address_____

Telephone _____

1. What does your child do best?

2. What does your child have most problems with?

3. If left alone, what will your child do? (How does your child spend most of his/her free time?)

4. What toys or other objects does your child like?

5. What are your child's favorite foods?

6. Is child on special diet? If yes, describe.

7. Does your child have allergies to foods or other materials? Which?

8. Is your child toilet trained? How much assistance does she/he require? How does your child indicate needs?

9. Does your child have medical problems that a teacher should be aware of? Seizures? Is your child on medication? When is medication given? By whom?

10. Is there a time during the day when your child functions best? Is least attentive?

11. Under what conditions does your child work best? (For example: sitting at a table, in a small space, with no distractions, etc.)

12. What behavior problems interfere with your child working? How frequently do these occur? Under what circumstances?

13. How are your child's behavior problems usually managed? (For example: time out, removal of toys, loud reprimand, ignoring.)

14. What reinforcement (reward) works best with your child?

15. Are there materials or activities that upset your child or that he/she is afraid of?

16. What are the names for parents, siblings, teachers, special friends, and pets that your child uses or relates to?

17. Please list any words that your child uses spontaneously (says, signs, or gestures without your saying or signing the word first) and appropriately.

CHAPTER 5

Assessment and Intervention Strategies for Children Who Use Echolalia

Patrick J. Rydell
Barry M. Prizant

Echolalia refers to the repetition of others' speech, repetition that may occur immediately after or significantly later than the original production of an utterance. Echolalia is characteristic of at least 85 percent of the children with autism who acquire speech (Prizant, 1987). The purpose of this chapter is to provide systematic strategies for communication assessment and intervention for children who use echolalia. Guidelines for assessment and intervention presented here are based primarily on a review of empirical studies and the authors' own experiences with children who use echolalia.

The first half of this chapter focuses on the assessment of echolalia within the context of a child's communicative abilities. Major components of a systematic assessment strategy will be introduced and described. Other chapters in this volume (specifically Chapters 4 and 7) offer additional methods of communication assessment that are relevant for children who use echolalia. Each assessment component will include specific guidelines that, while not exhaustive, should provide the interactant with sufficient information to structure appropriate intervention strategies for children who use echolalia.

The second half of this chapter will be devoted to intervention issues. Guidelines for intervention will parallel the assessment components found in the first half of the chapter. Due to the great variability observed in patterns of echolalia, the intervention section should not be viewed as a "cookbook" approach, but rather as a compilation of guidelines to individualize appropriate interventions based on the assessment outcomes and goals of communication programming.

DEFINITION AND NATURE OF ECHOLALIA

Differences in definition and lack of operationally defined criteria have resulted in inconsistent views of echolalic behavior of children with autism. Schuler (1979) indicated that the term "echolalia" typically is used to refer to a general class of speech repetition with few distinctions made regarding the degree of repetition or comprehension and intentionality underlying the production of echolalic utterances.

Since Schuler's observations, little progress has been made in reaching a consensus toward defining echolalic behavior. Immediate echolalia has been defined as "the meaningless repetition of a word or word group just spoken by another person" (Fay, 1969, p. 39). Fay noted that the use of the term "meaningless" is a necessary qualifier, although this judgment is most often based on inference. Roberts (1989) defined immediate echolalia as "recognizable imitation occurring within two utterances of the model" (p. 276). Delayed echolalia has been defined as the "echoing of a phrase after some delayed or lapse of time" (Simon, 1975, p. 1440). Similarly to Roberts and Simon, Prizant and Duchan (1981), Prizant and Rydell (1984) and Rydell and Mirenda (1991) used primarily structural criteria in their definitions of immediate and delayed echolalia (i.e., criteria specifying the degree of similarity between the model and repeated utterances). In contrast, Laski, Charlop, and Schreibman (1988) defined immediate echolalia as "inappropriate repetitions of words or phrases" (p. 394) and delayed echolalia as "non-functional repetitions [produced] out of context" (p. 394). Like Laski et al., Zyl, Alant and Uys (1985) and Prizant and Duchan (1981) viewed "relevance" as one dimension that varies within the category of echolalia, not as a criterion for defining echolalia.

The clearest distinction that has been made differentiates two general categories of echolalic behavior based on temporal latency between the original production of an utterance and the subsequent repetition. Immediate echolalia refers to utterances that are produced either immediately following or a brief time after the production of the model utterance. Delayed echolalia refers to utterances repeated at a significantly later time. The process involved with the production of delayed echolalia involves retrieval of information from some type of long-term memory, while for immediate echolalia, short-term memory is most often implicated (Hermelin & O'Connor, 1970).

Many researchers argue against viewing echolalia solely as meaning-less or inappropriate repetition. These researchers contend that echolalia is not always just rote repetition, but is at times produced with evidence of intervening rule-governed linguistic processes (Fay, 1967; Shapiro, Roberts, & Fish, 1970; Voeltz, 1977) as well as comprehension (Prizant & Duchan, 1981; Prizant & Rydell, 1984; Roberts, 1989). Telegraphic echoing and appropriate grammatical substitutions are forms of "mitigated echolalia," or echolalia produced with some change, and such forms are interpreted as denoting some degree of linguistic processing. These studies have expand-ed the category of echolalia from reflex-like parroting behavior to a contin-uum of behavior that, while clearly repetitive, does not involve only exact repetitions.

Research on echolalia addressing its functional value clearly reflects conflicting points of view. These range from descriptions of echolalia as pathological behavior without functional value, to considerations of echolalia as a socially motivated compensatory strategy serving the general function of maintaining social contact, to descriptions of echolalia as serv-ing specific communicative functions. Inherent in this diversity of view-points are the issues of the presence or absence of comprehension and com-municative intent underlying echolalic productions.

Researchers who view echolalia primarily as pathological behavior have applied a variety of approaches to the "remediation" of echolalia. Such procedures range from the use of the command "Don't echo" (Lovass, 1977) to replacement of echolalia with utterances such as "I don't know" (Schreibman & Carr, 1978) or other trained verbal responses (Fox, Faw, McMorrow, Davis, & Bittle, 1988; Durand & Crimmins, 1987). With few exceptions (e.g., Durand & Crimmins, 1987), this literature does not consid-er child differences apparent in the production of echolalia (e.g., situational and interpersonal determinants), functional usage in natural interactions, and its possible relationship to language and communicative growth. In fact, echolalia has been studied most frequently in highly controlled labora-tory contexts, not allowing for any consideration of its role in more natural social interactions. From this orientation, echolalia is rarely considered in reference to the expression of communicative intent or in reference to cog-nitive, communicative, and linguistic growth.

Other researchers (Fay, 1973; Fay & Schuler, 1980) have discussed the social value of immediate echolalia, noting that it may allow for social clo-sure and represent a primitive attempt to maintain social contact with oth-ers. While asserting that echolalia serves a general function of maintaining social contact, these researchers did not attempt to delineate specific social functions. A number of studies have attempted to explore specific social functions of immediate and delayed echolalia (Prizant & Duchan, 1981; Prizant & Rydell, 1984) (see Table 5.1). Prizant and Duchan derived seven functional categories of immediate echolalia based on videotaped analyses of 1,009 echolalic utterances of four children with autism.

▶**TABLE 5.1**

Functional
Categories of
Immediate and
Delayed Echolalia

I. IMMEDIATE ECHOLALIA INTERACTIVE FUNCTIONS	
Turn-taking	Turn fillers in a verbal exchange
Declarative[*]	Labels objects, actions, or location
Yes-answer[*]	Indicates affirmation
Request[*]	Requests objects or others' actions

II. IMMEDIATE ECHOLALIA NONINTERACTIVE FUNCTIONS	
Nonfocused	No apparent intent; often produced in states of high arousal
Rehearsal[*]	A processing aid; followed by utterance or action
Self-regulatory[*]	Used to regulate one's own actions; produced in synchrony with activity.

III. DELAYED ECHOLALIA INTERACTIVE FUNCTIONS	
Turn-taking	Turn fillers in verbal exchange
Completion	Completes familiar verbal routine initiated by others
Provide Info[*]	Offers new information not apparent from situational context
Labeling[*]	Labels objects/actions in environment (interactive)
Protest[*]	Protests or prohibits actions of others
Request[*]	Requests objects or other's actions
Calling[*]	Calls attention to oneself or maintains interaction
Affirmation[*]	Indicates affirmation
Directive[*]	Directs others' actions

IV. DELAYED ECHOLALIA NONINTERACTIVE FUNCTIONS	
Nonfocused	No apparent communicative intent or relevance to the context
Situational	No apparent communicative intent; appears to be association triggered by an object, person, situation, or activity
Self-directive[*]	Used to regulate one's own actions, produced in synchrony with activity
Rehearsal[*]	A processing aid; followed by utterance or action indicating comprehension of echoed utterance
Label [*]	Labels objects or actions with no apparent communicative intent; may be form of practice for learning language (noninteractive)

Prizant & Duchan, 1981; Prizant & Rydell, 1984
[*]Produced with evidence of comprehension

Children with autism were videotaped in naturalistic interactions over an eight-month period and were found to produce echolalic utterances that were interactive as well as noninteractive. The specific categories included: nonfocused, turn-taking, declarative, yes-answer, request, rehearsal, and self-regulatory. McEvoy, Loveland, and Landry (1988) and Zyl, Alant, and Uys (1985) later replicated in part the findings of Prizant and Duchan (1981). Prizant and Rydell (1984) also delineated fourteen functional categories of delayed echolalia based on systematic analyses of three children with autism. Procedures used to determine these categories were similar to those of Prizant and Duchan. Table 5.1 decribes these functional categories, which include delayed echoes used for a variety of social and cognitive purposes.

Although not specifically addressed in previous research, echoic utterances can be further differentiated based on the degree of conventionality with which the utterance is produced; that is, the extent to which verbal behavior is comprehended or understood by members of a language community, allowing for successful communication (Prizant & Rydell, 1993). Although echolalia has generally been considered as an unconventional verbal strategy, the authors feel that echoic productions should be viewed on a continuum from less to more conventional, based on the following criteria:

1. whether words in echoic productions are used with similar underlying meanings shared by other members of a community;
2. whether echoes are seen as relevant to the communicative context;
3. whether echoes are produced with communicative intent;
4. whether utterances add new or needed information to a conversational interaction;
5. the interactant's responsiveness to echoic utterances;
6. whether the echoic behavior interferes with a child's ability to attend to and participate productively in either communicative interactions or educational learning tasks; and
7. whether patterns of echolalia bring negative attention or otherwise stigmatize a child.

In summary, it is our contention that immediate and delayed echolalia is best described as a continuum of behavior in regard to exactness of repetition, degree of comprehension and conventionality, and presence of underlying communicative intent (Prizant & Rydell, 1993; Schuler & Prizant, 1985).

Echolalia and Language Development

Two positions can be identified regarding the role of echolalia in the process of communicative growth. One position is that echolalia is pathological behavior that stands outside the realm of cognitive and linguistic growth and may even interfere with such growth (Coleman & Stedman, 1974; Schreibman & Carr, 1978). Thus echolalia must be extinguished to allow for the acquisition and use of more functional communication. Interestingly, there is no evidence that extinguishing echolalic behavior has resulted in the acquisition of a more functional communicative repertoire.

An alternative position attempts to understand echolalic behavior within the context of a child's cognitive and linguistic growth. This position recognizes that movement from less conventional to more conventional communicative forms can be thought of as a developmental progression observed in children with and without disabilities (Prizant & Wetherby, 1987). The most specific position concerning the role echolalia may play in language acquisition was first posited by Baltaxe and Simmons (1977) and has since been expanded upon in greater detail (Prizant, 1983, 1987). Based on their research, Baltaxe and Simmons suggested that children with autism may acquire language by using a rote memory strategy, with subsequent segmentation of memorized linguistic forms. Prizant and Rydell (1984) found that their subjects frequently recombined and conjoined language chunks, a process analogous to young children's early movement from single to multiword utterances. Baltaxe and Simmons hypothesized that such segmentation of unanalyzed forms provided the basis for the acquisition of a rule-governed and generative linguistic system.

Prizant (1983) further hypothesized that echolalic behavior may play a role in the acquisition of linguistic function as well as structure among children with autism, and he emphasized that it is important to consider echolalic behavior within the larger context of the cognitive processing style of those children. That is, language acquisition in autism closely resembles what has been described as a gestalt style of language acquisition observed in typically developing children (Peters, 1983). Peters suggests that language learners fall along a continuum ranging from analytic processors to gestalt processors. Analytic processors acquire language with an appreciation of basic constituent structure and meaning and move through stages of increasing linguistic complexity (i.e., single words to two- and three-word utterances and beyond). Gestalt processors acquire language by memorizing and repeating multiword units, initially with limited linguistic comprehension. As noted, these "chunks" are eventually analyzed into their constituent components. Typically developing children demonstrate patterns reflecting each processing style, with some variability along the continuum (Peters, 1977).

It appears that children with autism who acquire spoken language may be limited to an extreme form of a gestalt processing style. In a gestalt processing mode, language may be processed as whole units rather than analyzed and segmented into meaningful components allowing for rule induction. An extreme gestalt processing strategy may help to explain other commonly cited problems in autism such as limitations in understanding and coping with unpredictable change, in inducing rules of hierarchical systems, and in understanding and developing social rule systems as well as in acquiring a flexible and generative language system (Prizant, 1983). Communicative and linguistic skills are especially likely to suffer because of the rapidly changing and contextually sensitive adjustments and repairs that are necssary for successful ongoing interactions.

ASSESSMENT

The systematic assessment of echolalia will be outlined in this section. Each assessment component is important in developing a comprehensive profile of echolalia within the context of a child's communicative system.

Assessment Considerations

Echolalia should be considered as a dynamic and integral part of a child's communicative functioning rather than an isolated and nonfunctional behavior. Echolalia should also be viewed as part of the child's total system of communication and considered in reference to the child's communication history, including evidence of progressive change with respect to functional, syntactic, and semantic usage (Prizant & Rydell, 1993). An assessment scheme for echolalic behaviors should also consider

1. situational determinants and antecedent conditions,
2. range of communicative intents and functions,
3. the range of verbal and communicative behavior other than echolalia,
4. the match between specific situations and type of echolalia,
5. the degree to which echolalia is understood by the communicative interactant and/or challenging to both the child and interactant, and
6. the relationship between echolalia and other communicative behaviors.

These considerations reflect current views on echolalia, which suggest that for many children with autism, echolalia is a legitimate compensatory verbal strategy that may be used for a variety of social and cognitive purposes and plays a significant role in the child's progression from automatic to more generative forms of language production.

Data Collection

The systematic assessment of echolalic patterns should begin with the collection of language samples, preferably using videotape across multiple settings. In collecting and transcribing language samples, the interactant should

1. use familiar routines, toys, and children;
2. create communicative opportunities (see Appendix 5.1 for examples);
3. request that the interactant communicate naturally, using both adult directive and facilitative styles (see the section headed Intervention for descriptions);
4. collect samples in a variety of settings that include different activities; and
5. document significant nonverbal as well as verbal behaviors.

A charting system is useful for transcription and analysis of echoic and other verbal behaviors. An example of a charting system that incorportates these assessment components can be found in Appendix 5.2.

Once all utterances and contextual variables have been transcribed from the videotape, a variety of analyses can be conducted and hypotheses formulated about the nature of the child's communicative system. If videotaping is not possible, audio taping or written transcription by a second observer is often useful. The following subsections delineate components for analyses.

Categorizing Echolalia and Other Verbal Behaviors

The initial focus in the analysis of echolalia is to identify and categorize echolalic utterance types according to the structural criteria that follow, while in turn differentiating it from other forms of both conventional and unconventional verbal behavior often used by children with autism. As we have noted, there are two primary types of echolalia: immediate echolalia are verbal repetitions produced immediately or soon after the production of the model utterance, and delayed echolalia are verbal repetitions produced at a significantly later time. Both types of echolalia can be further

▶ **TABLE 5.2**
Definitions of
Verbal Repetition
Strategies

I. *Immediate echolalia is repetition of speech that*
   • is produced either following immediately or within two turns of original production;
   • involves exact repetition (pure echolalia) or minimal structural change (mitigated); and
   • may serve a variety of communicative and cognitive functions.

II. *Delayed echolalia is repetition of speech that*
   • is repeated at a significantly later time—that is, at least three turns following original utterance, but more typically hours, days, or even weeks later;
   • involves exact repetition (pure echolalia), or minimal structural change (mitigated echolalia); and
   • may serve a variety of communicative cognitive functions.

III. *Perseverative speech is persistent repetition of speech that*
   • consists of a word, phrase, or combination of utterances that are imitated (echolalia) or self-generated;
   • is produced in a cyclical, recurring manner; and
   • is produced with no evidence of communicative intent or expectation of a response from the interactant.

IV. *Incessant questioning is repeated verbal inquiries that*
   • are directed toward the interactant;
   • are produced with communicative intent, often to initiate or maintain interaction with an expectation for a response; and
   • persist either immediately following a response or after a short respite even though a response was provided.

V. *Generative language is single words or utterances that*
   • are independently produced (nonrepetitions);
   • are produced as the result of the speaker's own linguistic rule system;
   • may be associated with more than one referent (are not context or referent specific);
   • demonstrate flexible language production by being combined and recombined with other words or phrases.

Prizant & Rydell, 1993

differentiated by whether they are exact repetitions of others' speech (pure echolalia) or produced with some modifications—that is, omissions, additions, or modifications of an interactant's model utterance (mitigated echolalia). Other verbal repetition strategies that may or may not be forms of echolalia include perseverative speech and incessant questioning, which tend to be produced in a more persistent, highly repetitive, or stereotypic manner and may be triggered by a preceding utterance, or specific environmental stimuli (e.g., objects, events, children). These verbal repetition strategies differ from generative forms of verbal behavior, which are flexible, creative, and derived from the child's own rule-governed language system. Table 5.2 provides categories and definitions of the various types of verbal strategies typically used by children with autism.

Research and the authors' experiences have suggested that echolalia is more likely to occur under specific environmental and interactional conditions, often as a compensatory means of communication. Higher incidences of echolalia have been noted to occur when children with autism are asked to participate in unfamiliar or challenging activities, during unstructured time, during transitions, and under highly obligatory interactions (e.g., when adults use high-constraint utterances and a directive verbal style). Difficulties in comprehending language and social situations are also associated with increased production of echolalia. Table 5.3 lists possible variables that may be associated with higher incidences of echolalia.

Research has demonstrated that echolalia is used for a variety of social, cognitive, and communicative purposes (Prizant & Duchan, 1981; Prizant & Rydell, 1984). Echoic utterances may be directed to a interactant (i.e., for attentional or instrumental purposes) or used for noninteractional/cognitive purposes (i.e., self-regulation, language rehearsal). Other forms may be

TABLE 5.3

Variables Associated With Higher Incidences of Echolalia

I. SITUATIONAL VARIABLES
- Unstructured, unpredictable, or transitional periods
- Unfamiliar tasks or situations
- Difficult or challenging tasks
- Stimuli presented in which the child is hypersensitive in audition, tactile, kinesthetic, vestibular and/or visual
- Emotionally arousing contexts or activities causing anxiety, fear, distress, elation

II. INTERACTIONAL VARIABLES
- Complex linguistic input
- High-constraint linguistic input
- Partner's directive interactional style

III. PERSON-SPECIFIC VARIABLES
- Gestalt style of language acquisition and use
- Language comprehension difficulties

highly automatic and nonfunctional without any reference to children or objects in the present context. Degree of interactiveness can be determined by body posture or orientation; by gaze behavior, including eye contact and gaze checks; by accompanying gestures including pointing or showing; and by quality of the utterance, such as loudness.

It is important to determine in general whether echoic utterances are produced with or without evidence of comprehension. The question of comprehension should not be determined on an all-or-none principle, but rather should attempt to discern the degree of comprehension associated with utterances. Evidence of comprehension can be determined by co-occurring nonverbal behavior that is clearly associated with echoic utterances. Such behavior provides clues as to the elements of utterances that may be understood. Nonverbal and interactional variables that help to determine degree of comprehension include the following: gestures such as reaching, pointing, showing, open-handed requests, movement to an object, or an action performed on an object immediately prior to, during, or following production of an echoic utterance; echolalia produced semantically contingent to prior discourse (produced subsequent to echoic response); and behaviors indicating the expectation of further action by the interactant (e.g., gaze check or subsequent verbal or nonverbal requests).

Communicative Intent

Probably the most important component in analyzing echoic behaviors is the determination of underlying communicative intent and the functions served by echoic utterances. These two assessment components can be differentiated as communicative intent and communicative function.

Communicative intent is the underlying purpose of a communicative act produced by a child. That is, what is the intended goal or effect of a communicative act? It may be said that acts are produced intentionally when a child has a plan in mind to achieve a specific goal or to have a specific effect on others. *Communicative function* is the actual effect of a child's behavioral act. Communicative function is dependent on the partner's interpretation of, and reaction to, the behavioral act.

In many cases communicative intent and the resulting communicative function are the same. For instance, a young child may echo, "Do you want a drink?" with the intention of requesting a drink, which in turn results in the interactant correctly interpreting and acting on this echo as a legitimate request. In other instances communicative behaviors may be interpreted as having a communicative function by the interactant without the child intending either to send that particular message or even to verbally interact with another child. For instance, a young girl may be producing the delayed echo, "Mommy, come here" while playing with dolls, with her back turned away from everyone in the room. The interactant may perceive this echo to have a "calling" function and go to the child. However, the purpose underlying the utterance may be a noninteractive labeling behavior in which the child was "practicing" or replicating a play activity. During the verbalization, the doll was referred to as "Mommy" without any intent of calling to, or interacting with, children who were present.

Careful and systematic analyses of communicative intent must be performed under a variety of conditions (Schuler, 1979). This is particularly true for echolalia if one is to determine the progression of echolalia from utterances produced without evidence of communicative intent to those produced with clear evidence of communicative intent and the range of that communicative intent.

Echoic utterances may be produced with differing degrees of communicative intent. Individual occurences can best be thought of as falling along a continuum of verbal production echoes with and without evidence of interactiveness and comprehension. Communicative intent underlying echolalia does not appear to be an all-or-nothing proposition (Prizant & Rydell, 1993) but rather is part of a progression from the absence of intent (i.e., reflexive, automatic, no awareness of goal) to clear intentionality in which communicative behaviors are coordinated and directed to others in the quest to accomplish a communicative goal (Wetherby & Prizant, 1989). Evidence of advanced degrees of intentionality can be seen in the child's use of repair strategies and the ability to reflect on the effectiveness of a communicative act.

Wetherby and Prizant (1989) have outlined the developmental progression of communicative intent in normal children, which is also useful in determining the degree of intentionality underlying echoic utterances in children with autism. A description of each category is followed by an example of this progression of communicative intent seen in autistic children who are echolalic.

1. *No awareness of a goal.* A child shows a diffuse fuss or reaction to a nonspecific situation to express an emotion such as frustration, anger, excitement, or pleasure. The autistic child is not directly involved in a purposeful activity (e.g, sitting in a beanbag chair) while engaged in behavioral and verbal perseverations without regard or attention toward interactants.

2. *Awareness of a goal.* The child reacts to an object or person by focusing attention to, manipulating the physical properties of, or vocalizing toward the person or object. The autistic child reaches for a cookie while producing the delayed echo, "Time for snack," but doesn't direct the utterance to others.

3. *Simple plan to achieve a goal.* The child focuses attention to and directs a motoric or vocal act toward a person. The autistic child reaches for the cookie and echoes, "Do you want a cookie?" directly to the adult as an affirmation after the person has shown him a cookie while asking, "Do you want a cookie?"

4. *Coordinated plan to achieve a goal.* The child uses intermediary objects or a combination of motoric and/or vocal behaviors and directs the act toward another person as evidenced by body orientation, eye gaze, or waiting for a response. For example, an autistic child and an adult are engaged in a turn-taking event such as rolling trucks back and forth on the floor. The child establishes eye contact and echoes, "Ready, set, go" as a request/directive. The adult subsequently rolls the truck to the child.

5. *Alternative plan to achieve a goal.* The child uses a modified form of a signal or uses an alternative strategy that is directed toward another person after at least one unsuccessful attempt to achieve a goal. The autistic child echoes, "Open the door." as a request to go outside after an unsuccessful attempt at opening a door. Following no response by the adult, the child looks at the adult and echoes, "Do you want to go outside?" thus using an alternative means to express intent through echolalia.

6. *Metapragmatic awareness to achieve a goal.* The child reflects on the means, success, or failure of a plan to achieve a particular goal.

The last category, metapragmatic awareness, is rarely observed in children who are primarily echolalic, but is more commonly seen in children who are primarily generative language producers. It has been our experience that most immediate and delayed echoes produced by autistic children fall within the first five categories.

Strategies for Assessing Communicative Intent

Several strategies may be useful in analyzing communicative intent underlying echolalia. The first involves conducting an interview with those children who are most familiar with the child and his/her communicative patterns. In Chapter 7, Quill discusses this format in greater detail. The primary purpose of an interview format is to develop a profile of how the child uses echolalia for communicative purposes across a variety of children and interactive contexts. Interview formats are also particularly useful in gathering descriptive information about the possible origins of delayed echoic responses, idiosyncratic patterns of usage, and interactive/contextual variables that may influence the production of echolalia. Table 5.4 outlines factors that may be useful in analyzing communicative intent.

In addition, specific communicative intents/functions may be determined for a child's echoic behaviors through videotaped analysis of the child and his or her interactants. Categories of pragmatic functions for immediate (Prizant & Duchan, 1981) and delayed (Prizant & Rydell, 1984) echolalia have proven useful in determining possible social and cognitive uses of echolalia by children with autism in naturalistic contexts.

Individual echoic utterances may also be differentiated according to whether they were produced as initiations or responses. By definition,

▶**TABLE 5.4**

Assessment
Factors in
Determining
Communicative
Intent

1. Communicative means. Actual nonverbal (gestures, gaze), vocal, and/or verbal (use of words, signs) signals used; the complexity and content of verbal acts should be specified.
2. Linguistic context of the behavioral act. Language produced prior to or following a communicative act determines semantic contingency or discourse structure.
3. Nonlinguistic context of the behavioral act. Consider the vocalizations, gestures, and facial expression that augment the communicative act.
4. Was the act interactive or noninteractive? Did the child address another person and/or an object or event? Consider nonverbal behaviors such as body orientation, eye contact, gaze checks, and visual regard toward a person, object, or event to clarify whether a behavioral act is intended to serve a communicative function or to serve a noninteractive physiological or emotional state.
5. Did the child await a response? Did the child display evidence of expecting a specific response to determine whether the child had a plan in mind and was attempting to accomplish a specific goal?
6. Nature of the adult's response. Did the adult's response serve an environmental and a social end of attending to the child, or a social end of attending to an object or event? The nature of the adult's response provides information as to the specific function that the act served.
7. The child's acceptance of or resistance to the subsequent adult response. Did the child accept or resist the adult's response? The child's reaction to the adult's response clarifies whether intent is expressed successfully or not.
8. Aspects of the situational contexts. Events occurring immediately before, during, or after the behavioral act further clarify intent or function.

Adapted from Wetherby & Prizant (1989)

immediate echoes are always produced in a respondent manner to a previously heard utterance and therefore cannot be differentiated according to this dichotomy. In contrast, delayed echoes are often used to initiate communicative acts (e.g., calls, protests, directives, requests) and/or to respond to or continue communicative exchanges (e.g., turn-taking, verbal completion, providing information, yes answer/affirmation). Labeling may be used in either an initiated or a respondent manner.

Echoic productions range from rigid repetitions of previous model utterances to mitigated forms that include a variety of structural changes (e.g, omissions, additions, reductions, transpositions, replacements of words or word order). These mitigated forms may reflect some degree of advancing linguistic processing and competence in the syntactic and semantic areas, and movement from a gestalt style of cognitive and linguistic processing to a more analytic style (Prizant, 1983). This same progression of more rigid to flexible verbal repetition patterns has been noted in the normal language acquisition literature (Clark, 1974, 1977; Kirchner & Prutting, 1987; Peters, 1977, 1983). Kirchner and Prutting have derived definitions and categories of verbal repetition strategies observed in normally developing children that are also useful in categorizing mitigated echoic forms.

INTERVENTION

Due to the idiosyncractic and unconventional nature of echolalia, it is essential that the information obtained in the systematic assessment of echolalia be used to develop highly individualized program targets, goals, and intervention strategies. It has been our experience that patterns of echolalia usage vary greatly depending on a number of social, cognitive, linguistic, and situational variables. Cookbook or highly prescriptive approaches are often not effective in that they tend to ignore internal and external variables and their interrelationships, which are essential in the planning and implementation of approaches to echolalia in intervention.

Intervention should not be the sole responsibility of one person, such as the speech-language pathologist, the teacher, or the parent. This often leads to fragmentation of programming in which developmental progress may be significantly compromised. Effectiveness of intervention is contingent on communication and cooperation among parents and professionals, who as a team need to acknowledge and understand the compensatory nature of echolalia and the role it plays in language development, social interactions, and learning.

The intervention strategies suggested here are derived from assessment results, and are multidimensional in nature (Prizant & Rydell, 1993). This approach involves both indirect and direct intervention strategies and acknowledges the interrelationships of internal and external factors and their potential influence on the production of echolalia. Although a multidimensional approach acknowledges that intervention goals in echolalia are highly individualized, several intervention foci should be considered based on the overall desired outcomes of increased communication effectiveness and conventionality:

1. Echolalia should initially be encouraged as legitimate communicative acts.
2. Echolalia should initially be encouraged for a variety of instrumental, social, and communicative purposes.
3. Echolalia should be encouraged for communicative purposes with a variety of children in a variety of contexts.
4. Rigid echoic productions (pure echolalia) should eventually decrease in proportion to more generative utterances (mitigated echolalia and/or creative utterances).
5. Echolalic utterances should eventually be replaced by generative utterances used for a variety of communicative purposes in a variety of contexts.

It may seem paradoxical to suggest an increase in the use of echolalia when the ultimate goal of communication intervention is generative language. However, intervention goals depend on the child's progression in language development; that is, echoic productions may be a viable and legitimate communicative option for some children at early stages of language development in which the establishment of a communication foundation is of primary importance. Eventually, intervention goals are designed to replace existing functional echolalia with generative utterances, that are more flexible and creative.

Indirect Intervention Strategies

Indirect strategies primarily involve increasing the level of communication among interactants regarding the child's use of echolalia, and the adjustment or fine-tuning of adult interaction styles, communicative context, and environmental stimuli. We will begin with the issue of communication among interactants.

Communication Among Interactants.   It is essential that all interactants are made aware of assessment results, descriptions of the child's echoic patterns, potential influencing factors on echolalic productions, and the compensatory nature that characterizes the child's use of echolalia. It is important that all children who interact regularly with a child understand his or her echoic productions in relation to the level of interactiveness, comprehension, rigidity/linguistic processing, and especially the underlying communicative intent. Without this background information, interactants may inadvertently miss or misunderstand intentional communicative acts produced by the child. Also, increased communication among interactants allows for the systematic fine-tuning of interactional styles and adjustment of contextual variables, elements that may be necessary to promote optimal and consistent communicative opportunities across environments.

Modification of Environment.   One factor associated with increased occurrences of echolalia is highly challenging environments that cause confusion or disorganization and thus compete with a child's use of communicative acts. For example, transitions between activities or classes, interruptions in routines, and unstructured time may cause a child to become agitated or emotionally aroused, especially when the child is unable to anticipate or predict the behavior and expectations of others or their role in the activity (Doss & Reichle, 1991). Cantwell, Baker, and Rutter (1978) and Charlop (1986) found higher incidences of echolalia in highly demanding or unfamiliar settings, including unfamiliar children and tasks. In some cases increased perseverative or noninteractive echoing may be a consequence or signal of emotional arousal, fatigue, or distraction (Schuler & Prizant, 1985). In other cases echoic utterances may be used to self-regulate and/or regulate the behavior of others in the environment so that consistency and order are regained. Interactants should attempt to modify the learning environment so that transitions and breaks can be anticipated well ahead of time. Visual, verbal, and auditory cues are helpful in signaling anticipated changes. Pictorial calendars and daily schedules are also useful to establish predictability of events of the day, as Nancy Dalrymple points out in Chapter 10. Systematic flexibility in programming and instruction are often useful in the classroom; however, abrupt changes in routine should be avoided.

Children with autism and other disabilities often have significant sensory processing difficulties in which particular auditory, visual, and tactile stimuli may cause disorganization, arousal, or possibly discomfort to the child. Environmental manipulations should be considered to dampen or modify the competing stimuli. This may serve to decrease the likelihood of echoic behaviors that are sometimes associated with increased sensory overstimulation.

Simplified Language Input.   Research has established the relationship between increased usage of echolalia and language comprehension difficulties (Carr, Schreibman, & Lovaas, 1975; Curcio & Paccia, 1987; Paccia & Curcio, 1982; Roberts, 1989; Schreibman & Carr, 1978; Violette & Swisher, 1992). Echoic utterances are more likely to be produced when the child does not understand preceding utterances. It is not uncommon for a child's comprehension level to be overestimated by interactants due to the apparent linguistic complexity of echoic productions. Thus the interactant's linguistic input may be presented at a level that is too complex for the child, increasing the likelihood of an echolalic response. For this reason it is important that the interactant use language input that is consistent with or slightly more advanced than the child's true language level as determined by the language sample analysis or from formal/informal language comprehension assessments.

Varied Adult Verbal Interaction Style.   Recent studies (Rydell, 1989; Rydell & Mirenda, 1991; Violette & Swisher, 1992) suggest that children with autism use verbal repetition strategies (echolalia) more in situations of high cognitive workload and demand, which has also been observed in normal developing children's use of imitation (Clark, 1974, 1977; Kirchner & Prutting, 1987; Peters, 1977, 1983). These studies found that the interrelationships among cognitive, social, and communication variables as part of adult verbal interaction styles influenced the production of both echolalia and generative language. Two primary types of adult verbal interaction styles were identified in these studies: directive and facilitative.

In adult *directive style* (Rydell & Mirenda, 1991) the adult controls the focus and direction of the verbal interaction the majority of the time, assumes the lead in conversation most of the time, and structures the nature of the child's contributions to the ongoing topic. The majority of the adult utterances are high constraint (i.e., directives, commands, "wh" questions used to elicit specific replies, yes-no questions, prompts eliciting specific verbal responses, attention-eliciting devices, negative corrective responses). The adult using a directive style uses verbal statements, gestures, or physical prompts that serve to specify either the specific form or content of a child's response; directive verbal statements, gestures, or direct guidance may identify two or more response options from which a student may choose.

In contrast, the adult *facilitative style* (Rydell & Mirenda, 1991) is an interaction style in which the child controls the focus and direction of the verbal exchange the majority of the time. The child is allowed to take the lead in conversation the majority of the time and is encouraged to contribute to the conversation in a variety of ways. The adult allows periods of silence before initiating a new utterance and the majority of adult utterances are low constraint (i.e., reflective questions, report questions, positive responses or acknowledgements, comments). When an adult uses a facilitative style, the adult's responses are similar in topography (imitations) or respresent a suitable expansion (elaboration) of a previously emitted child behavior and serve to deliver some object, activity, assistance, or attention for which the child has initiated (unprompted) a request. In addition, the adult uses motor/gestural or vocal/verbal behaviors that prompt a social/communicative response without specifying either the form (syntax) or content (semantics) of the response.

Adult directive styles, which place a higher degree of cognitive, social, and lingustic demands and constraint on children with autism, were found to increase the frequency of echoic productions compared to generative utterances. In contrast, the use of generative utterances was higher than echoic utterances under the adult facilitative style. Results suggest that under an adult directive style, echoic children tend to use a less sophisticated linguistic strategy (echolalia) that is more automatic and ritualized, thus requiring fewer cognitive resources for production. The use of a more sophisticated and creative linguistic process (generative language) may be more likely when demands and obligations are reduced, such as under an adult facilitative style. Clinical implications suggest that, for children who have available to them both generative and echoic utterances for communicative purposes, an adult facilitative style may provide increased opportunities for echoic children to attempt more sophisticated, generative linguistic strategies. Quill furthers this discussion in Chapter 7.

Modeling.   Given that the early communication of many children with autism may include echolalia or phrases "borrowed" from others, it is important to provide relevant language that relates to activities, objects, and children in the immediate context. It is often the case that children with autism intend to produce a communicative act but are unable to generate their own utterances. Thus they may depend on using the interactant's model utterances for their own purposes. Children who are in echolalic stages often repeat back verbatim what is said by others; therefore it is important to model utterances that are conventional and functional. For instance, use of utterances numbering seven to ten words in length should be avoided when the child is at the one-to-three-word generative level. The production of complex language creates additional processing difficulties for the child as he or she eventually converts the lengthy utterance into its constituent verbal units and gains greater understanding of word meaning and sentence structure (Prizant, 1983). Instead, modeled utterances should be at or near the level of linguistic complexity of the child to match his or her current level of linguistic competence and therefore increase the likelihood that utterances will be understood.

It may also be useful to provide model utterances from the child's, not the adult's, perspective during early stages of echolalia. These models would be provided for the child to use as forms for subsequent communicative purposes. For instance, if an intervention goal is to promote increased usage of verbalizations for behavior regulation in the natural environment, and the child indicates a desire for a drink, the interactant may want to model "I'm thirsty" or "Johnny's thirsty," which can be used in a conventional manner by the child in similar circumstances later on. A less effective modeling strategy would be to ask, "Are you thirsty?" The question may be echoed verbatim and appear as a less conventional communicative act in future similar circumstances.

Deixis and pronoun reversals (e.g., the pronouns I/you, you/me, my/your, etc.) may pose particular difficulties when modeling utterances in interpersonal interactions. Modeling utterances containing personal pronouns in small-group/turn-taking routines may be benefical to differentiate personal perspectives. The use of a softly spoken carrier phrase combined with a more vocally intensive model utterance may also help (e.g., "You say, 'I want the car'").

Direct Intervention Strategies

Intervention strategies may also be used to directly influence and promote developmental changes in echolalia over time. These approaches recognize the transitional nature of echolalia and that echoic utterances produced in early stages of language development are positive prognostic indicators for further language growth (Baltaxe & Simmons, 1975; Howlin, 1981; Kanner, 1973; Prizant, 1983). Developmental changes are characterized by a movement from automatic and rigid forms of echolalia to those that are more functional, generative, and conventional (Prizant, 1983; Prizant & Rydell, 1993).

Given the transitional nature of echolalia and the recognition of the role that echolalia plays in further language acquisition for many children, it is our experience that early goals of communication intervention should promote the child's use of echoic utterances for a variety of functional purposes. As the child gains in cognitive, social, and communicative potential, intervention goals then begin to focus on the systematic conversion from echolalia to generative utterances to meet the established and future communicative needs. This course of intervention recognizes that echoic children need to establish communicative competence early on by using an efficient verbal repetition strategy (echolalia), while acknowledging that a more conventional form of communication (generative language) is the eventual goal and desired outcome.

Responding to and Promoting Communicative Intent.   It has been established that echolalia may serve a variety of instrumental, cognitive, and social purposes for autistic children in naturalistic environments (McEvoy, et al., 1988; Prizant & Duchan, 1981; Prizant & Rydell, 1984; Rydell & Mirenda, 1991). Although echolalia is often produced in an unconventional and metaphorical manner, interactants who are familiar with a child's echoic patterns are often able to discern underlying intent by analyzing and pairing these verbalizations with their co-occuring nonverbal behaviors and environmental cues. In turn, interactants should promote the intentionality of echoic utterances used for communicative purposes through emphasizing the relationship between the child's echoic utterance and the environmental referents, verbally acknowledging the echoic communicative act and contingently responding to child's intent.

A more direct approach to modeling can be used to promote specific communicative functions. Specific routines may be set up to elicit the use of either echoic or generative utterances for a variety of communicative functions. Interactive routines can be devised to establish multiple "practice" opportunities for requesting, protesting, providing information, establishing joint attention or turns, and so on, while providing an appropriate verbal model that can be used for these and other similar episodes. Early intervention goals should consider expanding the number and variety of communicative functions that can be used by the child, and expanding the conditions (children, settings, etc.) under which the use can occur. Again, it is important to establish an effective communicative system early in intervention. This may require that a variety of communicative functions be served initially through nonverbal and echoic means, with eventual movement to more conventional linguistic forms.

Adult interaction styles may also be an important factor in responding to and promoting communicative intent and different communicative functions underlying echolalia. Results of a recent study (Rydell & Mirenda, 1991 and in press) suggest that children with autism use echolalia for different functional purposes under adult directive (including most adult high-constraint utterances) and adult facilitative (including mostly adult low-constraint utterances) styles. Results indicated that subjects' verbalizations increased significantly under the directive or linguistically constraining context in which a higher degree of obligation was placed on the child to respond in a particular manner. In these instances, the utterances were echoic and primarily used for turn-taking and responding functions. Under facilitative or less constraining situations in which adult utterances were used primarily to follow the child's lead, child echoes were used primarily as initations to request and provide information and to regulate the environment.

Implications of these studies suggest that interactants may elect to use an adult directive style (including high-constraint utterances) to promote increased verbalizations, but these utterances are more likely to be echoic and used as responsives or to fulfill their turn in a verbal exchange. If the intervention goal is to increase verbal initiations for behavior regulation and providing information, an adult facilitative style, including adult low-constraint utterances, may be a more appropriate strategy.

Advancing Linguistic Processing.   As previously noted, Prizant (1983) suggests that many children with autism acquire language through a gestalt style of linguistic processing in which words, phrases, or sentences are initially learned and retained in an unanalyzed manner. Initially, these acquired chunks of language, or echoes, tend to be processed superficially and are stored as units with direct and specific associations to the contextual cue or referent in which the utterances were first heard. Eventually, the echoic child applies more sophisticated linguistic processing strategies (analytic) in which previously unanalyzed echoic phrases are modified (additions, reductions, etc.) according to his or her emerging linguistic rule

▶ **TABLE 5.5**

Indirect and Direct Communication Intervention Strategies

I. INDIRECT INTERVENTION STRATEGIES
- Increase communication among all interactants regarding assessment results and intervention strategies.
- Modify environment to increase predictability and consistency while reducing highly confusing and arousing situations.
- Simplify language input to match child's level of linguistic processing.
- Vary adult verbal interaction style to reduce cognitive, social, and communicative demands and promote a variety of pragmatic functions.
- For early language users, model conventional and relevant utterances that can be easily borrowed and eventually converted into more sophisticated forms.

II. DIRECT INTERVENTION STRATEGIES
- Acknowledge and appropriately respond to echoic utterances that are used for instrumental, cognitive, and social purposes.
- Model conventional and appropriate utterances to promote specific communicative functions.
- Provide systematic modifications that serve to reduce, replace, or expand constituent parts of the echoed phrase to promote increased linguistic processing and creativity.
- AAC (augmentative and alternative communication) may be considered to augment verbal productions or replace challenging verbal behaviors.

system. Along this continuum of linguistic processing, the child moves from primarily using pure forms of echolalia, to mitigated echolalia, to eventual creative and flexible verbal productions.

The movement from pure echoic forms to mitigated echolalia signals advancing lingustic processing abilities (Fay, 1980; Shapiro et al., 1970). However, this conversion to more creative forms of utterance is often difficult for autistic children who are gestalt learners. Menyuk and Quill (1985) describe the difficulties these children face in acquiring and generalizing the meanings of words in that they acquire word meaning in absolute rather than relational terms. The differentiation and application of word meaning—especially words with multiple meanings, functional words, and relational or deictic words (e.g., verbs, adjectives, adverbs, prepositions)—pose far more difficulty than do referential words (names of objects, children, activities, etc.), which are more context specific and associated with a specific referent.

Increased flexibility in the application of word meaning and sentence structure (mitigated echolalia) may be intially demonstrated in gestalt learners in a variety of ways. Kirchner and Prutting (1987) have outlined a variety of means by which both normal language users and children with language delays demonstrate increased linguistic processing abilities through modification of previously unanalyzed units. Partial repetitions, reductions, replacements, and expansions have been documented as typical means by which these children combine and recombine semantic knowledge and linguistic chunks in new ways. An example of a mitigated utterance that includes both partial repetition and reduction might be as follows:

Original	"Do you want a cookie?"
Mitigation	"Want a cookie?"

A mitigated utterance characterized by a replacement and expansion might be this:

Original	"I want a car."
Mitigation	"I want a drink, juice."

Based on preliminary analyses by the current authors (Rydell & Prizant, 1992) using Kirchner and Prutting's classification system, mitigated echoic utterances of seven autistic children were characterized by similar modification strategies as those in Kirchner and Prutting's study. This suggests that children with autism may be using the similar modification strategies through mitigated echolalia as normal and language-disordered children use to modify their imitative responses.

Intervention strategies should take into account the dynamic nature of autistic children's echoic productions in their attempt to move the child toward more conventional and flexible uses of language production. Interventionists should provide direct and systematic modifications of the child's echoic utterance through verbal modeling in order to foster increased creativity in language production. Depending on the goals of therapy (semantic or syntactic flexibility), the interactant can provide systematic modifications that serve to reduce, replace, or expand constituent parts of the child's echoic utterance that more accurately reflects the current referent or activity. Since most of the autistic child's language learning is context specific, interactive routines should be developed in which specific elements of the interaction are systematically modified and verbal models provided that map these modifications. In this way comparisons, differentiation, and generalization in word meaning and sentence structure can be highlighted.

Augmentative and Alternative Communication (AAC).   AAC strategies may provide a viable option to assist children who use echolalia to communicate in more conventional ways. For some children who primarily produce highly unconventional verbal behaviors with little evidence of communicative intent (e.g., nonfocused or highly perseverative echoic patterns), nonspeech AAC strategies may serve as an efficient and conventional alternative means of communication, while reducing these echoic patterns and replacing challenging verbal behaviors. Nonspeech AAC strategies may also be used in combination with functional echolalia to develop a more comprehensive total communication approach, using both verbal and nonverbal means. Finally, AAC strategies may be useful in the acquisition of verbal language by helping young children transition from nonverbal to verbal systems (including echolalia), or by assisting some children in transitioning from echolalic to generative language stages. This latter issue is interesting, yet unstudied. For a comprehensive discussion of AAC and children who are nonverbal and/or use unconventional verbal behavior, see Reichle, York, and Sigafoos (1991) and Reichle and Wacker (1993).

A multidimensional approach to communication intervention is needed for children who use echolalia. Both indirect and direct intervention strategies, as summarized in Table 5.5, offer the interventionist systematic guidelines for adapting and fine-tuning individualized programs that meet the unique communication needs of children in various stages of echolalia.

SUMMARY

Since Kanner's early description of autism, echolalia has remained one of the most fascinating and poorly understood aspects of the communicative behavior of autistic children. Although differences of opinion still exist regarding the significance of echolalia, we believe that a significant body of research and accumulated educational/research experience points to specific approaches for assessment and intervention as discussed in this chapter. Assessment and intervention approaches should be multidimensional in nature, taking into account not only the specific patterns of echolalia, but also situational and interactive factors associated with its production. Finally, careful consideration should be given to its functional usage in communicative interactions and to how such patterns may contribute to communicative and linguistic growth over time. It is only through such analyses can we be effective in enhancing the communicative competence of children with autism.

REFERENCES

Baltaxe, C., & Simmons, J. (1975). Language in childhood psychosis: A review. *Journal of Speech and Hearing Disorders, 40*, 439–458.

Baltaxe, C. & Simmons, J. (1977). Bedtime soliloquies and linguistic competence in autism. *Journal of Speech and Hearing Disorders, 42*, 376–393.

Cantwell, D., Baker, L., & Rutter, M. (1978). A comparative study of infantile autism and specific developmental receptive language disorder—IV: Analysis of syntax and function. *Journal of Child Psychology and Psychiatry, 19*, 351–363.

Carr, E., Schreibman, L., & Lovaas, O. (1975). Control of echolalic speech in psychotic children. *Journal of Abnormal Child Psychology, 3*, 331–351.

Charlop, M. (1986). Setting effects of echolalia acquisition and generalization of receptive labeling in autistic children. *Journal of Applied Behavior Analysis, 16*, 111–126.

Clark, R. (1974). Performing without competence. *Journal of Child Language, 11*, 1–10.

Clark, R. (1977). What's the use of imitation? *Journal of Child Language, 1*, 341–358.

Coleman, S., & Stedman, J. (1974). Use of a peer model in language training in an echolalic child. *Journal of Behavioral Therapy and Experimental Psychiatry, 5*, 275–279.

Curcio, F., & Paccia, J. (1987). Conversations with autistic children: Contingent relationships between features of adult input and children's response adequacy. *Journal of Autism and Developmental Disorders, 17*, 81–93.

Dalrymple, N.J. (1995). Environmental supports to develop flexibility and independence. In K.A. Quill (Ed.), *Teaching children with autism: Strategies to enhance communication and socialization*. Albany, NY: Delmar.

Doss, S., & Reichle, J. (1991). Replacing excessive behavior with an initial communicative repertoire. In J. Reichle, J. York, & J. Sigafoos (Eds.), *Implementing augmentative and alternative communication: Strategies for learners with severe disabilities*. Baltimore: Paul Brookes.

Durand, V., & Crimmins, D. (1987). Assessment and treatment of psychotic speech in an autistic child. *Journal of Autism and Developmental Disorders, 17*, 17–28.

Fay, W. (1967). Mitigated echolalia of children. *Journal of Speech and Hearing Research, 10*, 305–310.

Fay, W. (1969). On the basis of autistic echolalia. *Journal of Communication Disorders, 2*, 38–47.

Fay, W. (1973). On the echolalia of the blind and the autistic child. *Journal of Speech and Hearing Disorders, 38*, 478–489.

Fay, W. (1980). Aspects of language. In W. Fay and A. Schuler (Eds.), *Emerging language in autistic children*. Baltimore: University Park Press.

Fay, W., & Schuler, A. (1980). *Emerging language in autistic children*. Baltimore: University Park Press.

Fox, R., Faw, G., McMorrow, M., Davis, L., & Bittle, R. (1988). Replacing maladaptive speech with verbal labeling responses: A case study promoting generalized responding. *Journal of the Multihandicapped Person, 1*, 93–103.

Hermelin, B., & O'Connor, N. (1970). *Psychological experiments with autistic children*. London: Pergamon Press.

Howlin, P. (1981). The effectiveness of operant language training with autistic children. *Journal of Autism and Developmental Disorders, 11*, 89–106.

Kanner, L. (1973). How far can autistic children go in matters of social adaptation? In L. Kanner (Ed.), *Childhood psychosis: Initial studies and new insights*. Washington, DC: Winston.

Kirchner, D. M., & Prutting, C. A. (1987). Spontaneous verbal repetition: A performance-based strategy for language acquisition. *Clinical Linguistics and Phonetics, 1,* 147–169.

Laski, K., Charlop, M., & Schreibman, L. (1988). Training parents to use the natural language paradigm to increase their autistic children's speech. *Journal of Applied Behavior Analysis, 21,* 391–400.

Lovaas, O. (1977). *The autistic child: Language development through behavior modification.* New York: Irvington Press.

McEvoy, R., Loveland, K., & Landry, S. (1988). The functions of immediate echolalia in autistic children: A developmental perspective. *Journal of Autism and Developmental Disorders, 18,* 657–668.

Menyuk, P., & Quill, K. (1985). Semantic problems in autistic children. In E. Schopler & G. Mesibov (Eds.), *Communication problems in autism.* New York: Plenum.

Paccia, J., & Curcio, F. (1982). Language processing and forms of immediate echolalia in autistic children. *Journal of Speech and Hearing Research, 25,* 42–47.

Peters, A. (1977). Language learning strategies: Does the whole equal the sum of the parts? *Language, 53,* 560–573.

Peters, A. (1983). *The units of language acquisition.* Cambridge, England: Cambridge University Press.

Prizant, B. M. (1983). Language and communication in autism: Toward and understanding of the "whole" of it. *Journal of Speech and Hearing Disorders, 48,* 296–307.

Prizant, B. M. (1987). Clinical implications of echolalic behavior in autism. In T. Layton (Ed.), *Language and treatment of autistic and developmentally disordered children.* Springfield, IL: Charles Thomas.

Prizant, B. M. & Duchan, J. F. (1981). The functions of immediate echolalia in autistic children. *Journal of Speech and Hearing Disorders, 46,* 241–249.

Prizant, B. M., & Rydell, P. J. (1984). An analysis of the functions of delayed echolalia in autistic children. *Journal of Speech and Hearing Research, 27,* 183–192.

Prizant, B. M., & Rydell, P. J. (1993). Assessment and intervention considerations for unconventional verbal behavior. In J. Reichle & D. Wacker (Eds.), *Communicative approaches to the management of challenging behavior.* Baltimore: Paul Brookes.

Prizant, B. & Wetherby, A. (1987). Communicative intent: A framework for understanding social and communicative behavior in autism. *Journal of the American Academy of Child Psychiatry, 26,* 472–479.

Quill, K.A. (1995). Strategies to promote social-communicative interactions. In K.A. Quill (Ed.), *Teaching children with autism: Strategies to enhance communica-tion and socialization.* Albany, NY: Delmar.

Reichle, J., York, J., & Sigafoos, J. (Eds.). (1991). *Implementing augmentative and alternative communication: Strategies for learners with severe disabilities.* Baltimore: Paul Brookes.

Reichle, J., & Wacker, D. (Eds.). (1993). *Communicative approaches to the management of challenging behavior.* Baltimore: Paul Brookes.

Roberts, J. (1989). Echolalia and comprehension in autistic children. *Journal of Autism and Developmental Disorders, 19,* 271–281.

Rydell, P. J. (1989). Social-communicative control and its effect on echolalia in children with autism. Unpublished doctoral dissertation, University of Nebraska, Lincoln.

Rydell, P. J., & Mirenda, P. (1991). The effects of two levels of linguistic constraint on echolalia and generative language production in children with autism. *Journal of Autism and Developmental Disorders, 21,* 131–158.

Rydell, P. J., & Mirenda, P. (in press). The effect of adult verbal style on echolalic communicative functions in children with autism. *Journal of Autism and Developmental Disorders.*

Rydell, P. J. & and Prizant, B. M. (1992). [A comparison of mitigated immediate echolalia in children with autism and verbal repetition strategies in normal language learners]. Unpublished raw data.

Schreibman, L., & Carr, E. (1978). Elimination of echolalic responding to questions through the training of a generalized verbal response. *Journal of Applied Behavior Analysis, 11,* 453–464.

Schuler, A. L. (1979). Echolalia: Issues and clinical applications. *Journal of Speech and Hearing Disorders, 44,* 411–434.

Schuler, A. L., & Prizant, B. M. (1985). Echolalia. In E. Schopler & G. Mesibov (Eds.), *Communication Problems in Autism.* New York: Plenum.

Shapiro, T., Roberts, A., & Fish, B. (1970). Imitation and echoing in young schizophrenic children. *Journal of the American Academy of Child Psychiatry, 9,* 548–565.

Simon, N. (1975). Echolalic speech in childhood autism. *Archives of General Psychiatry, 32,* 1439–1446.

Violette, J., & Swisher, L. (1992). Echolalic responses by a child with autism to four experimental conditions of sociolinguistic input. *Journal of Speech and Hearing Research, 35,* 139–147.

Voeltz, L. M. (November, 1977). *Rule mediation and echolalia in autistic children: Phonological evidence.* Paper presented at the annual meeting of the

American Speech and Hearing Association, Chicago, IL.

Wetherby, A. M., & Prizant, B. M. (1989). The expression of communicative intent: Assessment guidelines. *Seminars in Speech and Language, 10, 77–91.*

Zyl, I., Alant, E., & Uys, I. (1985). Immediate echolalia in the interactive behavior of autistic children. *Journal of the South African Speech and Hearing Association, 32, 25–31.*

SUGGESTED READING:

Reichle, J., & Wacker, D. (Eds.). (1993). *Communicative approaches to the management of challenging behavior.* Baltimore: Paul Brookes.

Schuler, A. L., & Prizant, B. M. (1985). Echolalia. In E. Schopler & G. Mesibov (Eds.), *Communication Problems in Autism.* New York: Plenum.

APPENDIX 5.1   **Communicative Temptations for a Communication Assessment**

1. Eat a desired food item in front of the child without offering any to him or her.

2. Activate a wind-up toy, let it deactivate, and hand it to the child.

3. Give the child four blocks to drop in a box, one at a time (or use some other action that the child will repeat, such as stacking the blocks or dropping the blocks on the floor); then immediately give the child a small animal figure to drop in the box.

4. Look through a few books or a magazine with the child.

5. Open a jar of bubbles, blow bubbles, and then close the jar tightly and give the closed jar to the child.

6. Initiate a familiar social game with the child until the child expresses pleasure, then stop the game and wait.

7. Blow up a balloon and slowly deflate it; then hand the deflated balloon to the child or hold the deflated balloon up to your mouth and wait.

8. Offer the child a food item or toy that he or she dislikes.

9. Place a desired food item in a clear container that the child cannot open; then put the container in front of the child and wait.

10. Place the child's hands in a cold, wet, or sticky substance, such as Jell-O, pudding, or paste.

11. Roll a ball to the child; after the child returns the ball three times, immediately roll a different toy to the child.

12. Engage the child in putting together a puzzle. After the child has put in three pieces, offer the child a piece that does not fit.

13. Engage the child in an activity with a substance that can be easily spilled (or dropped, broken, torn, etc.); suddenly spill some of the substance on the table or floor in front of the child and wait.

14. Put an object that makes noise in a opaque container and shake the bag; hold up the container and wait.

15. Give the child materials for an activity of interest that necessitates the use of an instrument for completion (e.g., a piece of paper to draw on or cut; a bowl of pudding or soup); hold the instrument out of the child's reach and wait.

16. Engage the child in an activity of interest that necessitates the use of an instrument for completion (e.g., pen, crayon, scissors, stapler, wand for

APPENDIX 5.1   (continued)

blowing bubbles, spoon); have a third person come over and take the instrument, go sit on the distant side of the room while holding the instrument within the child's sight, and wait.

17. Wave and say "bye" to an object and remove it from the play area. Repeat this for a second and third situation, then do nothing when removing an object from a fourth situation.

18. Hide a stuffed animal under the table. Knock, and then bring out the animal. Have the animal greet the child the first time. Repeat this for a second and third time, then do nothing when bringing out the animal for the fourth time.

Based on Wetherby and Prizant, 1989.

APPENDIX 5.2   Codes for Language Sample

Person

C   Child
A   Adult

Child Utterance Type

I   Immediate echo
D   Delayed echo
M   Mitigated echo
P   Perseveration
IQ   Incessant question
G   Generative

Child Initiation/Response

I   Initiation
R   Response

Adult Constraint

H   High
L   Low

Comprehension

Y   Yes
N   No

Interactive

Y   Yes
N   No

Communicative Intent

Mitigation Type

A   Reduced Repetition
A1   Partial repetition with
         reduction
A2   Partial repetition with
         reduction and replacement

B   Repetition with Replacement
B1   Partial repetition with
         replacement
B2   Partial repetition with
         replacment
         and expansion

C   Expanded Repetition
C1   Complete repetition with
         expansion
C2   Partial repetition with
         reduction and expansion

Immediate Echolalia

TT   Turn-taking
D   Declarative
YA   Yes answer
Rq   Request
N   Nonfocused
         R   Rehearsal
         SR   Self-regulatory

Delayed Echolalia

TT   Turn-taking
VC   Verbal completion
PI   Providing information
         LI   Labeling (interactive)
         P   Protest
Rq   Request
C   Calling
         A   Affirmation
         D   Directive
NF   Nonfocused
         SA   Situation association
         SD   Self-directive
         R   Rehearsal
         L   Label (noninteractive)

CHAPTER 6

Methods to Enhance Communication in Verbal Children

Diane D. Twachtman

This chapter addresses the educational needs of the more able child with autism who, having a basic language system, needs specific *pragmatic intervention* to increase the effectiveness of overall communication. The information presented is based on the assumption that language form and content (e.g., syntax and semantics, respectively) must be directly linked to pragmatic function (e.g., requests, protests) and social context in order to establish meaning, promote sense making, and maximize the development of literacy skills in children with autism. This chapter aims to enhance the reader's awareness and understanding of the unique perspectives that children with autism bring to their experiences. It is only through such knowledge that one may come to understand both their deficits in social understanding and what it is they need to know in order to process information and establish meaning. The overview will include a discussion of the language characteristics of verbal children with autism, as well as a brief look at informal assessment procedures to determine educational needs. Next, methodology to enhance communication in verbal children will be presented within the framework of the following: Setting the Stage, which focuses on creating a background of linguistic and nonlinguistic support; Facilitating Interactions, which addresses specific activities designed to increase the functional use of language and communication in context; and Orchestrating Success, which highlights the environmental manipulations, curricular modifications, and adjustments in adult interactive style which are necessary to ensure success.

UNDERLYING FEATURES OF AUTISM

A heart attack is recognized by one or more of the following symptoms: shortness of breath, pain across the chest or back, heaviness or weakness in the limbs, and pain radiating down the arm. It would be unfathomable, if not disastrous, to treat these symptoms as separate and distinct from one another. Approached from such a perspective, the physician might well recommend an inhaler for the breathing difficulty and a sling for the arm pain! The absurdity of this type of myopic, out-of-context treatment is immediately obvious when dealing with a medical problem. Unfortunately, out-of-context intervention is often standard operating procedure for dealing with children with autism. This occurs when symptoms of the disorder are viewed as discrete entities or, worse yet, as instances of willful behavior under the control of the child, rather than as manifestations of an underlying perspective and orientation that is different from our own and reflective of a system compromised by neurological impairment. Such an approach can severely compromise the development of a functional and flexible communication system. An understanding of, and respect for, the unique perspective of the child with autism is fundamental to the success of any intervention plan to increase the effectiveness of the child's use of language for communicative purposes.

An appreciation of the child's perspective presupposes an understanding of the way in which he or she views the world, for one's perception of objects, situations, and events shapes the perspective one develops regarding them. Conversely, it is just as true that one's perspective on the world colors one's perception of it. Children with autism, with their known sensory problems, often perceive environmental information in unusual ways. This atypical perception of information not only influences their perspectives, but also determines the character of their responses. Because of the nature of autism, with its deficits in social understanding and relatedness, these children generally attend to the inanimate and spatial characteristics of environmental stimuli, as opposed to those social features that better lend themselves to the establishment of meaning. A child with autism may be more interested in the configuration of the graphic symbols that make up the words in a story than he is in the meaning that the words convey.

This proclivity for a specific type of information also illustrates a very important concept that governs perception: salience. Individuals give their attention to that which they find most prominent. The notion of salience is an important one in the education of children with autism. On the one hand it has implications for the manner in which they make sense of the world, and on the other it serves as an important consideration in intervention. Generally speaking, as we have noted, it is the physical and/or spatial properties of objects, as opposed to the social dimensions of situations and events, that capture the attention of children with autism and provide the inducements for communication (Prizant & Schuler, 1987). Many reasons have been set forth to explain this phenomenon, the underlying theme of which centers about the child's difficulty in understanding a rapidly moving social world that demands flexibility and realignment of behavior in response to it (Courchesne, 1991; Mundy, Sigman, Ungerer, & Sherman, 1986). Correspondingly, the child's greater comfort with the object world reflects a cognitive style that deals more effectively with concrete, nontransient (i.e., stable over time) stimuli. Children with autism prefer visual-spatial information to information based on auditory and temporal properties, as Adriana Schuler noted in Chapter 1.

These characteristics of children with autism have led Sigman, Ungerer, Mundy, and Sherman (1987) to conclude that it is the lack of knowledge concerning other people in general, concomitant with the specific lack of recognition that other individuals have thoughts and feelings of their own, that underlie the social impairments of these children. This has profound implications for the development of a functional communication system. According to Geller (1989), a strong link between the child's social and linguistic knowledge is ultimately reflected in his or her use of language for interactive purposes. At issue, then, is the area of pragmatics, long recognized as an area of known deficit in autism. According to Owens (1988) the concept of pragmatics concerns the use of language for communication as opposed to the form in which it is structured.

Perspective-taking is that aspect of pragmatics that deals with children's ability to appreciate that other individuals have points of view that may differ from their own (Geller, 1989). There are three broad areas of perspective-taking: perceptual, involving the child's ability to understand that others may perceive things differently; cognitive, involving the child's ability to understand that others may have different ideas and intentions; and linguistic, involving the child's ability to adjust the form, content, and purpose of the utterance to suit the needs of the situation and/or listener (Geller, 1989). The notion of perspective-taking is fundamental to the concept of theory of mind, described by Frith (1989) as encompassing the ability to understand the relationship between external conditions and internal states of mind. Deficits attributed to this phenomenon have been hypothesized for individuals with autism (Baron-Cohen, Leslie, & Frith, 1985; Leslie & Frith, 1988) and are felt to exert a profoundly negative impact on the child's ability to derive meaning from the social world. Implications for the understanding and use of language are obvious, given that the establishment of meaning is fundamental to appropriate language usage (Genishi, 1988).

A common error made by those who seek to enhance communication in verbal children with autism is that of focusing on lexical elements and/or language form and structure apart from the underlying problems in social cognition, of which perspective-taking is but one component. While this orientation may lead to a superficial expansion in vocabulary and length of utterance, its narrow focus does not lead to an increase in actual communicative competence as defined by Schuler (1989). Such competence intertwines social with linguistic skills and allows children to use language functionally and flexibly. Consequently, if the goal of greater competence in communication is to be realized, intervention strategies must address ways of strengthening the child's underlying social knowledge, rather than merely focusing on overt language behavior. In addressing this important issue, Prizant and Wetherby (1989) specifically discourage the separation of speech and language from the sociocommunicative base that underlies their use.

In developing strategies to enhance communication in verbal children with autism, it is important to keep in mind those methods and procedures that take into account the children's social knowledge, cognitive styles, preferred learning modes, and unique perspectives. Such strategies are likely to meet with greater success than those that do not consider these factors and focus instead on overt speech and language behavior apart from the variables that influence it.

The methodology described here is designed to increase the effectiveness of overall communicative competence and communicative interactions in particular. The parameters of functionality and flexibility of language use are considered to be of utmost importance in determining the success of intervention procedures.

LANGUAGE CHARACTERISTICS OF VERBAL CHILDREN

Four-year-old Ryan was getting ready for bed one evening. His mother was helping him get into his pajamas when all of a sudden he looked down at a large red scab on his leg. He began to rhythmically chant, "South America, South America." At first his mother considered Ryan's reaction to be a bizarre, irrelevant response. She thought about the incident throughout the evening. The next morning she decided to follow up on a hunch. She asked Ryan's preschool teacher if the class was doing a lesson on South America. The teacher pointed to the map on the wall. To the mother's delight and surprise, the map of South America had the very same configuration as the scab on Ryan's leg!

Seven-year-old Ian was asked to write a story about how to make a friend. He wrote: "Atoms, cells, eyes, nose, mouth, arms, legs. P.S. Then say hello." When questioned about his "friend" Ian said, "That's what a friend is made of."

Twelve-year-old Michael was asked to write a book report. In the blank space next to Name of Book he wrote, *The Emperor's New Clothes*. Next to Author he inscribed, "The person who wrote it."

All three children typify what school districts are beginning to recognize as the subgroup of children with autism, those whose strengths and presentation of symptoms challenge both the traditional view of autism and the boundaries of its definition. In reality, the only *new* thing about these children is the growing awareness that their symptomatology does indeed reflect the neurological impairment associated with autism, as opposed to oppositional and/or emotional disorder. Variously described as verbal, capable, more able, and most commonly as high functioning, these children are often of normal to above-average intelligence.

As the anecdotes demonstrate, these children do possess a language system. They are able to use verbal and/or written language to express themselves. There is something decidedly idiosyncratic in their understanding and use of language that not only distinguishes it from that of their normally developing peers, but also interferes with the "readability" of the their messages. The Ryan anecdote illustrates the metaphoric use of language often seen in children with autism. Here the child makes an association between or among things that has a private meaning for him. Unless, like Ryan's mother, the listener has some understanding of the unique perspective of the child with autism, what is in reality a high-level association—the similarity between the configurations of the scab and the map—is likely to be dismissed as a bizarre, irrelevant remark.

Ian and Michael illustrate yet another characteristic of language use in verbal children with autism, literalness. In both cases the children respond to the literal meaning of the information requested, as opposed to the implied meaning; that is, writing a story about friendship and giving the name of the author, respectively. One reason for this is that in both illustrations the implied meanings encompass a social orientation, an area of known difficulty in children with autism; hence the literal as opposed to a social interpretation.

Although verbal children with autism share their common deficits in *using language for communicative purposes*, they nevertheless constitute a diverse group. They vary from minimally verbal to verbose. In addition, problems in perspective-taking not only manifest themselves quite differently across individuals, they also impede the children's ability to understand the listeners' needs and to use this information to modify their behavior to fit a given situation. Difficulty with perspective-taking has been linked to the oft-cited unilateral, pedantic speech that characterizes many high-functioning children with autism. These children can speak ad infinitum on a topic of interest to them, with no apparent recognition of cues from the listener regarding lack of interest and/or need for additional information.

Language behavior associated with problems in perspective-taking varies according to the child's orientation. For example, difficulty with cognitive perspective-taking is illustrated by the child who says "Band-aid

South America," inferring that the adult understands that it is the scab shaped like the map of South America that is the object of the child's request. Similarly, difficulty with perceptual perspective-taking is exemplified by the child who, reading a book at some distance from an adult, points to a term in the book and says, "What is this word?" inferring that the adult can see what the child himself is seeing. Finally, linguistic perspective-taking difficulty can be seen in the child who, referring to himself, says, "You want a cookie," revealing a failure to shift from a listener-appropriate pronoun to a speaker-appropriate pronoun.

As these examples illustrate, deficits in the acquisition and use of language for communicative purposes represent the peculiarities in cognitive function that are associated with autism. Consequently, it is imperative that the latter be taken into account in designing intervention programs that are individualized to their needs. The language characteristics described in the following discussion will be addressed within the context of the cognitive peculiarities that give rise to them.

Prizant & Schuler (1987) postulate a gestalt processing style that results in the rote learning of unanalyzed, holistic chunks of auditory and visual information. This type of cognitive style is both rigid and inefficient in that it does not allow for the fluidity in the extraction of meaning that is associated with a more analytic approach. The child's use of immediate and/or delayed echolalia is an example of gestalt processing style. In the former case, the child repeats precisely what has just been uttered (e.g., Mother: "Do you want a cookie?" Child: "Do you want a cookie?"). In the case of delayed echolalia the repetition occurs some time later. This can vary from several minutes/hours to several days or weeks. Mitigated echolalia is the term used to refer to repetitions that the child has varied in some way, ostensibly to reflect his or her growing awareness of the structure and/or function of language (e.g., Father: "Do you want a cookie?" Child: "Want a cookie."). From an intervention standpoint, echolalia serves specific communicative functions that can be shaped into more creative language use. For a comprehensive treatment of the functions of immediate and delayed echolalia, review Patrick Rydell and Barry Prizant's discussion in Chapter 5.

Duchan and Palermo (1982) describe a number of characteristics of language use in children with autism that they feel reflect problems in thematization, the cognitive process by which an individual makes sense of his world. They apply this theory to a number of phenomena associated with autism. Perseveration, the ongoing repetition of utterances, is viewed as locking onto a theme. They characterize stimulus overselectivity as a cognitive trait that reflects the child's narrowly construed focus on a specific aspect of a larger theme. For example, the child with autism who over focuses on spinning the wheels of a Matchbox car, as opposed to playing with the object in the manner in which it was intended, is evidencing the phenomenon of stimulus overselectivity. The latter has significant implications for the child's ability to derive meaning from his environment, since an inordinately narrow focus of attention impedes one's ability to learn about the affordances of objects and to develop an understanding of the social world. The child's use of language invariably reflects this narrow focus. Problems at this level undoubtedly contribute to the child's propensity for literal interpretation and his or her concomitant difficulty with abstract, socially determined information.

In contrast, metaphoric language use has been characterized by Duchan and Palermo (1982) as a theme-content problem reflective of too wide a focus. In this case the child makes a connection between or among things that are unrelated to one another, hence the idiosyncratic association underlying the use of metaphoric language.

Schuler and Prizant (1987) discuss the use of reenactment strategies by children with autism, as "nonverbal communicative analogue[s] of later gestalt language forms" (p. 307). Here the child performs the various behaviors that have led to the achievement of specific ends in the past, ostensibly because he or she does not know how to bring about those outcomes through more conventional means. The use of these strategies reflects the child's lack of understanding of social causality, the knowledge that he or she can do something to effect a change in outcomes. In some instances the use of metaphoric language may represent a verbal reenactment strategy. In this case the child repeats an utterance that he has associated with the achievement of a goal in the past in an effort to bring about the same end in the present. For example, a child who hears his mother say, "Don't spill it" as he is handed a soda, may repeat that utterance in the future as a request for a beverage.

ASSESSMENT CONSIDERATIONS

First and foremost, assessment and intervention are viewed not as sequential elements in the evaluation and education of children with autism, but rather as ongoing, interdependent processes. This view is driven by the multidimensional, educational purpose of assessment. It provides information that can be used in designing intervention plans and to monitor and evaluate the effectiveness of programming.

There are a number of ways to gather information regarding the child's speech, language, and communication development: case history, standardized testing and direct observation. One method involves obtaining information through record review and case history. The value of this information is that it affords a view of the developmental course of skill acquisition across domains (i.e., cognitive, social-emotional, language, etc.). Additional information can be obtained through the use of standardized testing procedures.

Because children with autism evidence developmental discontinuities that may go unrecognized in norm-referenced procedures, caution is in order when assessing the speech, language, and communicative needs of these children through the use of standardized testing procedures. In addition, the very problems that these children exhibit in areas of social cognition and communication/language, create a kind of "cultural barrier" that can contaminate test results. Consequently, while standardized testing procedures may be useful for some purposes, and in fact may have limited usefulness for purposes of intervention planning, employment of standardized measures should always be accompanied by more descriptive procedures. Informal observation procedures and formal testing should not be viewed as competing methodologies, but rather as components of the assessment of children with autism that, taken together, can provide complementary and relevant information for use in program planning.

Direct Observation

In order to be maximally effective, observation procedures should be carried out across environments and activities. Informal observation procedures should focus on obtaining information regarding the following parameters: communicative intent, syntax, semantics, comprehension and discourse features.

Communicative Intent.   The first step is to determine whether or not the child intends for a particular utterance to convey a specific meaning or whether it is simply self-stimulatory in nature. Next, determine the specific purpose or function of the utterance. Nonverbal behaviors should also be assessed, as they can serve as powerful "communicators" of internal states in children who lack the linguistic and pragmatic sophistication to employ more conventional means.

Syntax.   The next step is to determine the child's understanding and use of the syntactic elements of language and take note of his or her appreciation for the structural dimensions of language and the rules for combining words in order to convey meaning (Lund & Duchan, 1983). Length of utterance and the types of grammatical constructions employed by the child are important factors to consider. Caution should be applied in determining whether the utterances used by the child represent rule-governed utterances that are truly within his or her repertoire, or whether they reflect the repetition associated with echolalia.

Semantics.   The next step is to determine the status of the child's lexicon—that is, the individual's personal dictionary of concepts and words and the meanings they represent (Owens, 1988). In addition to looking at the range of vocabulary employed by the child, it is also important to determine the semantic categories represented by that vocabulary (e.g., objects, actions, locations), the child's knowledge of abstract relational meanings (e.g., prepositional concepts), and his or her understanding of shifting referents that reflect perspective-taking. Determine whether the child understands that word meanings sometimes vary depending on who is speaking, placement with respect to listener and speaker, and the particular time at which the utterance is said. For example, I becomes you, depending on who is speaking; here becomes there, depending on the position of the speaker or listener; and today becomes yesterday vis-a-vis the passage of time.

Comprehension.   While the predominant focus is on the linguistic elements of language, it is important to determine the child's ability to understand nonverbal cues such as gestures and other socially determined behavior. In addition, it is essential to obtain information concerning the child's level of symbolic representation: understanding of specific vocabulary and ability to process verbal information both with and without accompanying cues.

Discourse.   The separation of function, form, and meaning is an artificial one for the purpose of enabling the reader to better understand the relative contribution of each feature to the child's overall understanding and use of communication and language. In actuality, there is a great deal of overlap among these parameters. Since the more able child with autism is a language user, albeit an atypical one, assessment must extend beyond these attributes and encompass the communicative context and the verbal and nonverbal features of discourse as well. Communication is a dynamic event that takes place in a context that, by its nature, transforms the message into something qualitatively different from the mere sum of its static parts. The concept of communicative competence, with its holistic emphasis, speaks eloquently to this dynamic transformation.

Communicative Context. Context denotes the event, situation, and/or activity in which an utterance is embedded. From the perspective of meaningfulness, it is imperative that the child's use of language not be separated from the context in which it occurs, for according to Peck (1989), context and meaning are inextricably intertwined. Determine whether the child's language use is context bound; that is, whether it is restricted to the specific situations and/or persons in which the utterance was originally learned.

Nonverbal Features of Discourse. Features of nonverbal communication in discourse vary from the general to the specific. The former includes such physical dimensions as proxemics (i.e., issues related to social distance and the maintenance of appropriate space) and postural considerations, including those having to do with orientation to the communicative partner. Affective features of nonverbal communication center about the effective use of eye gaze for interactive purposes, the appropriateness of facial expression relative to the content of the communicative situation, and the use of head nods to convey specific intent. Finally, the more frankly communicative dimensions include gestures and paralinguistic features such as intonation and stress patterns that accompany verbal communication. Together, these features constitute the body language that accompanies and profoundly influences the "message value" of verbal discourse. As such, the degree to which they either support or detract from the communicative event is considered an integral part of the assessment process.

Verbal Features of Discourse. Verbal communication in discourse is determined by three main factors: topic, turn-taking, and perspective-taking. Topical considerations include the assessment of such issues as topic initiation and maintenance and topic manipulation. The latter subsumes the ability to both change the subject appropriately and use a variety of topics in conversation. It also includes the concept of topic shading, described by Brinton and Fujiki (1989) as a subtle shifting of focus from one topic to another that is in some way linked to the original subject matter. Turn-taking ability in verbal communication is closely related to the concept of topic manipulation. In assessing this parameter, it is important to determine the degree to which the child initiates and allocates turns, as well as the degree to which turn interruptions constitute a source of disruption during discourse. In observing turn-taking ability, it is also important to assess the child's level of competence in the understanding and use of conversational repair mechanisms. These are devices that allow listeners to signal lack of understanding and/or seek clarification so that speakers can make revisions to accommodate listener needs. Finally, perspective-taking, particularly as it relates to the child's ability to modify the content and style of his speech and language behavior to suit the needs of the listener, constitutes an important area of assessment for children with autism, given their recognized deficits in this area of discourse.

By integrating the information derived from the assessment of the communicative context and the verbal and nonverbal features of discourse with that of the information gathered from the assessment of function, form, and content, it should be possible to piece together a picture of overall communicative competence. For a more in-depth look at the specific features addressed here, see Brinton and Fujiki (1989) and Owens (1988).

SETTING THE STAGE

Maria Montessori introduced the concept of the prepared environment to underscore the importance of constructing a milieu that is eminently responsive to the developmental and educational needs of the children within it. The underlying principle is simple: children's learning may be enhanced within an environment that is optimally suited to their needs.

Not only does this principle apply in the case of children with autism, it is deemed an essential precondition for enhancing their communication and language development, given their recognized need for structure and predictability. Conversely, Ferrara and Hill (1980) found an increase in behavioral disorganization when children with autism were placed in unpredictable situations in which the contingencies governing behavior were not clear-cut.

Given that children with autism do not exhibit a natural proclivity toward engaging in sociocommunicative interactions, it is incumbent on the adults in their environments to come up with creative ways to foster such interaction. The best way to accomplish this is to utilize the child's interests and strengths to create motivating situations designed to promote the use of language for interactive purposes. The principle is a simple one. If the child focuses on trains, use trains to focus the child!

An example of the effective use of this approach concerns two children, ages 8 and 9, with high-functioning autism. Using traditional methods and materials, teachers had little success remediating their specific problems in linguistic perspective-taking or increasing their language use in interactive contexts. Since both children were enormously interested in Nintendo, the decision was made to use it to engage them in sociocommunicative interactions and to utilize that context to teach them about perspective-taking and the use of appropriate pragmatic devices to regulate verbal exchanges. A creative school psychologist responded by setting up Nintendo Club. She included typical peers and employed a boardroom format, with specific rules for participation. The latter is considered an essential element for children with autism, since it maximizes their understanding of the parameters of a given situation, and lends an overall structure to the activity. Progress was observed not only in the children's level of participation in interactive exchanges, but also in their use of repair strategies and specific pragmatic devices related to perspective-taking. In addition, both of their teachers reported increased competence in communication within their respective classroom settings, as a result of their involvement in this activity.

Creating a Background of Support

As a prerequisite for improving their response to it, children with autism must be shown how to make maximal sense of the social world. It is necessary to provide concrete environmental supports to increase their understanding and prompt communicative exchanges, and to adjust the environmental arrangement of activities and events to promote the establishment of meaning.

The social world is based on abstract cues and subtle nuances organized according to time dimensions that are transitory. As discussed previously, children with autism have specific difficulty in dealing with a rapidly moving social world. They also evidence a preference for concrete stimuli that remain stable over time (e.g., pictures, graphic symbols, objects). The use of concrete environmental supports provides an ideal framework for addressing the needs of children with autism because

1. supports can help stabilize an ephemeral social world;
2. supports can increase the salience of socially derived information so as to render it more noteworthy;
3. supports can help the child derive greater meaning from his environment;
4. supports can help the child to conform his behavior to more conventional standards; and
5. the use of supports is consistent with the child's cognitive style and j

Further, because of their social deficits, it has been hypothesized that children with autism may not use the same information for learning appropriate behavior that their normally developing peers use. They appear to use information based on the physical properties of objects rather than information that is socially determined (Shah & Wing, 1986). Consequently, anything that can concretize and distill abstract social information will not only render that information more salient, but also serve to increase the child's understanding of situational requirements and prompt specific responses to meet the needs of a given situation.

The establishment of meaning is further enhanced when the environmental arrangement of events follows a logical sequence in which one activity follows naturally from another. Specifically, children with autism function with greater success and with less anxiety in an environment that is orderly, understandable, and predictable both in terms of its macrostructure (i.e., general arrangement of activities, events, and materials) and in terms of its microstructure (i.e., inclusion of specific concrete supports). With regard to the former, the use of learning stations at the preschool and elementary school levels is one way of juxtaposing a specific activity with a clearly defined environmental space. Centers should be well-labeled and should include literacy artifacts consisting of items containing print related to the particular center in order to capitalize on the skills and interests that children with autism often evidence in this area, and to further promote the development of literacy skills.

A literacy-rich environment should contain the following types of materials: charts demarcating daily jobs, calendar information, a daily schedule, choice boards, labels and printed signs, bulletin boards, and the use of picture/word cue cards to aid in the processing of auditory information and to help direct behavior. The latter can also be incorporated into a system of rules that the high-functioning child with autism can use to monitor his behavior in specific situations. In terms of its microstructure, the environment should contain a number of concrete supports designed to maximize the child's understanding, and to provide a road map for specific responses. The following items are considered essential environmental supports for use with high-functioning children with autism.

Nonlinguistic Supports

A daily schedule is a tool that enables the child to keep track of the day's events and activities and at the same time helps him or her to develop an understanding of time frames and an appreciation of environmental sequences. Horizontal arrangements provide the child with practice in the left-right orientation used in reading. It is essential not only that the child be encouraged to check the schedule at the beginning and end of each activity, but also that he or she be provided with a method for indicating completion of a task. Change symbols can be incorporated into the daily schedule to enable children with autism to understand that something unexpected will take the place of the regularly scheduled activity. For example, if play rehearsal is to take the place of library time on a particular day, a generic symbol such as a jagged line representing a lightning bolt, or the word CHANGE itself, could be placed above the appropriate time slot, so that the alteration in schedule could be discussed in advance and anticipated by the child. The picture and/or graphic symbol of library could then literally be replaced by that of the auditorium cue. This type of concrete support can also aid the child in making transitions from one activity and/or place to another.

The use of an activity schedule promotes understanding of the environmental arrangement of activities and events and enables children to anticipate change and deal with it better. In addition, the daily schedule provides an ideal frame of reference within which to discuss past, present, and future events and to stimulate questions and conversations related to the day's activities. The visual symbols used for the schedule can serve as prompts to stimulate such discussion.

Color can be used to heighten understanding of information and to cue specific responses, while objects, pictures, and/or graphic symbols can be used to concretize abstract social information to render it more meaningful. The use of these devices not only capitalizes on the child's visual strengths and preferences, but also increases the saliency of information by remaining stable over time. Additional uses for these items include the prompting of verbal responses and the regulation of behavior. It should be noted that manual signs and natural gestures, though technically not considered concrete representations, can be used to stabilize auditory input and assist in the processing of verbal information.

The three accompanying vignettes offer examples of how concrete visual supports can be used to increase the autistic child's understanding of concepts and situational requirements, and how such information can be used to facilitate more appropriate responses from the child.

VIGNETTE   Bobby is playing a board game with Sarah, a typical peer in his kindergarten class. Bobby has little understanding of the concept of turn-taking, as he continually tries to take turns at inappropriate times. Verbal exhortations from Sarah and his teacher to wait his turn have not been effective in changing this behavior.

Solution: The amorphous concept of turn-taking can be rendered more meaningful through the use of a colored circle with the words "My Turn" written on it. This concrete tool can be used to demarcate each child's turn. It can also be used to prompt appropriate verbal responses. For example, when the turn marker is in front of Bobby, he can be asked whose turn it is. The graphic symbol on the circle prompts the correct response. When the circle is in front of Sarah, he can be prompted to answer the same question with the response, "Sarah's turn." This symbol can also be used to teach conversational turn-taking. Its use in different activities and settings can help to facilitate generalization.

VIGNETTE   Erich, a highly verbal child, is often disruptive in his regular second-grade setting because of his constant questioning while his teacher is trying to give directions to the class. Verbal directives to raise his hand or wait to ask his question have not helped him modify his behavior.

Solution: A concrete visual symbol can help Erich conform his behavior to the requirements of the situation. A circle that is green on one side and red on the other can be used to indicate when it is appropriate to speak and when it is important to remain silent—red side up for silence, green side up for talking. Similarly, if Erich has difficulty making judgments regarding when and when not to speak in other situations and settings, the same types of support can be used to direct behavior in those circumstances and environments as well, thus helping to facilitate generalization.

Linguistic Supports

In addition to the use of concrete environmental supports, it is also important to "index" the environment for the child, by pointing out information that he or she is likely to miss otherwise. The child can then be cued to generate a more informed response, based on the greater understanding of environmental situations and events. For example, given the nature of the autistic disorder and its effect on the understanding of social and emotional cues, it is imperative that this type of information be highlighted so as to render it more meaningful to the student.

Too often there is an inordinate emphasis on prompting children with autism to respond to situations appropriately, without the slightest regard

> **VIGNETTE**   Jennifer is in the seventh grade and an honor roll student. She does very well on tests requiring specific, memorized information. Essay tests are a real problem for her. She simply does not know how to approach the information from an organizational perspective.
>
> *Solution:* Semantic organizers are particularly beneficial for children with autism, as they capitalize on the children's cognitive strengths in the visual domain and provide a methodological framework for organizing information. Jennifer can be helped to organize the task by being given an annotated outline that calls for specific information in a particular order. This can serve as a "grid" or template for writing assignments. An annotated outline that delineates specific information for inclusion in the essay can bypass organizational problems that impede the student from accessing and expressing the information she has. The specificity of this outline can not only provide opportunities for practice, but also guide the student's thinking and help prepare her to employ more generic outlines later. For further information regarding the use of semantic organizers, see Pehrsson and Robinson (1985).

for whether they have any understanding of the situation or event to which they are expected to respond. It should be apparent that it is virtually impossible to generate skilled, socially appropriate responses to situations that one finds inexplicable. At best, these responses will be situation specific and/or cue dependent. The principle underlying behavioral responsence is a simple one: the quality of the output (response) is directly related to the quality of the input (understanding of the situation/event). Consequently, it is vitally important to increase the child's understanding of environmental and behavioral information in order to provide a "meaning link" between the behavior observed and the appropriate response to it. For example, in addition to increasing understanding of social and emotional information, caregivers should also highlight information that enables the child to develop anticipatory skills and the more social pragmatic functions of communication. Finally, the coding of feelings and the encouragement of perspective-taking is best achieved experientially, in the contexts that give relevance to them, as opposed to didactically, separate and apart from the events and situations that infuse them with meaning. Table 6.1 summarizes this technique.

The importance of laying a sturdy foundation for the development of speech, language, and communication skills cannot be overestimated. Increased comprehension can not only help to reduce anxiety in children with autism, but also set the stage for higher quality communicative interactions. Conversely, premature emphasis on expressive requirements, without regard to helping children with autism understand the events and

▶TABLE 6.1

Ways to "Index"
the Environment

1. Point out *social* information:
   "Look, Timmy's waving at you. Can you wave back?"
2. Point out *emotional* information:
   "Mary got hurt. Look, she's crying, poor Mary. Can you tell Mary 'I'm sorry'?"
3. Point out *anticipatory* information:
   "Look, Joey's going to throw the ball. Put your hands up."
4. Structure the *commenting* function:
   "Look at the bird eating birdseed. The bird must be hungry."
5. Code *feelings* and *reactions*:
   "Ryan's very angry at Joey for taking the ball. Tell Joey, 'Give me that ball.'"
6. Encourage *perspective-taking*:
   "Ryan likes his pickle. Look, Joey hates his pickle. Look at Joey. Joey's making a face that says 'I hate this pickle.'"

situations that give rise to them, places those children at risk for the development of isolated, out-of-context skills that will be of minimal benefit to them.

The use of linguistic and nonlinguistic supports capitalizes on the visual strengths of children with autism, enabling them to make maximal sense out of their environments. This is important from the perspective of increasing their understanding of environmental expectations, and helping them to use that information to conform their verbal and nonverbal behavior to situational requirements. These tools help concretize abstract, socially determined information, rendering it more stable and more understandable to children who have problems making sense of this type of input. They also afford the adult interactant with a relatively unobtrusive visual means of cueing the child in appropriate responses. This feature is particularly beneficial in integrated settings, as it ameliorates the undue attention associated with more intrusive verbal prompts.

FACILITATING INTERACTIONS

Despite sophistication at the structural level of language in some of the more verbal children with autism, there is often failure at the level of discourse. Discourse is an inclusive concept that encompasses the intermingling of pragmatic, linguistic, social, and cognitive factors (Mentis & Thompson, 1991). Failure at this level manifests iself in the child's inability to use language effectively for social interaction purposes. These children tend to be responders as opposed to initiators in situations requiring verbalization. Overall, they would be characterized as passive communicators (Fey, 1986). Knowledgeable regarding use of the technical aspects of language form and structure, they are profoundly impaired from the perspective of communication. Given this particular profile, an important consideration in communication programming would be to increase the child's level of participation in social contexts and at the same time address the development of the pragmatic functions that allow him access to the social world. The methodology needs to integrate linguistic and pragmatic elements within the natural environment to promote the understanding and use of communication and language in the contexts in which they would normally occur.

Given the ease with which typical children develop speech, language, and communication skills, it is not surprising that such a commonplace achievement is easily taken for granted. An appreciation for the underlying complexity that permeates communicative exchanges can be achieved only through examination of the dynamics involved in the process. Consider the following baseball card dialogue between two young boys:

BOY 1:   "I'll trade you a Roger Maris and a Yogi Berra for a Mickey Mantle."

BOY 2:   "Naw! But I'll give you a Mickey Mantle for a Carl Yastrzemski."

These two boys are communicating a wealth of information about their grasp of the sociocommunicative process and the underlying substrates that give rise to it. That is, they exhibit skills that traverse the developmental domains that address sensorimotor, cognitive, socioemotional, and language behavior. From the speech and language perspective, they demonstrate the ability to comprehend and express language, and they convey an impressive command of grammar, syntax, and knowledge of vocabulary and semantic relationships. Pragmatically, the two boys evidence an understanding of the complexities regarding the various forms of perspective-taking. Cognitive perspective-taking, the knowledge that another person may have different thoughts and ideas, is seen in their ability to recognize that their card preferences differ from one another. Perceptual perspective-taking, the knowledge that someone else may perceive things differently, is implied in their separate views regarding the subjective value the desired cards hold for each of them. They also demonstrate knowledge of linguistic perspective-taking, the abilty to modify one's language to suit the listener's needs. This is observed in their flexible use of both speaker- and listener-approriate pronouns, I and you, respectively. These young boys also demonstrate an understanding of the complexities, often subtle in nature, that underlie interactive, communicative exchanges. To begin with, they exhibit both the ability to focus jointly on the same subject, and the ability to maintain the topic to convey their intentions. Turn-taking and reciprocity is demonstrated in their back-and-forth verbal exchange. Relatively sophisticated negotiation skills are reflected in the boys' use of the following: the quid pro quo principle, the idea that one must give something to get something; the art of compromise; and the use of strategies to "sweeten the deal," the suggestion of giving two cards for one. The latter also reveals their understanding of value, in that they evidence appreciation for the relative worth of specific items. Knowledge of possession is observed in the proprietary interest that each boy evidences in his respective cards. The boys also demonstrate awareness of the rules of social propriety in that they use words to request, rather than physical aggression to usurp. Finally, the entire dialogue is made possible by the boys' understanding of the principle of social causality; that is, their recognition that they can engage in behavior to effect a change in another person. Clearly, then, what may superficially appear to be commonplace and trivial (i.e., a brief two-line dialogue), is in reality a complex, richly textured sociocommunicative tapestry in which cognitive, linguistic, affective, and social processes play major roles (Twachtman, 1992).

Expand the Pragmatic Base

It should be apparent from the baseball card dialogue that communication is a dynamic process into which language is imbedded. Therefore a breakdown requires an approach eminently respectful of the complexities involved in that process, particularly if the goal is communicative competence. To enable children with autism to gain greater flexibility in the use of language for interactive purposes, it is necessary to expand their repertoires of pragmatic functions, as opposed to concentrating efforts on the amplification of language form and structure. This can be accomplished best by promoting the use of language in the actual settings in which it would normally occur and by employing naturalistic procedures, contingencies, and reinforcement to encourage and facilitate its continued use.

Given the cognitive peculiarities, rigid learning styles, and specific impairment in social understanding that characterize children with autism, the language they exhibit is not necessarily used for communicative purposes. Apart from language used for purely self-stimulatory reasons, Prizant and Schuler (1987) distinguish between cue-dependent responses and those that are truly communicative acts. Cue-dependent responses are context bound. They tend to be inflexible and nontransferable to other settings. Prizant and Schuler argue against the training of situation-specific responses on the basis that functional communication is marked by flexible use across contexts. Children with autism can ill afford to learn a set of out-of-context, prompt-dependent verbal behaviors that give the appearance of skillfulness in the absence of actual competence, particularly since the issue of generalization of skills is always problematic for them.

This type of purposeless learning can be avoided by emphasizing the development and expansion of communicative function (i.e., the pragmatic base) as the foundation onto which language form and content (i.e., syntax and semantics, respectively) are mapped. For according to Bates, Benigni, Bretherton, Camaioni, and Volterra (1979), communicative functions develop prior to the acquisition of forms to express them. Further, addressing the development of communication and language behavior within the natural environment not only promotes both the establishment of meaning and the generalization of skills (Willard & Schuler, 1987), but also meets the criterion of ecological relevance, the degree to which the skills learned are considered functional within the child's daily life.

Research has demonstrated that children with autism do not evidence the variability or flexibility in the use of the pragmatic functions of communication that typical children do (Wetherby & Prutting, 1984). Specifically, they tend to employ communicative functions that serve instrumental as opposed to social purposes (Prizant & Schuler, 1987; Watson, 1987; Willard & Schuler, 1987); that is, those that relate to need satisfaction rather than those that relate to social interaction. Given the preeminence of function over form and structure, an important first step in facilitating interactions is to expand the child's repertoire of pragmatic functions in contextually appropriate environments.

After determining what functions the child is using and ascertaining the circumstances under which they are employed, situations can be set up, and/or opportunities created, to expand their use across people and settings prior to venturing forth into new areas. The idea here is to move from the familiar to a topographically similar, though unfamiliar, situation. For example, if the child characteristically requests food items but tends to wait for other objects, it would be prudent to expand requests to a variety of objects, across settings and people, before addressing the more "social" requests for assistance, information, attention, and the like.

There are several parameters to consider in the selection of additional pragmatic functions if the latter are to become an integral part of the child's functional repertoire. One of the most important of these is developmental appropriateness. For example, instrumental functions develop prior to social functions in children with autism and, as such, would serve as a good starting place. For example, requesting objects and asking for information are easier for the child with autism to understand and do than the more social functions such as commenting. Another parameter to consider is that of meaningfulness and/or relevance. While words such as *please* and *thank you* are unquestionably important to adults, their social nature and abstract quality probably do little to enhance sense-making for the child with autism. A third factor to consider, and one that is particularly important in dealing with these children, concerns the issue of control. Functions that enable a child to gain greater control and influence over his or her life are, by their nature, naturally reinforcing. For example, saying "No," and "May I have a break?" not only empower the child, but also mitigate against behavioral outbursts stemming from frustration and feelings of powerlessness. Finally, an important factor to take into account is that of interdependence; that is, pragmatic functions that enable the child to interrelate with others in his environment undoubtedly contribute to the child's sense of well-being. For example, knowing how to ask for help does more to enhance the quality of the child's life than does the act of labeling objects within the environment.

Inducements designed to promote the idea of communication as a vehicle for social interaction can serve as powerful tools to control one's world. They address the expansion of pragmatic functions through environmental restructuring (e.g., the use of obstacles, the violation of routines and object function, the withholding of needed materials, and the like). For example, communication can be encouraged by staging problem-solving situations in which the child needs to request specific items in order to carry out a particular task. Another type of inducement involves having someone walk into a room with an unusual item. When the child sees the item the interactant immediately prompts, "Say, what is that?" Observation and timing are extremely important. The key to getting the most out of this technique is to observe the child closely and provide the prompt before frustration occurs. One of the major advantages of using this type of technique is that it makes maximal use of typical peers and others as interlocutors to both model and cue appropriate responses. It should be noted that activities and materials can be designed to suit all age levels.

Provide Dialogue Scripts

The whole-language movement in education, with its emphasis on theme building and meaning making (Norris & Damico, 1990) provides an ideal context in which to enhance communication in verbal children with autism. Despite the fact that high-functioning children with autism often exhibit the phenomenon of hyperlexia—high-level reading skills within the context of significant impairment in the development of language and communication—this skill is not usually functional from the standpoint of comprehension. The use of print within a specific context, repeated and expanded on over time, can help to establish connections between words and their referents, thereby increasing comprehension skills in these children. In addition, graphic symbols or print in the form of dialogue strips used in combination with pictures and other nonlinguistic supports can provide the child with ready-to-use language in contextually relevant situations. Opportunities for practice in different settings can help to facilitate generalization.

This approach has a number of benefits for children with autism. First and foremost, it takes advantage of their gestalt processing and rote learning styles by giving them chunks of appropriate language that require no analysis to work in given situations. Second, it minimizes the cognitive load with respect to their limited capability for generative, spontaneous language. Third, it provides a structured, contextually relevant, and predictable interactive routine in which to expand knowledge and learn specific vocabulary. Fourth, it takes advantage of their visual strengths. Finally, it offers a kind of oasis in which successful interactions may take place (Twachtman, 1990).

This methodology emphasizes a holistic approach to the enhancement of communication in verbal children with autism. Activities can be adapted for use with children across the age range. They illustrate ways to build interactive scripts around normally occurring environmental routines, as well as ways to utilize interactive scripts in contrived situations designed to increase the functional use of language and communication in context. For the most part, activities incorporate an experiential, whole-language, integrative approach to skill development, based on the emphasis that approach places on the importance of meaningful experiences in the construction of knowledge. It should be noted that theme building across activities, which is an integral part of whole-language approaches, is felt to be especially beneficial for children with autism, given that it provides structured opportunities to maximize the development of literacy skills and at the same time fosters continuity and promotes generalization.

Build Interactive Scripts Around Routines

It is well established that children learn language within the context of routines with their caregivers (Bruner, 1983; Dickinson & McCabe, 1991; Kirchner, 1991; Snow, 1981). In fact, according to Dickinson and McCabe, children's verbal performances are greatly enhanced by the the use of routines. Snyder-McLean, McLean, Etter-Schoeder, and Rogers (1984) introduced an augmented version of this interactive technique that they called the joint action routine (JAR) for use with children who evidence impairments in language and communication skills. JARs can be set up around such normally occurring environmental events and activities as snack/mealtime, food preparation, sports activities, leisure/play activities, going to the store/restaurant, and doing laundry. The requirements for implementation of the routines, though critical, are easily achieved. On the part of the participants there must be both a common purpose that undergirds the activity and joint attention to the items and events that support it. In addition, carefully delineated roles should be carried out within a logical and predictable sequence, in order to maximize sense making and lay the groundwork for systematic variation later. Interactive routines not only can expand a child's length and number of utterances over the course of involvement with the activity, but also generate greater interest in interacting with peers as well as increased competence in the area of play. For additional information on the implementation of joint activity routines and play routines, the reader is encouraged to see Snyder-McLean et al. (1984), as well as the discussions of Quill and Pamela Wolfberg in Chapters 7 and 8 of this book.

Act Out Children's Stories

At the early childhood and early elementary levels, nursery rhymes such as "Little Miss Muffet" can be acted out with props. In addition, stories such as "The Three Bears" and "Little Red Riding Hood" can initially be told orally, using props. For example, in the former story the following props would be needed: three bears, a Goldilocks doll, three toy chairs, three bowls, and three toy beds. The adult can tell the story as he or she manipulates the objects according to the story line. Later, children can provide dialogue as they act out the scenario. There are many advantages to using this approach. First, the three-dimensional visual supports are more concrete (and probably more interesting) than the unidimensional pictures in a book. Second, telling the story in this fashion enables the adult to slow down the pace, use repetition, and simplify the language input to meet the individual needs of these children. Third, the activity provides an interactive context in which children may participate both verbally and actively. Fourth, this approach maximizes understanding and sense making. Fifth, using this technique makes the eventual introduction of the book format more meaningful. Finally, exposure to this type of activity provides vocabulary and language structure that may be used in novel ways by children in their future play activities.

Engage in Reciprocal Reading

This activity may be thought of as a special case of the joint activity routine. According to Kirchner (1991) reciprocal book reading can be used as a context for language intervention by extrapolating from patterned children's books to create reciprocal (two-way) discourse activities. While several different types of patterns are used in these books, those based on repetitive language patterns in which phases or sentences are repeated at intervals throughout the story are among the most common. *Brown Bear, Brown Bear, What Do You See?* by Bill Martin provides an excellent example of this type of pattern. Other categories of patterned literature include those containing rhyming patterns and those containing repetitive-cumulative patterns in which the base literary unit is not only repeated in each new series of events, but also enlarged on as the story progresses. *The Very Hungry Caterpillar* by Eric Carle provides a prototypical example of the latter. Finally, books with predictable story lines that allow the reader to forecast future events also fit into the category of patterned children's literature. *I Know an Old Lady Who Swallowed a Fly* by Nadine Bernard Westcot provides an example of this type of book. In discussing the merits of using reciprocal reading as a context for language intervention, Kirchner (1991) cites the case of a 4-year-old boy with Asperger's syndrome (considered a diagnosis along the autistic continuum) in which generalization of language patterns to play contexts occurred spontaneously as a result of utilizing this type of approach. For more information on the use of this technique see McCracken and McCracken (1979, 1986) and Tompkins and Webeler (1983).

Build Themes Across Activities

Books around a particular theme can serve as a prelude to a variety of activities. Consider fire engines, for example. A trip can be taken to the firehouse. Using props (e.g., firefighter's hat, rope to simulate hose), sequences in the book can be acted out. Dialogue strips and other visual supports (e.g., signs, graphic symbols) can be employed to prompt contextually rele-

▶**TABLE 6.2**
Strategies to
Facilitate
Interactions

1. Expand the pragmatic base.
2. Provide dialogue scripts.
3. Build interactive scripts around routines.
4. Act out children's stories.
5. Engage in reciprocal reading.
6. Build themes across activities.
7. Encourage replica play.
8. Videotape discourses.
9. Provide referential communication tasks.

vant language use. Later, cutouts depicting people and fire engines can be used in combination with the visual supports to provide additional opportunities for language use in magnet and/or flannel-board activities. This approach not only helps infuse meaning into stories, but also provides a context and format for play activities in which the child can actually apply the vocabulary and language forms in situations designed to foster their use. Finally, repeated exposure to theme building across contexts and activities is an ideal way to promote the meaningful generalization of skills in children who have difficulty seeing commonalities among situations and events.

Encourage Replica Play

Dollhouse miniatures as well as standard toys can be used to represent activities and events. Adults can act out specific sequences and model the language and social behavior required by the situation. They can also provide a paced dialogue to connect the child's actions to the words that describe them at a level of complexity adapted to the needs of the child. Example: A 5-year-old boy named Ryan was playing with a miniature replica of a boom box as his mother manipulated a small father-figure doll saying, "That's too loud. Turn that down." Ryan directed his attention toward the doll and said, "No. You sit down!" Puppets can also be used for this purpose. It should be noted that all of the activities noted here can be used with older children by selecting situations and materials that are age appropriate.

Videotape Discourse

Video instrumentation can be used in a variety of ways with children at all age levels. It is particularly effective for the more verbal children, given that they can both view and model the verbal behavior demonstrated in the videotape footage. Shadden (1983) employed this technique with language-impaired children. She reported gains in the area of pragmatics, despite the fact that the latter was not specifically targeted in her project. Charlop & Milstein (1989) used video modeling to teach conversational speech to children with autism. They found that this technique was effective in increasing conversational skills in these children. They also found that there was generalization of skills to new topics of conversation, and that these gains were maintained over a fifteen-month period.

There are two main ways in which videotapes can be used with children with autism: self viewing and peer viewing. The latter can be particularly useful in demonstrating the appropriate use of language, communication, and social skills in selected situations. Utilizing typical peers as role models to act out scenarios, these situations can be contrived to provide the specific type of sociocommunicative input deemed appropriate. After a great deal of repetition, children with autism can be encouraged to engage in the same role plays with typical peers. With practice, variation on the themes and elaboration of the language and communicative requirements can occur over time.

Provide Referential Communication Tasks

A prototypic pragmatic intervention technique that can be used to great advantage with verbal children with autism at all age and functioning levels is that of the referential communication task. Also known as barrier games, these activities customarily involve two children seated across from one another with a set of identical materials in front of them and an opaque screen (barrier) between them. One child, designated the sender, directs the other child, designated the receiver, to perform various functions with the materials. Switching roles enables the child with autism to gain experience in both the receptive and expressive dimensions of language. As the receiver of directions, the former sender will perform the same task that he or she earlier directed the partner to perform. Thus a visual model is available for comparison and performance check on completion of the activity. For example, if dollhouse miniatures are used, the child receiving the message can be directed to "put the shoe under the bed," "put the cup on the table," and so on. Increased language complexity can be achieved by varying the materials and thus the communicative requirements of the situation. To encourage the the use of repair strategies—that is, using language to prevent and/or restore communicative breakdown—introduce two tables: a round one and a square one or one that is larger than the other. The direction to "put the cup on the table" will now require a request for additional information: "which table?".

Not only do referential communication tasks provide rich, meaningful contexts in which to use language for interactive purposes, they also enable children to use language to direct the behavior of others, to employ repair strategies in meaningful ways, and to develop increased knowledge of language concepts, vocabulary, and structure. Further, they are ideally suited to fostering structured, communicative interactions between children with autism and typical peers. For additional information on the use of referential communication activities, the reader is encouraged to see Glucksberg & Krauss (1967).

ORCHESTRATING SUCCESS

Given that communication does not exist in a vacuum, but rather is imbedded in the context of the events and interpersonal relationships that help define and shape it, the success of language and communication efforts is directly related to variables that exist outside the child's realm of expertise and control. Consequently, if meaningful gains in the use of language for communication are to be achieved by children with autism, adults must match their teaching styles to their students' learning styles and be willing to address all the variables involved in communicative breakdown. Fundamental to this concept is the notion of following the child's lead in terms of his or her interests and adjusting and/or augmenting curriculum to increase relevance and promote success.

At its simplest level, communication is a two-person (dyadic) event. When a breakdown occurs in that process, it should be interpreted as a two-person phenomenon, requiring a two-person solution. This type of orientation encourages adult interactants to examine factors within themselves that may be contributing to communicative breakdown—speaking in long sentences, for example, or waiting an insufficient length of time to accommodate the child's processing ability. It also directs attention toward other factors outside the child, such as environmental overstimulation. The advantage of this type of orientation is that it is multidimensional and focused on a variety of possible contributory factors, as opposed to unilateral and focused solely on the child. Such a comprehensive perspective fosters a mental set on the part of adults that encourages them to modify and/or adjust their teaching strategies and interactive styles to accommodate the needs of children with autism, thus increasing the chances of greater success in the latter's use of language for interactive purposes.

Given the severity of the deficits in social understanding and communication that result from neurological impairment in children with autism, the adults in their environment must assume responsibility for making necessary adjustments and modifications in three critical areas: the environment, adult interactive style, and curriculum.

The Environment

The environment can either encourage communicative interactions, or discourage them. Constable discussed the idea of creating a communicative context to facilitate the use of language for interactive purposes (Peck, 1989). This concept is not only vitally important in programming for children with autism, but actually needs to be expanded. Environmental opportunities should be augmented and/or specifically created to increase saliency and to cue verbal responses. Specifically, the adult should construct an environment that is set up to create in the child a need to communicate in order to obtain desired items and/or make certain things happen. McClowry & Guilford (1982) refer to this phenomenon as that of "dynamic disequilibrium" and note that its purpose is to facilitate greater responsivity.

**Adult
Interactive Style**

There are many aspects of adult interactive style that can either facilitate communication or impede it. Table 6.3 contains some of the style variables that are important to consider in working with children with autism as well as the types of adjustments that can be made to promote increased communication in these children.

The ideal adult interactive style is facilitative rather than directive (McDonald, 1989) because by its very nature it involves sensitivity and attunement to the child. The goal is to adjust one's communicative style to accommodate the needs of the child. It is important to note that small adjustments in style on the part of the adult can yield large communicative dividends for the child. For example, simply waiting a sufficient amount of time for the child to process information demonstrates that a response is expected and sets the stage for its emergence. Rhetorical communication, however—that is, perfunctory language input in the absence of behavior that demonstrates expectation of a response—communicates to the child that a reply is unnecessary. Adjustments in adult interactive style help promote child-initiated verbal interactions in children who tend to respond to communication more readily than they attempt to initiate it. Finally, it is important to emphasize that adjustments in interactive style are the responsibility of the adults and/or typical peers in the environment, since such modifications involve perspective-taking, an area of known difficulty in children with autism. For a comprehensive treatment of this subject, see Quill's discussion in Chapter 7.

Curriculum

The curriculum can serve to support language and communication development. This is a particularly important area of consideration for those children with autism who are being educated in the mainstream, since rigid adherence to the standard curriculum can be inimical to their educational interests. Consider, for example, a child with autism who feels compelled to make the McDonald's arches for the letter "M" in writing assign-

▶**TABLE 6.3**
Features of Adult
Interactive Style

1. Phasing:	time interactions to occur synchronously
2. Adaptive:	adjust paralinguistic features
3. Facilitative:	promote initiations through environmental and interactional setups
4. Elaborative:	expand upon the child's behavior to reach the next level
5. Initiating:	entice attention to capture the teachable moment
6. Controlling:	direct through the use of environmental supports and augmentative cues

Schaffer, 1977

ments. A rigid teacher who insists that the child form a perfectly proper "M" can raise a major control issue that leads to the child becoming discouraged about all writing assignments. A sounder approach would be to recognize that the child's compulsive adherence to the arches is part of the autistic impairment (e.g., perseveration, insistence on sameness) and to adjust the requirements of the situation to accommodate the behavior pattern. This approach does not preclude continued efforts to provide incentives for behavioral change; it merely discourages power struggles over relatively unimportant issues that can lead to frustration for everyone involved.

Curricular adjustments are often necessary to accommodate the child's lack of comfort with sensory experiences. These situations can be exploited to demonstrate to the child how he or she can use language to control uncomfortable environmental experiences. For example, the child who finds handling glue in an art project aversive should be encouraged to communicate this to the teacher. Accommodations in the child's level of participation in the task vis-a-vis the expressed discomfort can go a long way to reinforce the use of this type of language to control his or her world.

There are times when curricular modifications can increase the relevance of academic assignments for children with autism. For example, incorporating the child's interests into class projects can go a long way toward increasing the child's level of attention and participation in them. These are important factors in promoting increased interest in sociocommunicative interaction.

Finally, curriculum should serve the child. It should include information and materials that are meaningful and relevant to him or her. Too often children with autism are forced to endure a curriculum that they find irrelevant and meaningless. If the goal of individualized education is to be realized, it is essential that teachers and clinicians modify the curriculum to accommodate the needs of the child with autism.

SUMMARY

More able, verbal children with autism present many challenges to educators. Ironically, the very strengths in expressive language that they exhibit, often impede the functional and flexible use of language for interactive purposes. Impressed by their strengths, teachers too easily assume an underlying conceptual and pragmatic framework that is simply not commensurate with the superficially sophisticated language behavior. Building skills on so shaky a foundation is tantamount to constructing a house on quicksand. Neither end product serves the purpose for which it is intended: functional use.

The phenomenon of delayed echolalia illustrates the tyranny of the child's strengths and the misunderstanding it causes. Children who exhibit this type of echolalia sometimes memorize parts of dialogues from television or motion picture scripts that they echo later, often in situations with similar defining characteristics. Their concomitant use of appropriate paralinguistic features—for example, those governing stress patterns and tone of voice—lends an air of authenticity to these utterances, and furthers the appearance that they are spontaneously generated by the child. It is easy to see how such an assumption can cause adults to overestimate the ability of these children, leaving open the possibility of subjecting them to linguistic demands they are not able to meet.

Problems in the social use of language can also arise from product-oriented approaches that stress the proliferation of language forms, irrespective of the child's underlying social understanding governing their use. This type of unilateral focus on the superficial form and structure of language, in the absence of an appreciation for the richness and complexity of the processes that give rise to it, promotes the training of situation-specific, cue-dependent responses that glorify form over function (and substance, as well!). Such an orientation leads to a preoccupation with length of sentence and number of words in the child's vocabulary, completely disregarding his or her actual needs in the sociocommunicative domain. Reducing the dynamic, multidimensional process of communication to that of mindless insistence on requiring the child to "say the whole thing" not only sets children with autism apart from typical peers, but also makes communication a stressful event.

The methodology set forth in this chapter to enhance communication in verbal children emphasizes process over product. As such, it addresses the child's needs from a holistic perspective that is sensitive to the interdependence among the linguistic, pragmatic, social, and cognitive factors that are an integral part of the communicative process. The training of situation-specific, robotic responses is discouraged in favor of promoting the functional use of language in the natural environment, in order to promote sense making and to meet the goal of communicative competence. Further, the emphasis on providing language-based experiences across settings, activities, and people promotes generalization of skills, an area of notorious difficulty for children with autism.

Finally, this methodology is eminently respectful of the unique perspectives that children with autism bring to their experiences. Specifically, adults are encouraged to take the perspectives of children with autism in order to understand their needs and to create programs that are individualized to their learning styles, strengths, and interests.

"If my possessions were taken from me with one exception, I would choose to keep the power of communication, for by it I would soon regain all the rest" (Daniel Webster).

REFERENCES

Baron-Cohen, S., Leslie, A. M., & Frith, U. (1985). Does the autistic child have a "theory of mind"? *Cognition, 21*, 37–46.

Bates, E., Benigni, L., Bretherton, I., Camaioni, L., & Volterra, V. (1979). *The emergence of symbols: Communication and cognition in infancy.* New York: Academic.

Brinton, B., & Fujiki, M. (1989). *Conversational management with language-impaired children.* Rockville, MD: Aspen.

Bruner, J. S. (1983). *Child's talk.* Oxford, England: Oxford University.

Charlop, M. H., & Milstein, J. P. (1989). Teaching autistic children conversational speech using video modeling. *Journal of Applied Behavior Analysis, 22,* 275–285.

Courchesne, E. (Speaker). (1991). *A new model of brain and behavior development in infantile autism* [Cassette recording]. Silver Spring, MD: Autism Society of America.

Dickinson, D., & McCabe, A. (1991). The acquisition and development of language: A social interactionist account of language and literacy development. In J. F. Kavanagh (Ed.), *The language continuum: From infancy to literacy.* Parkton, MD: York.

Duchan, J. & Palermo, M. (1982). How autistic children view the world. *Topics in Language Disorders, 3,* 10–15.

Ferrara, C. & Hill, S. (1980). The responsiveness of autistic children to the predictability of social and nonsocial toys. *Journal of Autism and Developmental Disorders, 10,* 51–57.

Fey, M.E. (1986). *Language intervention with young children.* San Diego: College-Hill.

Frith, U. (1989). *Autism: Explaining the enigma.* Oxford, England: Basil Blackwell.

Geller, E. (1989). The assessment of perspective-taking skills. *Seminars in Speech and Language, 10*(1), 28–41.

Genishi, C. (1988, November). Children's language: Learning words from experience. *Young Children,* pp. 16–23.

Glucksberg, S., & Krauss, R. (1967). What do people say after they have learned to talk?: Studies of the development of referential communication. *Merrill-Palmer Quarterly, 13,* 309–316.

Kirchner, D. M. (1991). Reciprocal book-reading: A discourse-based intervention strategy for the child with

atypical language development. In T. M. Gallagher (Ed.), *Pragmatics of language: Clinical practice issues.* San Diego: Singular.

Leslie, A. M., & Frith, U. (1988). Autistic children's understanding of seeing, knowing and believing. *British Journal of Developmental Psychology, 4,* 315–324.

Lund, N. J., & Duchan, J. F. (1983). *Assessing children's language in naturalistic contexts.* Englewood Cliffs, NJ: Prentice-Hall.

McClowry, D. P., & Guilford, A. M. (1982). Normal and assisted communication development. In D. P. McClowry, A. M. Guilford, & S. O. Richardson (Eds.), *Infant communication: Development, assessment and intervention.* New York: Grune & Stratton.

McCracken, M. J., & McCracken, R. A. (1979). *Reading, writing, and language.* Winnepeg, Canada: Peguis.

McCracken, R. A., & McCracken M. J. (1986). *Stories, songs, and poetry to teach reading and writing: Literacy through language.* Winnepeg, Canada: Peguis.

McDonald, J. D. (1989). *Becoming partners with children: From play to conversation.* San Antonio: Special Press.

Mentis, M., & Thompson, S. A. (1991). Discourse: A means for understanding normal and disordered language. In T. M. Gallagher (Ed.), *Pragmatics of language: Clinical practice issues* (pp. 199–227). San Diego: Singular.

Mundy, P., Sigman, M., Ungerer, J., & Sherman, T. (1986). Defining the social deficits of autism: The contribution of non-verbal communication measures. *Journal of Child Psychology and Psychiatry, 27,* 657–669.

Norris, T. A., & Damico, T. S. (1990). Whole language in theory and practice: Implications for language intervention. *Language, Speech, and Hearing Services in Schools, 21,* 212–220.

Owens, R. E. (1988). *Language development* (2nd ed.). Columbus, OH: Merrill.

Peck, C. A. (1989). Assessment of social communicative competence: Evaluating environments. *Seminars in Speech and Language, 10*(1), 1–15.

Pehrsson, R. S., & Robinson, H. A. (1985). *The semantic organizer approach to writing and reading instruction.* Rockville, MD: Aspen.

Prizant, B. M., & Schuler, A. L. (1987). Facilitating communication: Theoretical foundations. In D. J. Cohen & A. M. Donnellan (Eds.), *Handbook of autism and pervasive developmental disorders.* New York: Wiley.

Prizant, B. M., & Wetherby, A. M. (1989). Enhancing language and communication in autism: From theory to practice. In G. Dawson (ed.), *Autism: Nature, diagnosis & treatment*. New York: Guilford.

Quill, K. A. (1995). Enhancing children's social-communicative interactions. In K. A. Quill (Ed.), *Teaching children with autism: Strategies to enhance communication and socialization*. Albany, NY: Delmar.

Schaffer, R. (1977). *Mothering*. Cambridge, MA: Harvard University Press.

Schuler, A. L. (1989). Preface. *Seminars in Speech and Language, 10*(1).

Schuler, A. L. (1995). Differences in learning and development. In K. A. Quill (Ed.), *Teaching children with autism: Strategies to enhance communication and socialization*. Albany, NY: Delmar.

Schuler, A. L., & Prizant, B. M. (1987). Facilitating communication: Prelanguage approaches. In D. J. Cohen & A. M. Donnellan (Eds.), *Handbook of autism and pervasive developmental disorders*. New York: Wiley.

Shadden, B. B. (1983). Videotape applications in pragmatic intervention with language-impaired children. *Journal of Childhood Communication Disorders, 6*(2), 71–84.

Shah, A., & Wing, L. (1986). Cognitive impairments affecting social behavior in autism. In E. Schopler & G. B. Mesibov (Eds.), *Social behavior in autism*. New York: Plenum.

Sigman, M., Ungerer, J. A., Mundy, P., & Sherman, T. (1987). Cognition in autistic children. In D. J. Cohen & A. M. Donnellan (Eds.), *Handbook of autism and pervasive developmental disorders*. New York: Wiley.

Snow, C. (1981). The uses of imitation. *Journal of Child Language, 3*, 205–212.

Snyder-McLean, L., McLean J., Etter-Schoeder, R., & Rogers, N. (1984). Structuring joint action routines: A strategy for facilitating communication in the classroom. *Seminars in Speech and Language, 5*, 213–228.

Tompkins, G. E., & Webeler, M. (1983, February). What will happen next? Using predictable books with young children. *The Reading Teacher*, pp. 489–502.

Twachtman, D. D. (1990, Summer/Fall). Communication for the nineties. *The Advocate*, pp. 17–20.

Twachtman, D. D. (1992). *Ethics-based student educational experience matrix*. Manuscript submitted for publication.

Watson, L. R. (1987). Pragmatic abilities and disabilities of autistic children. In T.L. Layton (Ed.), *Language and treatment of autistic and developmentally disordered children*. Springfield, IL: Charles C. Thomas.

Wetherby, A. M., & Prutting, C. (1984). Profiles of communicative and cognitive-social abilities in autistic children. *Journal of Speech and Hearing Research, 27*, 364–377.

Willard, C. T., & Schuler, A. L. (1987). Social transaction: A vehicle for intervention in autism. In T. L. Layton (Ed.), *Language and treatment of autistic and developmentally disordered children*. Springfield, IL: Charles C. Thomas.

Wolfberg, P. (1995). Enhancing children's play. In K. A. Quill (Ed.), *Teaching children with autism: Strategies to enhance communication and socialization*. Albany, NY: Delmar.

CHAPTER 7

Enhancing Children's Social-Communicative Interactions

Kathleen A. Quill

More than half a century ago, Leo Kanner (1943) described autism as a trilogy of features: extreme aloneness, a desire for sameness, and islets of ability. This constellation of features continues to characterize the syndrome and guide treatment decisions today. The wisdom of Kanner's observation of "extreme aloneness" is appreciated in ongoing efforts to understand the central social impairment. Current theories suggest that social development in autism is constrained by an inability to derive meaning from people and social contexts in a flexible way (Frith, 1989). Children with autism reveal a limited understanding of people's motivations, perspectives, and feelings. And, as they struggle to understand the meaning of interpersonal relationship, its expression through communication is compromised. Put simply, it is difficult to communicate with a partner you do not understand. Yet children with autism demonstrate what does make sense to them in their "desire for sameness" and "islets of ability." A desire for sameness seems to be a plea for order amid social chaos. Routine, predictability, and order exist in the world of objects and less in the world of people. A key element of treatment, then, is to make people and social interactions more predictable and better understood. Similarly, Kanner noted "islets of ability" in rote memory and the recollection of complex visual patterns and sequences. Although these abilities cannot compensate for social impairments, they can be used in treatment as a catalyst toward social understanding.

The purpose of this chapter is to offer a set of strategies that use the children's learning preferences as a means to promote their understanding and participation in social-communicative interactions with adults and peers. The chapter will define the dimensions of interaction, describe the challenges facing children with autism, and apply our understanding of the children's abilities to a system for assessing and promoting social-communicative interactions.

PRINCIPLES OF COMMUNICATION ENHANCEMENT

This approach to communication enhancement embraces three fundamental beliefs about social interactions and intervention:

1. Social communication is a reciprocal, dynamic relationship based on mutual understanding, enjoyment, and benefit.
2. Impairments in social-communicative interaction are related to cognitive differences.
3. The child's active involvment in naturalistic contexts promotes social-communicative interactions.

Social communication is a reciprocal, dynamic relationship based on mutual understanding, enjoyment, and benefit. A level of sensitivity about how children with autism perceive the social world is integral to engaging in meaningful, pleasurable interactions. Communication is enhanced by understanding the children's social perspective and communication efforts. With this knowledge, the adult or peer interactant can create motivating opportunities for social-communicative engagement. The more competent communicator can structure interactions to increase the child's understanding and use of language and enhance participation in the social dynamic.

Impairments in social-communicative interaction are intertwined with cognitive differences. The development of social-communicative interactions involves a complex interplay of abilities in cognitive, language and social domains. The relationships across the various domains are so apparent that any effort to provide intervention in one area must consider all the other systems. Strategies to enhance social-communicative interactions must take into account cognitive strengths and differences. In this regard, adults with autism have provided insights about their learning style that have profound treatment implications (Grandin, 1995; Grandin & Scariano, 1986; Williams, 1992). The insights of Temple Grandin and Donna Williams are used in this chapter as a framework for understanding the treatment strategies. The discussion includes steps to systematically observe and assess the child's social and communication behaviors and then to organize interactions through interactant modifications, environmental supports, and interactive predictability.

The child's active involvment in naturalistic contexts promotes social-communicative interactions. For over a decade, models of communication enhancement have emphasized transactional approaches (McLean & Snyder-McLean, 1978; Bloom & Lahey, 1978; Koegel, O'Dell, & Koegel, 1987). While these models are philosophically sound, there has been ongoing debate as to the application of transactional approaches for children with autism. A polarity of viewpoints is offered by proponents of the two basic treatment approaches: the behavioral model and the transactional model. These two approaches share common beliefs about the nature of autism but quite divergent views about the process of learning to communicate and how it translates into treatment. The behavioral model is based on principles of operant conditioning along with specificity of purpose, goals, and activity structure. It is the prevailing approach to language and communication intervention. Skill development is defined as mastery of a series of discrete subskills. The model emphasizes precision and organization during instruction. This includes the arrangment of the learning environment, use of prompting and shaping techniques, and attention to immediate reinforcing feedback. The difficulties associated with using a behavioral model for communication enhancement relate to the artificial nature of the instructional setting, the role of the child as a passive responder to adult-initiated interactions, and the lack of a clear link between language programming and the social uses of language. As a result, communicative spontaneity and meaningful application of acquired skills is often compromised by this approach. In contrast, the transactional approach is framed within the natural ecology of interactions. The model uses social pragmatics as a theoretical base and the influence of adult-child interactions on the normal process of communication development. It is based on the belief that children acquire language and communication by using it, not through practicing its separate parts. Transactional approaches emphasize naturally occurring situations as the context for instruction, child-directed instructional activities, and the adult's role as a conversation facilitator. The difficulties associated with the use of this model for children with autism relate to the open-ended quality of the instructional setting, the reliance on the child's initiations to guide the interaction, and the lack of clarity as to the adult's role. However, intervention strategies that combine the beneficial components of behavioral technology with the developmental knowledge of the interactive process can structure meaningful interactions for children with autism to enhance their social-communicative competence.

THE NATURE OF SOCIAL-COMMUNICATIVE INTERACTIONS

Instances of social and communication interaction are varied and complex. Social interactions can be reciprocal communication or group events, like many forms of play. A social situation may require individuals to coordinate roles in a turn-taking fashion or participate concurrently, as when everyone does the same thing at the same time. Communication can be direct or indirect, verbal and nonverbal. Speech, written language, gestures, facial expression, physical proximity, emotion, and virtually every behavior has the potential to communicate and promote interaction. While the purpose of social interaction is pleasurable and active engagement with others, the specific function or purpose of communication is to influence change and have an impact on others in some way. As such, communication is a social act, but not all social acts are communicative in nature.

The Development Interaction

The development of interactive skills involves an interface of cognitive, language, and social parameters. Characteristics of preverbal social communication include joint attention, imitation, and the use of vocalizations and gestures to engage and regulate an adult's behavior. Before the emergence of language, children are able to initiate social contact, observe others, and maintain focused attention with another through vocal or object play. They engage in turn-taking, imitate simple actions or vocalizations, and use a variety of means to call attention to themselves and regulate another person's behavior. The ability to understand the effect one's behavior has on others influences communicative knowledge and social relatedness (Bates, 1976). With the emergence of language, children develop a variety of verbal and nonverbal means to express a range of communicative functions. They satisfy basic needs, exert control over the environment, establish social relationships, ask for information, share experiences, and express individuality through language. As conceptual and linguistic competencies develop, these skills are used in the context of social discourse. The complex dimensions of conversation, such as maintaining appropriate topics, considering another's perspective, and balancing speaker-listener roles, are learned and refined throughout childhood. At the same time, children must flexibly use nonverbal features such as vocal quality, eye gaze, and physical proximity to support participation in the conversation. Refinement of these discourse skills across different social contexts and conversational partners is a lifelong developmental process. See Bates (1976), Bruner (1975), Muma (1986), or Wells (1981) for a comprehensive exploration of communication development.

The Social-Communicative Challenges of Autism

Temple Grandin and Donna Williams are two highly respected women with autism. Their personal insights into the nature of the disorder contribute greatly to an understanding of the social-communicative challenges facing children with autism. Williams (1992) explains:

> I found social contact hard to understand or respond to, people's intentions and motivations (p. 111). . . . the inconsistencies in my perception of the world resulted in the loss of meaning from these experiences (p. 207).

Observes Grandin:

I thought of my childhood, the confusion, the effort to communicate, the conflict. . . . Now, as a teenager, communication should be established, but the chasm of misunderstanding was deep (Grandin & Scariano, 1986, p. 82).

Social-communicative interactions are the instrumental force that propels a child's growing cognitive, linguistic, and social knowledge and sense of self. Children devoid of these social experiences are locked in a world of confusion and isolation. Children with autism struggle to understand the intents, internal states, and meaning behind people's social, communicative, and affective behavior and are therefore profoundly impaired in the ability to participate in social-communicative interactions (Frith, 1989). This constrained ability to analyze and integrate information in a cohesive and flexible manner underlies their pattern of social impairment. If unable to extract meaning from social events in a flexible way, the children are left with a series of fragmented social experiences that are manifested as ritualized, context-specific behaviors. This aptly describes the nature of the autistic disorder. The children associate a particular social context with a specific response. They seem less able to analyze the parameters of similar situations in order to respond flexibly and often have difficulty generalizing social-communicative behaviors to related situations. As a result, the dynamic and unpredictable quality of typical social interaction is problematic for them.

The profile of social-communicative impairments in autism is characterized by deficits in early cognitive-social skills and an aberrant developmental pattern of language use, both in terms of the range of communicative functions expressed and atypical discourse skills (Paul, 1987). Children typically show limited use of joint attention and social referencing, the basic means of social engagement. Most communicative efforts serve instrumental functions such as requesting or rejecting, not the social functions of sharing information and feelings (Wetherby, 1986). They understand and use communication that has a clear and immediate effect on the environment, while the social means to draw attention to oneself and engage others eludes them. The use of requests ("I want juice") or rejections ("no, I don't want that") is linked to tangible contextual cues (the desired/undesired item) and adult consequences (give/remove item). In contrast, communication that is more social typically does not have explicit cues. Because clear contextual cues guide their communication, the absence of social communication is not an unwillingness to share information but a difficulty extracting relevant information from a social context.

A stereotypic, routinized style of interaction dominates the children's discourse skills. Situation-specific language, repetitive or perseverative questions, preoccupation with a narrow range of topics, and routine scripts typify conversation (Prizant & Schuler, 1987). The complex, ongoing adjustments and modifications inherent in conversation challenges the most able children with autism. Because of a constrained ability to consider the perspective of another during conversation, they show a limited awareness of speaker-listener roles and have difficulty maintaining topics and repairing conversational breakdowns. This is coupled with a poor understanding of the meaning conveyed by nonverbal cues such as facial expression, body posture, and paralinguistic features. The task of teaching children to become attuned to the meaning of the multiple dimensions of social-communicative interaction is a formidable responsibility.

The Ecology of Interactions

The term *ecological* in this context refers to the totality of individual and environmental factors that account for the success or failure of social-communicative interactions. In the case of autism, there is a tendency to attribute problems solely to the individual. It is too easy to link the cognitive, linguistic, and social differences to the failures in social-communicative interaction. Yet children may display problems because of a lack of congruence between their abilities and unique features and the demands of the social situation and social partners (Simpson, 1991).

The study of child language acquisition has demonstrated the importance of environmental factors to the developmental process, specificially the adult's role in shaping social interactions. Most notable is the work of Bruner and his colleagues (Bruner, 1975; Ratner & Bruner, 1978) who emphasize the function of interactive routines between adult and child as the framework within which language and communication is acquired. Interactive routines are a limited, sequential, and predictable set of contextually meaningful utterances that allow a child to anticipate and insert appropriate responses. Such routines provide interactive turns that are clear and reversible. Routines provide reciprocal interaction patterns that represent the turn-taking aspect of conversation. Routines assist a child's understanding of his or her active role in the social dynamic. Through consistent experiences with a variety of routines, a child learns to assign meaning to the language forms and communicative behaviors used within each interaction.

In addition to interactive routines, adults modify their style of language input to engage in reciprocal exchanges with a child (Snow, 1977). This modfied input, referred to as "motherese," includes syntactic simplicity; redundancy; exaggerated prosody; and reference to objects, activities, and events in the child's immediate environment. The adult's fine-tuned speech, which is based on a desire to be understood and elicit information from the child, highlights the social nature of communicative interactions.

Certainly, then, the social context and interaction styles of adults (and peers) need to be modified for the child with autism in order to develop successful social-communicative interactions. New information, language forms, and social behaviors are most readily acquired in the context of established interactive routines and modified language input. This basic construct put forth by studies of child language becomes the framework for designing appropriate intervention contexts.

ASSESSMENT

Assessments are intended to provide careful and systematic attention to the child's communication abilities as well as the characteristics of the environment and interactive partners (Peck, 1989).

In Chapter 2 of this volume, Grandin reminds the reader that being a successful teacher "requires an understanding of how people with autism think and feel" (1995, p. 33). Donna Williams (1992) also emphasizes this point: "Gain the child's trust and . . . . accept who and where he or she is" (p. 201).

The focus of assessments is to identify the relationships between the child's communicative behavior, the interactant's communicative behavior, and aspects of the interactive context. In this way the assessment process is directly linked to the intervention goals of social-communicative competence. Traditional normative assessment tools that examine skills independent of context are not sufficient here. The analysis of social-communicative interactions requires systematic classifications of observations in natural and contrived contexts. In particular, the objective of the assessment process is to determine when interactions occur, what is communicated, how the child communicates, and what characteristics of the context and interactant affect the child's abilities. Particular attention is given to the kinds of opportunities the child has to initiate communication and the contexts that motivate these interactions. Such an analysis of social-communicative interaction is descriptive rather than developmentally hierarchical, and it is independent of language ability. Although this discussion of assessment strategies makes specific reference to children who have acquired a symbolic system for communication, the assessments can be applied across the broad spectrum of communicative abilities observed in autism. The observational tools can be used flexibly with children who are nonverbal, and with those who demonstrate emergent language, echolalia, and more advanced language levels.

There are a wide variety of factors to be considered in the qualitative assessment of social-communicative competence in children with special needs (Peck, 1989; Prizant & Schuler, 1987). In an attempt to offer a practical and informative system that addresses the major assessment goals, four basic tools are suggested to record observations in natural and contrived settings, develop intervention strategies, and evaluate specific changes in the child's social-communicative interactions. These are a Communicative Means-Functions Questionnaire, a Natural Communication Sample, a Language Comprehension Inventory, and an Interaction Analysis. Table 7.1 summarizes the variables to be considered when analyzing social-communicative interactions.

Communication Questionnaire

It is often useful to begin the assessment process by interviewing one or more adults who are close to the child. The Communicative Means-Functions Questionnaire (Appendix 7.1) is an adapted version of interview protocols developed by Schuler, Peck, Willard & Theimer (1989), Wetherby & Prizant (1989), and Finnerty & Quill (1991). The purpose of the questionnaire is to identify how the child communicates (means) and for what purposes (functions) across a variety of situational contexts. This information provides a capsulized view of the scope of the child's language and communication abilities. Questions are organized according to twenty-six communicative functions, with sample situational contexts presented for each function. The assessed functions include a variety of requests, negations, comments, and expressions of feelings. The sample situations are meant to guide the interview, and it is expected that additional questions will be raised during the process. The interviewer describes a situational context that is an opportunity for communication: for example, "He sees another child playing with one of his favorite toys" (an opportunity to request peer interaction) or "You offer him a food that he doesn't like" (an opportunity to refuse). Then the interviewer asks, "What does the child say or do?" Because the question is posed in this way, any descriptions of the child's verbal and nonverbal communicative means can be recorded. Communication may include nonstandard nonverbal behaviors such as

▶**TABLE 7.1**

Assessing Social-Communicative Interactions

I. COMMUNICATIVE MEANS-FUNCTIONS QUESTIONNAIRE
  • Inquire about a range of communication contexts
  • Identify communicative function
  • Describe communicative means
  • Describe repair strategies

II. NATURAL COMMUNICATION SAMPLE
  • Record child-initiated communication
  • Record context, communication means and function

III. LANGUAGE COMPREHENSION INVENTORY
  • Assess factors which enhance comprehension: linguistic, speaker, contextual
  • Describe routinized patterns
  • Assess generalization across speakers and settings

IV. INTERACTION ANALYSIS
  • WHO initiated
  • WHERE positioned
  • WHY communicated
  • WHAT communicated
  • HOW communicated
  • WHEN communicated
  • Child response

---

tantrums and running; standard nonverbal behaviors such as reaching and pointing; nonstandard verbalizations such as echolalia; and standard verbal behaviors using either speech, sign, or other augmentative communication system. When the child uses verbal means, the interviewer then asks for two or more examples of what the child might say in the given context. It is important also to assess the child's ability to persist in his or her communication efforts and "repair" the communication attempt in each situation by asking the respondent "What does the child do if you ignore his or her first communication attempt?" The information gathered through the questionnaire summarizes the child's range of communicative means, range of communicative functions, ability to use the same communicative behavior for multiple purposes, ability to use more than one means to convey each function, repair strategies, and communication differences across familiar adults.

Communication Sample

A Communication Sample is an adaptation of a standard language sample. Whereas a language sample collects 50 to 100 utterances used by a child in order to gather information about syntactic competencies, a Communication Sample records 100 different episodes of unelicited child-initiated communication to obtain information about the child's communication competencies. Samples may be recorded over a day or a week, at home or at school, depending on the communicative abilities of the individual child. A Communication Sample records the situational context, the communicative utterance or behavior observed, and the communicative function inferred from the context and child's behavior. A portion of a Communication Sample of a child named Brian is shown in Table 7.2.

Once the Communication Sample is collected, communicative utterances and behaviors are analyzed and compared to the information gathered through the Communication Means-Functions Questionnaire. Since a major goal for the child is flexible use of many interactive functions, the relative frequency of the twenty-six communicative functions is then calculated to see what the child prefers to talk about and note the functions that are absent from the sample. If a pattern emerges—for example, a high fre-

▶**TABLE 7.2**
Communication
Sample

Situation	Communication	Function
Time to go to bed	"No bed"	Protest
Spills his drink	"Brian, what happened?"	Comment/mistake
Wants peer's swing	Grabs child	Request permission
Struggles to open	Hands to adult: "come here"	Request help
Wants video	"Wanna watch Sesame"	Request permission
Sees item in book	"What's this name?"	Request information
Plays blocks	Looks at peer: "put it on"	Comment/activity

quency of requests and an absence of comments—then the low-frequency functions are targeted for intervention. The sample also reveals motivating contexts that become opportunities to further expand communication. If desired, the level of structural complexity (syntactic and semantic) can be analyzed with the sample (Lund & Duchan, 1983) along with an analysis of the echolalic utterances (Prizant & Duchan, 1981; Rydell & Prizant, 1995).

Language Comprehension Inventory

A major question for educators and parents is the child's level of language comprehension. To enhance social-communicative interactions, it is critical to identify the conditions under which the child consistently responds to language information in order to modify language input and aid in comprehension. Terms like "not paying attention" and "noncompliant" are often used to describe a child's responses to verbal input. It is better to assume that the child responds when he or she understands and knows how to respond. While formal assessments may estimate the child's vocabulary and comprehension of different grammatical structures, the most relevant information about a child's comprehension can be gathered through a Language Comprehension Inventory of observations in the natural setting. The goal of the inventory is identification of the conditions under which comprehension occurs; the method is systematic observation of specific variables that influence comprehension. Again, the key element is to identify when the child is successful!

Comprehension can be influenced by linguistic complexity, the interactant's presentation of information, and contextual cues. Sentence complexity, information linked to the here-and-now, the interactant's use of gesture, pace of speech, the familiarity of the situation, and motivational factors all contribute to the child's understanding. To complete the inventory, the child' responses to specific words, phrases and sentences in a variety of contexts are recorded, and the variables that influence comprehension are noted (see Table 7.3)

Through the Language Comprehension Inventory, the linguistic, interactant and contextual cues that support the child's comprehension are discovered. Routinized or scripted response patterns that may or may not reflect comprehension can be examined more carefully through the inventory questions. Because of the gestalt learning style observed in many children, generalization of language comprehension across speakers and settings is also taken into account. The child's preference for particular persons, and its effect on language comprehension can be identified through the inventory. It is not atypical for a child to respond to a specific question or statement in one context, or with one person, and not another. The intervention goal is to expand comprehension across settings and persons through the use of those identified factors that contribute to the child's success.

▶**TABLE 7.3**
Language
Comprehension
Inventory

I. WHAT LINGUISTIC FACTORS ENHANCE COMPREHENSION?
  • Sentence length
  • Sentence type
  • Semantic relevance to here-and-now

II. WHAT SPEAKER FACTORS ENHANCE COMPREHENSION?
  • Proximity to child
  • Use of accompanying gestural cues
  • Tone of voice
  • Use of repetition
  • Amount of time given for child to respond

III. WHAT CONTEXTUAL FACTORS ENHANCE COMPREHENSION?
  • Motivating context
  • Familiar routines
  • Specific adults or peers as interactants
  • Use of concrete referents
  • Use of visual supports

IV. DOES CHILD SHOW ROUTINIZED RESPONSE PATTERNS?
  • Echolalic patterns
  • Scripted responses

V. DOES COMPREHENSION OF MESSAGE GENERALIZE ACROSS
    SPEAKERS/SETTINGS?

**Interaction
Analysis**

The most revealing information is obtained from the Interaction Analysis. The primary intent of the Interaction Analysis is to assess the relationship between the characteristics of the interactant and the social-communicative competence of the child. Studies have shown that the level of communicative behaviors in children with autism vary significantly across familiar and unfamiliar adults (Bernard-Opitz, 1982) and different styles of interaction (Mirenda & Donnellan, 1986). For example, children demonstrate more initiations and responses when adults support the conversation by using comments and elaborations than when the adults direct the conversation through questions (Duchan, 1983). By using the Interaction Analysis to compare a child's social-communicative interactions in a variety of motivating contexts with familiar adults and peers, it is possible to recognize features of the interactant that enhance the child's communicative competence and identify needed modifications in the interactant's style.

Begin by selecting two or more motivating activites that include a variety of communicative opportunities for the child and familiar adult or peer. A videotape of the activity is needed for a systematic analysis of all the interactional variables, although portions of the analysis can be completed by using audio tapes and/or naturalistic observations. A five- to ten-minute tape of an activity usually provides enough data for useful analysis. The focus of the Interaction Analysis is the social-communicative behaviors of the interactant, both in terms of how the adult responds to the child and how the child responds to the adult. The Interaction Analysis is structured to examine single exchanges during dyadic interactions rather than longer conversations. The Interaction Analysis form and guidelines can be found in Appendix 7.2.

As indicated on the Interaction Analysis form, the taped interactions are transcribed, listing each interactant communicative utterance and any of the following features that apply:

1. WHO initiated the topic
2. WHERE the interactant is positioned in proximity to the child
3. WHY the interactant is communicating with the child
4. WHAT form the interactant uses (e.g., question, statement, direction)
5. HOW the message is communicated
6. WHEN the child responds (elapsed time)
7. The child's response

The information gathered helps determine what features of an interactant's style enhance continuation of a child's interaction and what features produce no response or shift the child's attention to a new topic. For example, statements that are contingent on the child's focus of attention may maintain interactions, while recurring patterns such as directions with no response, or question-answer routines, can be identified as less effective and subsequently guide changes in the adult/peer style of interaction. Patterns of interaction that allow for increased child communication can be identified as successful means for enhancing social-communicative interaction and applied across adults, peers, and settings.

Drawing from all the forementioned assessments as well as other informal observations, social-communicative interaction goals and objectives are developed. Intervention planning is approached differently for each child, given the wide range of communicative abilities observed in autism. For the child at an early stage of communication development, the goals are to expand the communicative means used to initiate and respond, and expand communicative functions expressed. Intervention for children with language includes the use of multiple means to express each function, the ability to generalize communicative skills across settings, and the ability to inititate and maintain interactive exchanges with various adults and peers. Intervention for the child with more advanced language skills focuses on the development and refinement of verbal and nonverbal discourse skills.

PROMOTING ADULT-CHILD INTERACTION

The core challenge for a child with autism is to extract meaning from what others are saying, doing, and feeling (Wing, 1988). The primary role of others is to create meaningful and mutually beneficial interactions.

Williams (1992) urges people to "relate to such children always in terms of how those children perceive the world" (p. 201) and suggests that focus be on the experience, with social contact secondary. In Chapter 2, Grandin reminds us: "People with autism desire emotional contact with other people but they are stymied by complex social interaction" (1995, p. 44).

Designing meaningful interactions to promote social and communicative effectiveness can be approached somewhat like directing a theatrical play. Each social interaction might be viewed as a mini production. In theater, the responsibility of the director is to understand the play's central theme, set the stage, organize the props, analyze each actor's role, know the script, and demonstrate to the actors how to successfully express key lines in the narrative. The design of activities to promote interactions among children with autism follows these same basic principles. With an understanding of the child's communicative abilities through assessment, social-communicative interaction is fostered by organizing activity routines, modifying interaction style, and providing environmental supports. Table 7.4 sumarizes the variables to be considered when promoting social-communicative interactions.

Activity Routines

An activity routine is an interaction pattern that follows a logical sequence and predictable set of communicative responses (Snyder-McLean, Solomonson, McLean, & Sack, 1984). Quite simply, it is a predictable sequence of interactive turns—that is, a conversational script of what to do and what to say within the context of a meaningful situation. The benefit of activity routines for promoting social-communicative interaction is reflected in the words of Donna Williams (1992):

> My behavior puzzled others, but theirs puzzled me, too. It was not so much that I had no regard for their rules as that I couldn't keep up with the many rules for each specific situation (p. 47). . . . my favorite teacher was a gentle voice that seemed somehow predictable (p. 69). . . . security I found through pattern and rhythm (p. 206).

The form of an activity routine parallels the ritualized patterns of interaction that are prominent in the interactions between adults and very young children discussed earlier. The interaction routines provide a limited and predictable set of contextually meaningful messages that allows the child to anticipate and insert appropriate responses. Through consistent experiences with an activity routine, the child learns to assign meaning to the language and communicative behaviors used within the interaction and thereby understand and use them. Once the child can participate in an established, predictable interaction, expansion and flexibility are systematically introduced into the activity.

Using the work of Snyder-McLean et al. (1984) as a guide, there are a series of steps to be taken in the design and implementation of activity routines.

Motivating Activities.   Motivating, naturally occurring activities set the stage for structuring activity routines. There are two ways to select contexts: (1) focus on contexts where the child is already motivated to communicate, and (2) select situations that have a clear theme or purpose. Most daily experiences have inherent routines. Bedtime, mealtime, story time, playtime and other daily events all present opportunities to develop activity routines. A predictable sequence of actions and communicative behaviors can be created artificially within any activity. Snyder-McLean et al. suggest beginning with activities that produce a clear end product such as cooking and art projects or turn-taking games. The key element is to assure that the activity requires joint focus and interactive, rather than parallel, communication from the child.

Clear Goals.   Begin with clearly defined communication goals to organize the interactive activity routine. Look at how the activity or situation naturally occurs for other same-age peers to identify the specific communicative intents that can be imbedded into the activity. Examine the common questions and comments expressed by other children within the activity. For example, during snack time, there are opportunities to request items, request assistance, refuse, comment when handing items to a peer, and indicate when finished. While building blocks, a child might request an action, label the building materials, comment on an action, and call attention to her or his building. Target the specific communicative functions (request toy from peer, comment on action) to be included within the activity routine and the means (word, phrase, communicative behavior) for the child to express them. Build on the child's current communicative intents and forms.

Activity Sequence.   Determine the sequence of actions or steps within the activity. Activity routines such as art have a natural sequence built in, while artificial routines need to be established in activities such as general play. The rigidity of the initial routine varies with the child's behavioral repertoire. The structure of the activity routine must provide predictability and tangible verbal and/or nonverbal and/or contextual cues to mark each step of the routine.

A "Script."   Having identified the specific phrase/sentence structures and vocabulary to be used, determine when to model these various communicative behaviors for the child. Establish a pattern of messages that predictably occur at set times during the activity sequence. Structure the script so that the child can link a message with an event and learn "what to say" in that specific context.

The framework for designing scripted interactions is the same for simple turn-taking games and elaborate conversational scripts. The length, complexity, and variety within the activity script will vary with the communicative competency of the child. For some children, there will be a limited range of phrases and words used; for others, the script will be more expansive. The degree to which the child has difficulty initiating, becomes frustrated in loosely structured activities, is confused by unanticipated social-communicative messages, and is highly reliant on particular prompts influences these decisions. The level of structure built into an activity routine depends on these factors. A consistent set of turn-taking actions and communicative behaviors allows the child to anticipate, regulate and practice interactions.

Shared Roles.   The majority of the script should be shared information—that is, what the adult/peer says or does is equally appropriate for the child to say or do in the same context. The interactant's language and communicative behavior is paired with objects and ongoing events, which allows the child to learn the form, function, meaning and social value of the interaction simultaneously. The interactant *mirrors* the child's verbal and nonverbal communicative behaviors and encourages the child to do the same.

Repetition.   A degree of repetition is needed in order for the child to understand and participate in the activity routine. Repetition does not mean repeating the same message over and over again, but rather limiting the range of comments, questions, and nonverbal communicative behaviors that occur within the interaction. These messages are repeated while following the initiations and responses of the child. The level of simplicity or complexity of a routine is defined by the number and variety of interactive turns. Simple routines may entail multiple repetitions of the identical three-step sequence during one activity, while a more complex activity routine may have a dozen components in the sequence. A high degree of repetition will enhance familiarity and participation.

Flexibility.   If activity routines were merely fixed scripts, then the child would be learning only rote responses in cued situations. The value of the activity routine is that it provides a framework for systematically introducing new elements to the context. The most critical element in designing activity routines is the ongoing process of revision and expansion. As the child masters the activity routine as reflected by increased participation and child-generated interaction, variations and additions to the action sequence and script are introduced and modeled for the child. Variations within the activity routine can be the addition of new steps within the activity, elaboration of the number of core messages included in the script, the intentional omission of a step and/or message, or changes in the sequence or materials. The systematic expansion of activity routines, termed *scaffolding,* is central to supporting the child's growing communication development (Bruner, 1975). Elements of one familiar routine must also be systematically built into other activity routines. Planned flexibility across different activity routines offers the child opportunities to successfully use learned communication under different conditions and with various interactive partners. It is important to remember that the child's level of engagement is the primary criteria for determining when to expand the activity routine. Children are typically engaged when they are motivated and understand the purpose and meaning of the social dynamic. When a child does not understand the meaning behind the messages and events in the situation, the activity needs to be clarified and/or simplified.

▶ **TABLE 7.4**
Promoting Social-
Communicative
Interactions

I. ACTIVITY ROUTINES[*]
- Motivating, naturally occurring activities
- Clearly defined communication goals
- Predictable sequence of actions or steps
- Organized script
- Shared roles
- Planned repetition
- Plans for expansion and flexibility

II. MODIFIED INTERACTION STYLE
- Joint attention
- Proximity to child
- Messages linked to present context
- Messages linked to child's actions
- Model what to do and what to say
- Complexity matches child's comprehension
- Degree of repetition
- Use of pausing
- Simultaneous speech and gesture
- Exaggerated paralinguistic cues
- Simultaneous use of interactant and environmental supports

III. ENVIRONMENTAL SUPPORTS
- For organization
- To enhance comprehension
- To cue communication

[*]Activity routines adapted from Snyder-McLean et al. (1984)

Modified Interaction Style

The challenges children with autism face when trying to engage in reciprocal interactions is best understood when their social perspective is considered. Explains Williams (1992):

> Words were no problem, but other people's expectations for me to respond to them were, as this would have required my understanding what was said (p. 4). . . . My response to what people said to me would often be delayed as my mind had to take time to sort out what they had said. The more stress I was under, the worse it became (p. 69).

Grandin offers a similar perspective:

> Sometimes I heard and understood, and other times speech reached my brain like the unbearable noise of an onrushing freight train (Grandin & Scariano 1986, p. 149).

> I have difficulty remembering long strings of verbal information. . . . I can't follow the rhythmic give and take of conversation . . . remembering what people say hampers my social interactions (Grandin, 1991, p. 90)

The primary intent of interaction is to communicate with the child at his or her level of social-communicative competence. A modified style of interaction can ensure and maintain interaction. The following considerations help create a reciprocal relationship with the child.

Who is establishing joint attention?   There is a tendency for adults to control interactions with language-impaired children through language that focuses the child's attention, then asks questions or commands the child to do something. Given that the purpose of conversation is to share information, it is important to use language that focuses on what is happening at the moment. Select language appropriate to the child's comprehension skills. Talk about the child's actions to establish joint reference, and comment on one's own parallel actions to reinforce language meaning. For the more able child, it is essential to interpret others' feelings and thoughts, intent and perspective.

Where are you positioned in proximity to the child?   The most effective interactions occur near the child. Children with autism are often easily startled so it is helpful to enter their space gently, observe their behavior for a moment in silence, and then convey a message. Establishing joint attention on an object or action is more important than maintaining a vacuous eye gaze.

Why are you communicating?   The communicative function of messages spoken to the child needs to parallel his or her targeted goals. The adult's role is to model for the child what to do and what to say, while jointly participating in the activity. Information should be semantically relevant to the ongoing experience.

How is your message conveyed?   The adult's role is to make all the subtle elements of conversation more explicit. Exaggerate the verbal and nonverbal components of conversation to increase the likelihood that the child will extract meaning from the message. A melodic tone of voice, dramatic facial expressions, and gestures add clarity to the message. Slow down the pace such that nonverbal cues are fixed in space and time like a movie in slow motion. Some children respond to dramatic personalities, appearing to understand the social dynamic best when it is exaggerated. Other children seem to respond best to individuals who speak slowly, calmly, and in a highly predictable manner. In both cases the clarity with which information is presented is the key element. Keep in mind that the quality of the language input must take into account the chronological age of the child. As the child gets older, nonverbal discourse strategies need to be assessed for age appropriateness.

When is there time to respond?   The child is often struggling to make sense of the information and to integrate the context, social intent, and meaning behind verbal and nonverbal messages. Adults and peers help children by pausing after delivering a message. Pausing gives the child time to integrate the information and respond—that is, to organize and retrieve a response. Multiple repetitions of a message, especially when paraphrased, may be overwhelming and confusing for the child. Become comfortable with silent pauses within a conversation.

What are you saying?   The semantics of the language input should reflect and mirror the ongoing events. This includes talking about the child's or interactant's activity while systematically restating and expanding on the child's communicative behaviors. For the more able child, it is essential for the interactant to clarify the thoughts and feelings of others in an effort the support the child's understanding of social perspective.

The syntactic complexity of the language input should reflect the comprehension abilities of the child. For example, framing questions in a fill-in-the-blank form ("The cat is where?") often produces more correct responses than posing questions in standard form. A simpler syntactic structure appears to reduce the processing load on the child. Information from the Language Comprehension Inventory can be used to assess the level of linguistic complexity that enhances the flow of interactions.

When the child is not attending, it is important to determine whether he or she is distracted or does not understand the events of the moment. Assumptions about what the child understands risks failure and frustration. The child's behavior and responses to a variety of input styles guide the type and form of needed modifications. Assume that the child is doing the best he or she can at the moment!

Environmental Supports

The task of promoting both understanding and spontaneity in the social dynamic may require incorporating a strategy that takes into account the children's preference and cognitive strengths in processing of non-transient, visual-spatial information (Schuler, 1995). Both Temple Grandin and Donna Williams note this learning preference:

> All my thinking is visual. . . . Memories play like a movie on the big screen of my mind. . . . I remember very little of what I hear unless it is emotionally arousing or I can form a visual image (Grandin & Scariano, 1986, p. 135).

> I became fascinated by words and books, making outside order out of inner chaos (Williams, 1992, p. 42).

Even with the predictability of activity routines and the clarity of the interactant's modified style, children with autism often fail to achieve spontaneous use of acquired communication skills. The use of environmental supports, particularly exposing the child to written or graphic language symbols within the context of activity routines and other interactive contexts, is one way to address this learning preference. Many young children demonstrate a precocious ability to read words without instruction (Whitehouse & Harris, 1984); others learn to recognize orthography and written language with little difficulty, while others demonstrate language via augmentative systems. While the ability to encode written language does not necessarily imply comprehension, exposure to both spoken and written language increases the opportunity to develop comprehension. Therefore it is suggested that a multimodal language input of speech paired with written or graphic language symbols be adopted to enhance both an understanding of verbal language and use of acquired communication skills. The symbols can be in the form of printed words, pictographic symbols, or pictures, hereafter referred to as written language. The complexity of the written language varies across children and contexts, varying from a single graphic symbol that represents an activity to detailed written scripts that remind the child what to say. The simultaneous presentation of spoken and written language enhances the child's ability to focus attention on the message, organize and extract meaning from the language, and respond more efficiently (Quill, 1991b). This strategy parallels current approaches to reading acquisition that dominate literacy reform today, and recognizes that all forms of language competence—listening, speaking, reading, and writing—develop concurrently (Weir, 1989).

Written language can be used as an instructional tool in three basic ways: as a cognitive tool to organize the sequence of the activity routine or interaction; as a communication tool to cue the child's communication; and as a comprehension tool to clarify the information spoken to the child. These three strategies can be used independently or in combination.

For Cognitive Organization.   The more clarity there is about the rules and expectations of social-communicative interaction, the more successful the child will be participating. Written language can depict the sequence of actions and steps of the activity routine or social context. The rules, the steps, and the expectations of the social situation can be displayed in the form of a checklist or narrative. The visual display serves as a guide of the interaction sequence and can be as detailed as needed so long as it aids the child's ability to understand, anticipate, and participate more fully.

To Enhance Comprehension.   This strategy is most familiar to practitioners. The use of objects, pictures, and written language to supplement verbal instruction is common practice. Weaving written language supports into social-communicative interactions can be cumbersome; but if it aids a child's ability to understand the social dynamic, it's worth trying. The following strategies to cue communciation use are often the most effective means to enhance both comprehension and use.

To Cue Communication.   Written language can be used to serve as a reminder of what to say and/or what to do in a situation. It is an augmentative communication system for children at all language levels. The visual materials serve as a retrieval cue that is not dependent on the interactant's prompts and cues, thus fostering spontaneity. The range and complexity of written language to prompt communication and social behaviors is unlimited. It can be as simple as a single symbol available as a cue card to elicit a specific message, or as complex as a written script describing an entire social situation (Gray, 1995). A variety of communicative functions, including commenting and asking questions, have been taught to preschoolers with emerging language using simple written messages and were maintained once the cue cards were removed (Quill, 1993). The written language can be presented on communication boards that contain multiple messages appropriate to a particular activity routine or social situation. For children with more advanced language, conversational expectations can be outlined for them in writing and reviewed prior to participating in the social situation. A small erasable pad is a useful device for writing down messages for children when they are stuck at any time.

These environmental supports are intended as a catalyst to independence. As a communication skill or social behavior is acquired and used spontaneously, material adaptations are no longer needed in that context. Once children integrate their social role and the communication for a particular setting, they will naturally disregard the written prompts (Quill, 1993). Supports are then applied to the next social-communicative context, continually expanding the child's "bank of social-communicative scripts." With a growing understanding of the rules of interaction in a variety of contexts, flexibility and generalization will ensue.

PROVIDING PEER GUIDANCE

Access to peers who model the language forms and social conventions of interaction is crucial to promoting social-communicative interactions. However, the mere availability of peers does not constitute criteria for success; rather, a number of strategies need to be incorporated in the context of activity routines and naturally occurring situations to nurture peer-child interactions. In addition to the activity routines of which peers are naturally a part, peers require specific guidance to promote social-communicative exchanges. Peer guidance helps children recognize and respond to the verbal and nonverbal communicative behaviors of the child with autism. Peer guidance has proven successful in promoting increased social-communicative interactions in children who show low rates of initiations and responses to peers (Goldstein & Strain, 1988). Strategies focus on the peer's understanding of the child's communicative attempts, the peer's ability to initiate and respond to the child, and the peer's ability to maintain an interaction with the child. The adult's role varies with the age and abilities of the peers and child and might include direct instruction, modeling, and/or environmental supports.

Direct Instruction

Direct instruction teaches peers to use specific means to encourage and maintain interactions. First, peers need to become aware of the many forms of communication and begin to understand the communicative attempts of their autistic friends. Through discussion, peers learn that in addition to talking, pictures, objects, and written words are all forms of communication. They learn that facial expression, eye contact, gestures, and proximity all help convey a message. Peers become sensitive to the subtle ways some of their friends try to communicate, with and without words. They learn the importance of being a "good listener" as their friend tries to communicate, and they learn how to interpret nonstandard means of communication such as grabbing or throwing objects. Next, peers can be directly told how to get their friends to talk with them. Through role playing, peers are taught what to say and what to do to get a friend's attention, initiate and maintain an interaction. Depending on the needs of the particular child with autism, the peer practices what to do—such as stand close, point to or give/take an item, take the child's hand, tap the child's arm, or show the child an item. Teaching peers what to say focuses on talking about their own actions or the actions of their friend, repeating themselves simply, repeating what their friend says, and requesting clarification. Peers are shown how to persist if a friend does not respond, how to wait for a response, and how to ignore certain behaviors. The range and complexity of the peer guidance is contingent on the targeted communication goals for the child with autism.

Modeling

Modeling is often the most common role taken by the adult to promote interactions among children. In modeling, adults observe the social context and show the peer what to say and what to do in the context. Modeling is intended to provide explicit support to the peer. Modeling can be in the form of demonstration or verbal support. Adults can take an active role as coparticipants in the children's activity or serve as directors of interaction. Demonstration is easiest when the adult acts as a coparticipant. When serving as director of an activity routine or other social situation, it is helpful to provide verbal prompts to peers from the periphery or by standing behind the peer. It is important that the adult's role in the interaction is explicitly clear to both the peer and the child with autism.

Environmental Supports

Environmental supports can be used in conjunction with modeling or as an alternative to direct adult support. Environmental supports are charts or cue cards that summarize techniques for the peers. Environmental supports remind the peers what to do and say and can be a useful option when peers appear too dependent on the adult's model. It is a pictorial or written reminder of how to talk with a friend that is visually available for the peers and may be reviewed periodically.

The ultimate goal of peer guidance is for peers to incorporate these interactive techniques into their repertoire and no longer require adult support. Some peers rapidly alter their interactive style through informal observation and adult modeling, while other peers may require direct instruction and environmental supports. If peers receive little feedback from a child, adults should provide ongoing reinforcement for their efforts. The ultimate goal is to promote social-communicative interactions that are mutually enjoyable and beneficial for all the children.

SUMMARY

The hallmark characteristic of autism, an impairment in reciprocal social interaction, remains as fascinating and perplexing today as it was fifty years ago. Children with autism struggle through the maze of social contact, and the only way they can develop improved skills is through experiencing some success in social-communicative interactions. Although it is important to recognize the complexity of social relationships and communicative interactions, one approach to promoting interactions is through careful assessment and a combination of interactive routines, modifications in the interactant's communication style, and use of environmental supports. The assessment provides a framework for understanding the child's perspective. The routines offer a consistent interactive pattern that is predictable and therefore more secure. The modifications in the interactant's style take into account the conditions under which the child is most responsive, and environmental supports reflect the child's preference for visual clarity. These basic features mirror the learning preferences of children with autism and interface developmental and behavioral methodological considerations. It is only by accepting the child's perspective as valid and useful that treatment can begin to support his or her understanding of others' perspectives. With this as our beginning, we can enhance social communication and interpersonal relationships that are mutually beneficial.

REFERENCES

Bates, E. (1976). *Language in context: The acquisition of pragmatics.* New York: Academic.

Bernard-Opitz, V. (1982). Pragmatic analysis of the communicative behavior of an autistic child. *Journal of Speech and Hearing Disorders, 47,* 99–109.

Bloom, L., & Lahey, M. (1978). *Language development and language disorders.* New York: Wiley.

Bruner, J. (1975). The ontogenesis of speech acts. *Journal of Child Language, 2,* 1–19.

Dalrymple, N. (1989). *Learning to be independent and responsible.* Publication of the Indiana Resource Center for Autism.

Duchan, J. (1983). Autistic children are noninteractive: Or so we say. *Seminars in Speech and Language, 4,* 63–78.

Finnerty, J., & Quill, K. (1991). *The communication analyzer.* Lexington, MA: Educational Software Research.

Frankel, R. (1982). Autism for all practical purposes: A micro-interactional view. *Topics in Language Disorders, 3,* 33–42.

Frith, U. (1989). *Autism: Explaining the enigma.* Oxford, England: Blackwell.

Goldstein, H., & Strain, P. (1988). Peers as communication intervention agents: Some new strategies and research findings. *Topics in Language Disorders, 9,* 44–57.

Grandin, T. (1991). Autistic perceptions of the world. *Proceedings of the Autism Society of America Conference,* pp. 85–94. Indianapolis, IN: ASA.

Grandin, T. (1995). The learning style of people with autism: An autobiography. In K.A. Quill (Ed.), *Teaching children with autism: Strategies to enhance communication and socialization.* Albany, NY: Delmar.

Grandin, T., & Scariano, M. (1986). *Emergence: Labeled autistic.* Novato, CA: Arena Press.

Gray, C. (1992). *The curriculum system: Success as an educational outcome.* Publication of the Jenison Public Schools, Michigan.

Gray, C. (1995). Teaching children with autism to "read" social situations. In K.A. Quill (Ed.), *Teaching children with autism: Strategies to enhance communication and socialization.* Albany, NY: Delmar.

Hart, B., & Risley, T. (1982). *How to use incidental teaching for elaborating language.* Austin, TX: Pro-Ed.

Howlin, P. (1989). Changing approaches to communication training with autistic children. *British Journal of Disorders of Communication, 24,* 151–168.

Kanner, L. (1943). Autistic disturbances of affective contact. *Nervous Child, 2,* 217–250.

Koegel, R., O'Dell, M., & Koegel, L. (1987). A natural language teaching paradigm for nonverbal autistic children. *Journal of Autism and Developmental Disorders, 17,* 187–200.

Lund, N., & Duchan, J. (1983). *Assessing children's language in naturalistic contexts.* Englewood Cliffs, NJ: Prentice-Hall.

McLean, J., & Snyder-McLean, L. (1978). *A transactional approach to early language training: Derivation of a model system.* Columbus, OH: Charles Merrill.

Mirenda, P., & Donnellan, A. (1986). Effects of adult interactional style on conversatonal behavior in students with severe communication problems. *Language, Speech and Hearing Services in Schools, 17,* 126–141.

Muma, J. (1986). *Language acquisition: A functionalistic perspective.* Austin, TX: Pro-Ed.

Ochs, E., & Schiefflin, B. (1979). *Developmental pragmatics.* New York: Academic.

Paul, R. (1987). Communication. In D. Cohen & A. Donnellan (Eds.), *Handbook of autism and pervasive developmental disorder.* New York: Wiley.

Peck, C. (1989). Assessment of social communicative competence: Evaluating environments. *Seminars in Speech and Language, 10,* 1–15.

Prizant, B., & Duchan, J. (1981). The functions of immediate echolalia in autistic children. *Journal of Speech and Hearing Disorders, 46,* 241–249.

Prizant, B., & Schuler, A. (1987). Facilitating communication: Language approaches. In D. Cohen & A. Donnellan (Eds.) *Handbook of autism and pervasive developmental disorder.* New York: Wiley.

Prizant, B. & Wetherby, A. (1989). Enhancing language and communication in autism. In G. Dawson (Ed.), *Autism: Nautre, diagnosis and treatment*. New York: The Guilford Press.

Quill, K. (1991a). *Using graphic symbols in the communication training of nonverbal preschoolers with autism*. Unpublished manuscript.

Quill, K. (1991b). Methods to enhance student learning, communication and self-control. In *Autism Society of America Conference Proceedings*. Indianapolis.

Quill, K. (1993). *Using written cues in the communication training of verbal children with autism*. Manuscript submitted for publication.

Ratner, N. & Bruner, J. (1978). Games, social exchange and the acquisition of language. *Journal of Child Language, 5*, 391–401.

Rydell, P., and Prizant, B. (1995). Assessment and intervention strategies for children who use echolalia. In K.A. Quill (Ed.), *Teaching children with autism: Strategies to enhance communication and socialization*. Albany, NY: Delmar.

Schuler, A. (1995). Thinking in autism: Differences in learning and development. In K.A. Quill (Ed.), *Teaching children with autism: Strategies to enhance communication and socialization*. Albany, NY: Delmar.

Schuler, A., Peck, C., Willard, C., & Theimer, K. (1989) Assessment of communicative means and functions through interview: Assessing communicative abilities of individuals with limited language. *Seminars in Speech and Language, 10*, 51–62.

Simpson, R. (1991). Ecological assessment of children and youth with autism. *Focus on Autistic Behavior, 5*, 1–18.

Snow, C. (1977). The development of conversaton between mothers and babies. *Journal of Child Language, 4*, 1–22.

Snyder-McLean, L., Solomonson, B., McLean, J., & Sack, S. (1984). Structuring joint action routines: A strategy for facilitating communication and language development in the classroom. *Seminars in Speech and Language, 5*, 213–228.

Weir, B. (1989). A research base for kindergarten literacy programs. *The Reading Teacher, 42*, 456–460.

Wells, G. (1981). *Learning through interaction: The study of language development*. Cambridge, UK: Cambridge University Press.

Wetherby, A. (1986). Ontogeny of communicative functions in autism. *Journal of Autism and Developmental Disorders, 15*, 295–315.

Wetherby, A., & Prizant, B. (1989). The expression of communicative intent: Assessment guidelines. *Seminars in Speech and Language, 10*, 77–91.

Whitehouse, J., & Harris, J. (1984). Hyperlexia in infantile autism. *Journal of Autism and Developmental Disorders, 14*, 281–290.

Williams, D. (1992). *Nobody nowhere*. New York: Times Books.

Wing, L. (1988). The continuum of autistic characteristics. In E. Schoper & G. Mesibov (Eds.), *Diagnosis and assessment*. New York: Plenum.

APPENDIX 7.1   **Communicative Means-Functions Questionnaire**

Function	Sample communicative context	What does the child do/say?
Request attention	You are giving your attention to another child.	
Request affection	You approach child after child has been hurt.	
Request assistance	Child needs help putting on shoes.	
Request information	Child sees a picture of something or someone new.	
Request permission	Child wants to go outside.	
Request peer interaction	Child sees another child playing with one of his/her favorite toys.	
Request adult interaction	You tickle child a few times and then pause.	
Request food or object	Child wants a toy that is out of reach.	
Refusal	You offer child a food that he/she doesn't like.	
Protest	You want child to go to sleep and child doesn't want to.	
Cessation	Child wants to be finished with a meal or task.	
Greetings	A family member or friend comes to visit.	
Affirmation	You ask child if he/she wants a favorite toy.	

Finnerty & Quill, 1991

APPENDIX 7.1   (continued)

Function	Sample communicative context	What does the child do/say?
Comment: object	Child sees an interesting person or object in a book.	
Comment: action	You sit with child while he/she is playing with a favorite toy.	
Comment: mistake	Child accidentally spills his/her drink.	
Express humor	You laugh unexpectedly when child does something.	
Express confusion	Child is given a task that he/she does not understand.	
Express fear	Child sees or hears something that frightens him/her.	
Express frustration	Child is having difficulty completing a task.	
Express anger	You make child stop doing a favorite activity.	
Express happiness	Child is doing a favorite activity.	
Express sadness	Child experiences something sad.	

APPENDIX 7.2   **Interaction Analysis (sample assessment form)**

Child's name:_____

Interactant's Name_____ Date: _____

Context:_____Videotape sequence:_____

Adult/Peer Message	*Who*	*Where*	*Why*	*What*	*How*	*When*	*Child Response*

Codes:

Adult/Peer   Record what is said by adult/peer interactant
Message: Code each adult message for any of the following features
                  that apply

WHO: I=Adult initiated,   R=Adult response to child initiation

WHERE: N=Near child,   F=Far away from child

WHY: Communicative Function; e.g.,
                  R=Request,   C=Comment   N=Negation

WHAT: Q=Question,   C=Comment,   D=Directive
                  N=NewTopic,   E=Elaboration,   R=Repetition

HOW: G=With gesture,   I=Exaggerated intonation, P=SlowPace,
                  R=Referent present,   VC=VisualCue present

WHEN: How many seconds are given for the child to respond?

Child   Record child's response to adult/peer's message and code as:
Response: C= Continues topic, N=New topic,
                  O=Off topic,   NR=No response

Promoting Socialization

8

Enhancing Children's Play

Pamela J. Wolfberg

Children with autism commonly encounter problems entering into imaginative and social play activities with other children. Paucity of play is distinctly characteristic of autism and not easily disentangled from social, cognitive, and affective aspects of the disorder. The core features of autism, qualitative impairments in reciprocal social interaction and imaginative activity, and a markedly restricted repertoire of activities and interests, all denote problems in the social and symbolic dimensions of play (American Psychiatric Association, 1987). Children with autism typically lack the social sophistication necessary for pretending and coordinating play with other children. Limitations in social understanding make it especially difficult for them to relate to peers in play. They often fail to comprehend the rather unpredictable actions and perspectives of others. Unable to make sense of the social world, they become locked in a solitary world of literal meanings (Frith, 1989).

Peer play experiences are seen as especially critical for acquiring social knowledge (Bruner, 1986; Corsaro & Schwarz, 1991). While playing with peers, children develop friendships and learn a variety of key social strategies that are affiliated with increasing social competence (Hartup & Sancilio, 1986). The task to sustain social relationships and friendships with peers requires that children achieve interpersonal coordination in mutually enjoyed play activities (Parker & Gottman, 1989). Thus children refine a number of verbal and nonverbal social strategies to participate in increasingly complex and sophisticated collaborative play activities. For instance, in order to resolve conflicts over materials or play roles, children develop strategies for negotiation and compromise (Rubin, 1980). Children also learn to interpret subtle social cues to successfully extend invitations and gain entry into peer group activities (Dodge, Schlundt, Schocken, & Delugach, 1983).

Pretend play has special significance for children's social development. In a pretend framework, children mutually explore social roles and rules and construct shared meanings (Garvey, 1977). Since aspects of the social world and expectations about the behavior of people provide the main materials for social pretend play, children are able to test out hypotheses about possible interactions and relationships among humans. Moreover, pretend play permits more effective understanding of the perspectives of others and the adoption of a metarepresentational mode, capacities seen as critical for socialized thought (Leslie, 1987).

The purpose of this chapter is to present ways in which we as practitioners and parents can guide and support the imaginative and social play experiences of children with autism. Many of the strategies presented draw from work related to the integrated play groups project (Schuler & Wolfberg, 1992; Wolfberg & Schuler, 1993). Originated as a pilot program in an urban elementary school (Wolfberg, 1988), over a period of several years this project evolved and transformed under the collaborative efforts of many professionals, parents, and children. The ensuing integrated play groups model is the culmination of this collective effort.

THE INTEGRATED PLAY GROUPS MODEL

The integrated play groups model draws heavily on the work of Russian psychologist Lev Vygotsky (1966; 1978), who accorded play a central place in his overall theory of development. Vygotsky presumes that play is an inherently social and collective process. This emphasis on the social nature of play conforms to Vygotsky's main premise that the transmission of culture through social interaction is critical to the formation of mind. Vygotsky stresses the importance of social pretend play as a mechanism to construct shared meanings and appropriate social knowledge. He also considers solitary play social activity, since the themes, roles, and scripts enacted in play represent the child's understanding and appropriation of the sociocultural materials of society.

The integrated play groups model conceives of play as naturalistic and meaningful activity in which children of all ages make sense of the world through shared experiences. This notion of play departs from other interventions in which play serves merely as a context for social skills instruction, or as a set of discrete behaviors that can be taught in a directive step-by-step fashion. Rather than being directive, the integrated play groups approach provides a support system for peer play. Children faced with the task of learning how to play gain expertise while playing with other, more competent players in small groups organized around pretend play activities. Capitalizing on child initiations, an adult guides and mediates peer play activities. Novice players take on whatever roles they are capable of performing in play themes and scripts designed by more experienced players. Multiple opportunities are provided for the children to imitate and practice advanced play behaviors in collective activity.

The integrated play groups model combines Vygotsky's social constructivist theory with current knowledge of play, autism, and social integration. While it is not essential to become an authority on all of the theories that comprise the integrated play groups model, it is important to acquire at least a basic understanding of how these theories translate into practice. The aim of this chapter is to give parents and practitioners a working knowledge of play as it can be applied to assessment and intervention.

The chapter is divided into three interrelated sections. The first section focuses on understanding play as it relates to social and symbolic aspects of development. To begin, play is defined as a basis for application of the model. An overview of how play progresses in typical childhood development follows to serve as comparison for understanding play in autism. This section concludes with qualitative descriptions of play variations commonly observed in children with autism.

The second section of this chapter focuses on methods for observing children's play. It begins with an observational framework for classifying the social and symbolic dimensions of play in children with autism. To systematically record and evaluate play observations, practical strategies and tools derived from the integrated play groups project are offered.

The third and final section of this chapter provides strategies for enhancing children's play. It opens with an overview of methods for guiding children's participation in social and imaginative play activities. A number of strategies for designing supportive play environments are presented.

UNDERSTANDING PLAY

Supporting children in peer play experiences requires understanding play as it relates to social and symbolic development. While we usually have little difficulty deciding whether or not a child is playing, defining play is notoriously complex. Consensus on a precise definition of play is complicated by the various disciplines and approaches taken to investigate different aspects of play. Anthropology, sociology, psychology, and education vary greatly in terms of the motives and methodologies employed to study play. Thus it is commonly accepted that different types of play may need to be defined in different ways (Smith, Takhvar, Gore, & Vollstedt, 1986) and that definitions will vary according to the theoretical biases of a particular researcher (Rubin, Fein, & Vandenberg, 1983).

Most pertinent to enhancing play in children with autism are definitions that reveal concern for social constructive processes involved in the acquisition of play and their cultural significance (Bruner, 1986; Vygotsky,1966; 1978). Such perspectives take into consideration the transactional processes that lead to both social reciprocity and the formation of symbols. Sympathetic to this notion of play as an inherently social and collective process, we have adopted a working definition of play reflecting the convergence of multiple research perspectives (Garvey, 1977; Piaget, 1962; Rubin, et al., 1983; Smith & Vollstedt, 1985; Vygotsky, 1978). The following interrelated descriptive features serve to distinguish play from nonplay behaviors. Defining play in this way allows theorists and practitioners to recognize play behavior in children whose development may or may not be considered typical. These play descriptors are detectable across multiple developmental levels and contexts involving both interactive and independent forms of activity.

Play is *pleasurable* and commonly accompanied by signs of positive affect. Although not essential, smiling and laughter are often signs of a playful orientation. Children engaged in playful activities may exhibit other signs such as blissful humming or singing to themselves, or simply an intense focus on a particular play act.

Play involves *active engagement* in a freely chosen activity. Thus play is differentiated from passive states such as lounging, aimless loafing, boredom, and inactivity. Daydreaming, on the other hand, may be viewed as actively playing with ideas or inventing fantasy.

Play is *intrinsically motivated*, occurring without external demands or rewards. The goals of play are self-imposed rather than externally imposed by others. By the same token, since the rules of play are self-imposed, a distinction is made between play and organized games that have predetermined sets of rules. Moreover, there is greater attention on the process of play than on the attainment of a particular goal or outcome. There is an open-ended quality that distinguishes play from goal-directed activities such as work.

Play includes *flexibility* to do the unexpected, change the rules, and experiment with novel combinations of behaviors and ideas. Flexibility involves variations on themes through elaboration and diversification of existing behavioral repertoires. This quality of play may be contrasted with highly rigid and perseverative activity characteristic of stereotypic behaviors.

Play frequently has a *nonliteral* or "as if" quality that the involved players can easily appreciate. This characteristic is obvious in pretending when children treat an object as if it were something else. When children pretend, they give clear signals to indicate pretend versus not pretend. This nonliteral orientation may appear in other forms of play that do not involve pretending. For instance, play fighting can be distinguished easily from aggressive fighting.

**Play
Development**

Although descriptive characteristics allow theorists and practitioners to recognize play behavior, they do little to explain individual variation evident in play as children develop. Elucidating the course of play in typical development provides a context for understanding play in children whose development is delayed or discontinuous. Recognizing present and emerging developmental levels across multiple play and language dimensions is especially critical for designing the most appropriate assessment tools and intervention programs.

Beginnings of Play. Although it is difficult to determine when children first begin to play, playful behavior is apparent during the first few months of life when infants exchange gazes and take turns vocalizing with caregivers (Garvey, 1977). Moreover, infants as young as 8 weeks of age display signs of a playful orientation such as vigorous smiling and cooing when provided opportunities to interact with objects that provide contingent responses—for example, a mobile controlled by a string tied to the baby's leg (Watson, 1972). These types of play experiences involving joint attention and contingent responding reflect the highly transactional nature of play.

The play that develops between adult caregivers and infants during the first year of life appears to be the earliest form of social play. Prior to the age of 6 months, infants mainly play an appreciative role in adult initiated social games such as peek-a-boo and pat-a-cake (Ross & Kay, 1980). To engage the infant, adults often perform a sequence of actions contingent on the infant's response (Stern, 1974). For instance, adults display exaggerated and varied facial expressions, vocalizations, and tactile contacts to elicit such responses as smiling, laughing, and gazing.

As infants develop, they increasingly take an active role in social play. Laughing and smiling in anticipation of the actions performed by adults, they begin to discover rhythm in the give and take of social games. At first they hesitatingly take turns, relying on adult responses to carry out the sequence. To encourage greater participation, the adult regulates the amount of support provided to the child's advancing ability to initiate and sustain social play exchanges (Bruner & Sherwood, 1976). Eventually, babies take confident and regular turns and initiate familiar play sequences.

Following a relatively consistent sequence, social play directed toward peers also appears early in typical development (Hartup, 1983). Beginning around the age of 6 months, infants actively express interest in peers through directing natural signs such as looking, smiling, vocalizing, gesturing, and reaching out and touching. They begin to recognize familiar peers and respond to them in idiosyncratic ways (Hay, 1985). This is followed by a period in which babies engage in brief and fleeting encounters by offering and exchanging toys, mutually manipulating objects, and occasionally imitating each other's toy play (Vandell & Wilson, 1982).

Early play with objects progresses from repetitious and undifferenti-ated actions to predictable and organized play sequences. Initially, infants actively explore different objects by mouthing, reaching, and banging. While attending to single objects, they begin to apply appropriate actions schemes such as pulling, twisting, or turning knobs. Subsequently, babies begin to combine and use objects as containers to explore relational proper-ties. They eventually recognize familiar objects and use them in conven-tional ways—for instance, drinking water from a cup or combing hair.

Physical objects in the immediate environment commonly serve as vehicles for play exchanges (Vandell & Wilson, 1982). By approximately the age of 9 months, babies develop the capacity to establish a joint refer-ence to an object with another person by vocalizing, gesturing, showing, or giving objects. Though still unable to use language, they are able to com-municate an interest or desire for an object intentionally through purpose-fully attracting adult attention. They begin to seek out others actively to obtain an object out of reach or demonstrate how to manipulate the object correctly.

During this period, babies also learn to respond to the emotional cues of adults, a capacity known as social referencing (Sorce & Emde, 1981). An adult's emotional reaction to a particular object or event directly affects the baby's exploration of that object or event. For instance, babies will hesitate to carry out an action such as picking up a toy or leaving a particular area at which an adult expresses disgust or alarm. This stage of development reflects the baby's early capacity to form representations of people, things, and events. Hobson (1989) describes social referencing as significant not only as an entry point for the child's understanding that a given object or event can have meaning for self and others, but also for an appreciation of the multiple-meanings nature of symbolism. Thus mature forms of symbol-ic activity including pretend play are seen as rooted in the infant's experi-ence of a world of shared feelings and patterns of activity with others. This has profound implications for children with autism, whose lack of shared attention with caregivers is often one of the earliest signs of the condition.

Play in Early Childhood.   As children make the transition to symbolic play, a number of related abilities emerge reflecting the reorganization of thought. Symbolic play develops along several dimensions during early childhood, a period Singer and Singer (1991) refer to as the "high season of imaginative play." A number of theorists present a similar progression of symbolic play (Garvey, 1977; Rubin, et al. 1983; Nicholich, 1977; Westby, 1991). Primitive symbolic representations gradually become incorporated into play sequences with objects and people. Governed by internal repre-sentations of ideas, rules, or symbols, children assign new and novel mean-ings to objects. Increasingly, they use props in abstract and inventive ways where an object stands for something else, or where something totally imaginary is created. The thematic content of play reflects the increasing use of gestures and language to invent novel, elaborate, and integrated play scripts. Imaginative play themes become organized with greater coherence and complexity. Eventually children play by adopting roles of others and treating animate objects (e.g., dolls and stuffed animals) as if they could initiate their own actions.

It is at this particular juncture in play development that children with autism experience the greatest difficulty. Here it is necessary to make a distinction between two forms of symbolic play commonly referred to as make-believe, pretend, or pretense. The first form of symbolic play, emerging in typical development at around 18 months, is described as reality-oriented play or *simple pretense* (Harris, 1989). In this type of play, the child responds to an object's actual properties or expresses knowledge of its conventional use. Children initially rely on realistic props to reenact brief and isolated actions relating to familiar routines or events, for instance washing and feeding. Subsequently, children reenact the isolated actions of others such as cooking or cleaning. They later extend these simple play scripts to dolls and other people.

The second type of symbolic play, emerging between the ages of 2 and 3 years, is described as *advanced pretense*. The transition from simple to advanced pretense signifies the child's emerging ability to form representations of representations or *metarepresentations*. In this type of pretend play, children are able to disengage from reality and entertain nontruths. Initially, children organize play scripts around familiar events they have personally experienced. They intentionally incorporate appropriate materials for the activity into play scripts. For instance, putting a doll to bed with its pajamas, a blanket, and a pillow, and commenting on the activity: "Baby sleeping." The thematic content later reflects familiar experiences that adults commonly perform—for instance, grocery shopping with a baby doll. At this point, children begin to talk to dolls (e.g., "Baby go shopping") but do not yet project their feelings or desires on dolls.

Between the ages of 3 and 4 years, children rely less on realistic replicas or lifelike props to pretend and increasingly use language to narrate and plan play scripts. They can transform objects—for example, a block can represent a car. They also transform themselves into different play roles such as animating miniatures and dolls or dramatizing persons, animals, and things. Children eventually enact reciprocal role-taking by playing the part of two or more actors, such as a mother and a baby. Connecting several play scripts, children dramatize elaborate scenes in sequential and evolving play episodes.

Advanced pretense includes the growing capacity to conjure up mental states or imagine and simulate the feelings, desires, and beliefs of another. Recently evolving as an explanatory construct for autistic symptomatology (Baron-Cohen, Leslie, & Frith, 1985), this capacity is viewed as a precursor to the development of a fully mature theory of mind (Leslie, 1987). Failure to imagine and achieve insight into the perspectives of others has extreme consequences for a person's ability to make sense of the world. Thus the transition from simple to advanced pretense is a major turning point in the play development of children with autism.

In typical development, the increasing capacity to engage in advanced pretense and to use flexible and sophisticated language dominate the preschool and kindergarten years in the form of social pretend activities (McCune-Nicholich, 1981). Socially coordinated pretend play involves the ability to share a pretend framework requiring that children work together to maintain intersubjectivity as they collaborate on play scenarios (Bretherton, 1984). During this period, children may at first intensely watch one another in play and engage in parallel play activities beside other children. Gradually play interchanges increase in length, frequency, and complexity. Rules become much more complex as they are established during the course of play. Dramatic roles and thematic content are fueled by familiar aspects of the social world, popular characters, as well as pure invention and fantasy. As children mature, they increasingly use complex and sophisticated language to coordinate play roles. Moreover, they prefer playing in collaboration with peers to playing alone.

Play in Middle Childhood.   Societal constraints and expectations placed on children as they enter school have limited the study of play development past early childhood (Glickman, 1984; Singer & Singer, 1990). Children in middle childhood are commonly thought to abandon make-believe play for what are considered more advanced play endeavors (Piaget, 1962). Thus games and sports are the dominant play activities formally available to children in school and recreation programs while occasions for make-believe play activities are rare. Nevertheless, the impulse to pretend in middle childhood continues, particularly when opportunities for imaginative activities are made available (Bergen & Oden, 1988).

As compared to that of younger children, there appear to be qualitative differences in the style and content of older children's pretend play. Singer and Singer (1990) suggest that overt play is gradually and subtly transformed into private thought or fantasy. Thus children seek out playful activities to pursue their fantasies. Dramatic play with other children, dolls, and miniatures are common in the middle-childhood years. Some children create elaborate and detailed private imaginary worlds, or paracosms, that often extend well into adolescence (Cohen & MacKeith, 1991). Fantasy is also easily detected in the complex imagery produced in other representational activities such as art, writing, and storytelling. While older children's play scripts and creative expressions often reflect greater complexity and sophistication than those of younger children, they are frequently constrained by concerns for convention and peer acceptance (Gardner, 1989).

Children spend increasing amounts of time in peer play in middle childhood, away from the watchful eyes of adults (Hartup, 1983). There is a greater focus on establishing stable friendships and affiliations with peer groups. Children typically form friendship alliances with others who share common interests and status. Play groups tend to be homogenous with respect to age and gender, while membership status is typically hierarchically arranged (Parker & Gottman, 1989). Older males tend to engage in more organized large-group play activities such as sports, while females tend to prefer more intimate activities with one other person or a small group of friends (Lever, 1976).

Older children display greater sophistication in the use of both verbal and nonverbal social-communication strategies to coordinate play activities with peers. Successfully extending invitations to others to play and joining peer groups at play requires a kind of social finesse that is evident among socially competent or popular children as opposed to children who are frequently rejected (Putallaz, 1983; Putallaz & Gottman, 1981). The ability to gain entrance into ongoing play group activities requires an initial understanding of the group's frame of reference. Socially competent children are thus able to employ a sequence of strategies that reflect an ability to understand the group's perspective to gracefully enter the play activity. These include the ability to gradually approach an activity, hover on the periphery of the group, mimic and comment on the activity, gradually move closer, and wait for an invitation or for a natural break to enter the group without disrupting the players (Dodge et al., 1983). Mastering the skills necessary for group entry is of critical importance for children with autism and others who frequently encounter peer rejection.

Play Variations in Children With Autism

The play of children with autism is especially striking when contrasted with the richly imaginative and social nature of play in typically developing children. Despite considerable variation in the form and content of play, there are certain qualitative characteristics that seem fairly consistent within the population of autism. Overall, they lack the spontaneous and flexible qualities characteristic of play. Symbolic pretense and social engagement are conspicuously absent in play activities (Ricks & Wing, 1975; Wing, Gould, Yeates, & Brierly, 1977). When left to their own devices, they commonly impose rigid and perseverative play routines (Boucher, 1977; Frith, 1989). Some children engage for several hours in a single repetitive play sequence extending over months or even years. Once established, many children with autism express considerable resistance to a play routine being disrupted.

Children with autism display patterns of play that differ among children and change within children over time. The tendency to manipulate objects in a stereotyped fashion is a frequently cited characteristic (Tiegerman & Primavera, 1981). As compared to typical children, children with autism engage in higher rates of manipulative forms of play and in fewer distinctly different combined play acts involving objects (Tilton & Ottinger, 1964). Object manipulations range from quite simple, self-directed play acts to highly physically coordinated, complex, and elaborate play routines (Wing & Attwood, 1987).

While some children with autism present more conventional play with objects (Lewis & Boucher, 1988), mature forms of symbolic pretense rarely spontaneously emerge (Baron-Cohen, 1987). Overall, they tend to exhibit less time and diversity in advanced play skills, fewer functional play sequences, and fewer symbolic play acts related to dolls and others (Mundy, Sigman, Ungerer, & Sherman, 1987; Sigman & Mundy, 1987; Sigman & Ungerer, 1984). Reality-based pretend play that is object-directed (e.g., stirring a pot on a play stove), self-directed (e.g., holding a telephone to one's ear), or doll-directed (e.g., bathing and feeding a doll) is often repetitive and literal. Language, gestures, and sound effects that are indicative of imagination are rarely spontaneously incorporated into these types of play sequences.

Some children with autism enact play routines that resemble advanced forms of pretend; however, evidence of flexible imagination including the attribution of mental states to people, characters, or animate objects is rare (Leslie, 1987). For instance, they may repeatedly construct and reconstruct the same intricate layout of buildings and roadways but never actually incorporate novel elements into the construction. Others may recreate the role of a certain fictional character, such as a television star, or reenact a particular theme or event over and over with minimal variation. Play themes comprising peculiar fascinations or obsessions with especially anxiety-producing events, such as natural disasters or death, are void of dramatic expression and emotionality.

Children with autism also commonly experience difficulties engaging in mutually supported play activities with peers. Some children avoid peer interaction and are unresponsive to social overtures. Others may be passively led into play but rarely initiate play on their own. Still others actively approach peers for the purpose of play but do so in an awkward and idiosyncratic fashion (Wing & Attwood, 1987). Limitations in social understanding, particularly in the ability to share another's perspective, form a gap between the child with autism and potential playmates. The social nuances necessary for entering a play situation and coordinating activities with one or more peers are especially difficult for children with autism to imitate and comprehend. They cannot easily convey their intentions or desire to play with other children through conventional communicative means. Thus social initiations to join an activity are frequently misinterpreted or overlooked by peers. Interpreting the intentions of others poses a similar dilemma for children with autism, resulting in their failure to respond to the social bids extended by peers.

Peer groups also play a significant role in perpetuating problems associated with play in children with autism. Typical children's failure to appreciate the perspectives and idiosyncrasies of children with autism widens the gap between them. Since children with autism play and act in ways that deviate from the familiar, peers often form social perceptions regarding them as peculiar or socially maladroit. Children with autism may therefore become victims of teasing and purposeful exclusion from peer play activities (Frith, 1989). While typical children also may feel genuine compassion for children with autism, they may overwhelm them with solicitous displays to enlist them in play. Peers may inadvertently cross the threshold of a particular child's sensory tolerance compelling that child to retreat or withdraw.

As a result of the reciprocal influences of play transactions with peers, children with autism tend to remain on the fringes of peer groups. As they spend increasing amounts of time in isolation from typical playmates, they seek refuge in ritualistic activity. Without the availability of playmates to share, expand, and negotiate play routines, these rituals become firmly established and increasingly resistant to change. Familiar play rituals may well provide children with autism a safe haven in which to establish order and make sense of an otherwise threatening and unpredictable social world. Yet there is an overwhelming sense that these seemingly aimless repetitive motions and gestures are efforts to communicate and be a part of the world of children's play. Donna Williams (1992), a remarkable woman with autism, describes the irony of this situation through accounts of her own childhood play:

> Other children played school, mothers and fathers, doctors and nurses. Other children skipped ropes and played with balls or swap-cards. I had swap-cards. I gave them away in order to make friends, before learning that I was supposed to swap them, not give them away (p. 22).

> [My mother] bought me a doll's pram. I ventured outside my room with it, dragging it repetitively up and down the stairs without much interest in what I was doing. I was acting normal, wasn't I? (p. 39).

OBSERVING CHILDREN'S PLAY

An important first step in guiding children's play experiences is becoming a keen observer of the social and symbolic dimensions of play. Systematically documenting and evaluating observations is one way to detect patterns and relationships in play behavior that might otherwise go unnoticed. Many play assessments currently used in education and psychology delineate social and symbolic forms of play within a normative framework. While identifying play skills typical of different ages and developmental stages may be useful for targeting specific problems, these types of assessments often fail to take into account individual variations in play. Based on the assumption that play is a linear process involving the accumulation of separate skills, these types of assessments do not easily translate into interventions for children who exhibit discontinuities in development.

Assessments of children with autism must be especially sensitive to the subtle qualities rather than obvious deficiencies observed in their play. Recognizing play development as a transformational process rather than as a series of successive stages allows us to alter our perceptions of normalcy. In this way, we interpret all behavior, even unconventional expressions in play, as purposeful and adaptive, as meaningful attempts to initiate independent and social play activities. Observations of child initiations in play, even in unusual forms, may serve as indices of present and emerging abilities in play. Assessing play in this way is essential for guiding our decisions as to how to intervene on behalf of the children learning to play.

Table 8.1 presents a framework for identifying characteristics associated with the symbolic and social dimensions of play. The symbolic dimension of play includes play acts that are directed toward objects or signify specific events. These range from simple exploration of objects to more complex imaginative play schemes. The social dimension of play focuses on the child's distance to and involvement with one or more children. These include peer-directed social behaviors progressing from brief and fleeting encounters to coordinated and sustained interactions. While each set of characteristic behaviors appear to follow a relatively consistent developmental sequence, they are not regarded as mutually exclusive stages of development.

Taking the time to observe and reflect on how children play beside and with other children fosters a greater understanding and appreciation of each child's unique play characteristics. Observing children in a variety of natural play contexts is especially helpful for developing individual and group portraits. To get a holistic view of the social play context, we suggest that you periodically "play anthropologist" when guiding children in playgroup experiences. That means allowing yourself to stand back and watch the children play without intervening. While you will most certainly be tempted to jump in and give support where needed, if you resist this temptation you will gain invaluable insight into the behaviors of the children in their "natural habitat." You can even learn a great deal from the ways in which children resolve their own conflicts without adult assistance. We have also found it helpful to videotape play group sessions as a way to not only assess children's play group experiences, but also evaluate yourself as you guide the children in play.

Provided as Appendix 8.1 and Apendix 8.2 at the end of this chapter are two observation tools that we have developed for integrated play groups. They will help you record and evaluate your observations in a relatively uncomplicated manner.

▶**TABLE 8.1**
Framework for
Observing
the Dimensions
of Play

Symbolic Dimension of Play	Social Dimension of Play
No interaction Child does not touch or play with toys. The child engages in self-stimulatory behavior that does not involve toys (e.g., stares at hands, rocks body, waves or flaps arms or hands, stares at toys).	*Isolate* Child appears to be oblivious or unaware of others and may occupy self by watching anything of momentary interest, playing with own body, or playing alone (e.g., child wanders, gets on and off chair, sits quietly, plays with back to peers).
Manipulation Exploratory play with toys ranging from simple to quite complex interactions. There is an apparent motivation to control the physical world. Child shows an interest in toys, but does not use them in conventional ways (e.g., holds and gazes at toy; mouths, waves, shakes, or bangs toys; stacks blocks or bangs them together; lines up objects).	*Orientation* Child has an awareness of the other children as evidenced by looking at them, their play materials, or activities. Child does not enter into play (e.g., child quietly watches other children, child turns whole body facing children).
Functional Complex and conventional use of toys in which there is a definite dependency of one response on another. There is a quality of delayed imitation while actions are performed that includes simple pretense (e.g., puts teacup to mouth, puts brush to hair, connects train sections and pushes train, arranges pieces of furniture in dollhouse, builds a building with blocks).	*Parallel/proximity* Child plays independently, beside rather than with the other children. There is simultaneous use of the same play space or materials as peers. There may be occasional imitation, showing of objects, or alternation of actions with peers (e.g., one child plays with a ball sitting close to another child who plays with a train; one child brushes a doll's hair while another pushes a doll in a carriage).
Symbolic/pretend Child pretends to do something or to be someone or something else with an intent that is representational. Advanced pretense involves role-playing and includes movements, vocalizations or verbalizations which are substituted for real objects (e.g., child makes hand move to mouth signifying drinking from tea cup; makes a puppet talk; uses a toy person or doll to represent self; uses block as a car accompanied by engine sounds).	*Common focus* Child engages in activities directly involving one or more peers including informal turn taking, giving and receiving assistance and directives, and active sharing of materials. There is a common focus or attention on the play (e.g. each child plays with blocks sharing blocks, each plays with dolls and touch each other's dolls, they take turns playing bean bag toss).

Definitions for symbolic play dimension derived from Fenson & Schell, 1986; McCune-Nicholich, 1981; Piaget, 1962; and Smilansky, 1968. Definitions for social play dimension were adapted from Parten (1932).

Appendix 8.1, the Play Preference Inventory, is a whole-group observation tool designed to record the play preferences of every child, including both novice and expert players. The inventory provides a place to record each child's preferred play materials, interactions with objects, play activities, play themes, and playmates. The information gathered will help you identify patterns of play interests shared by different members of the group.

Appendix 8.2, the Profile of Individual Play Characteristics, is an observation tool for recording a novice player's demonstrated play behaviors and preferences. The profile includes a section to indicate and describe the symbolic dimensions of play, social dimensions of play, and communication strategies, as well as preferred play activities, materials, and playmates.

ENHANCING CHILDREN'S PLAY

Through a carefully tailored system of social support, we can provide children with autism meaningful and successful peer play experiences. To bring about most competent forms of play necessitates combining a number of important methods within the social arena of play groups. Guiding participation in play and designing supportive play environments are central to enhancing and refining social and imaginative play.

Guided Participation

Guided participation in play refers to your role in guiding novice and expert players to participate in increasingly socially coordinated and sophisticated play activities. To concurrently mediate social exchanges and extend individual play themes, your job is to monitor individual and group behaviors, interpret social and symbolic play initiations, build on play initiations through modeling and coaching social interaction and play schemes, and ultimately transfer the onus of support to the expert players. While emphasis is placed on guiding children's participation in social play, one should not dismiss the importance of solitary play. As a natural extension of social play experiences, children often pursue solitary play activities as a way to practice, consolidate, and appropriate newly acquired skills. The methods used to achieve this system of support are described in more detail as monitoring play initiations, scaffolding interactions, social-communication guidance, and play guidance.

Monitoring Play Initiations.   Carefully monitoring initiations in play through ongoing observations is a pivotal feature of the integrated play model. Object-, self-, and other-directed play initiations, even when they take unusual form, reflect present and emerging proficiency in play. By determining each novice player's range of individual competence as supported by experts, we can begin to make decisions about how to mediate individual and collective play activities. Based on your ability to recognize, interpret, and respond to the play initiations of the novice players, you can match the amount and type of support to each child's zone of proximal development. According to Vygotsky (1978), the zone of proximal development refers to the distance between the child's developmental level as demonstrated in independent activity and potential developmental level as demonstrated under adult guidance and in collaboration with more capable peers. Monitoring initiations in play allows you to navigate the play experiences of each child playing beside and with other children. Play initiations become the point of departure for novices and experts to collaborate in mutually enjoyed activities.

Scaffolding Interactions.   Scaffolding, by definition, refers to the provision of adjustable and temporary support structures. Through scaffolding interactions in play groups, you adjust the amount of external support you provide in relation to the children's play needs. Initially, most children require a great deal of assistance while they acclimate to the experience of being in play groups. As the children grow increasingly comfortable and competent in their play, you gradually lessen this support and withdraw from the play group. Remaining readily available on the periphery of the group, you offer the children a "secure base" from which to explore and try out new activities. At the same time, you continue to monitor play initiations and provide assistance whenever necessary.

To illustrate how to scaffold interactions, we delineated three levels of support that may fluctuate at any given time in play groups. At times you may need to provide support at one of the three levels for an entire session. At other times you may need to vacillate among the three levels. Children in play groups with little prior experience may require a great deal of direction and support for extended periods. Children who are familiar with one another or simply demonstrate a natural proclivity to play together may need very little support. Still others may change from one moment to the next, requiring that you continually oscillate among the three levels of support illustrated in Table 8.2

Level 1 is Modeled and Directed Play. Your role at this level is similar to that of a director of a stage performance. To set the stage for play, you are in the play area actively interpreting play initiations, arranging play materials, assigning roles, and directing children to engage play partners and set up play events. While monitoring play initiations, you continually search for play themes that will allow every child—every novice and every expert—to have a satisfying role in the play experience. You may model various ways to invite and engage peers and to use props creatively in play. The table illustrates modeling and directing children to collaborate on an initiated play activity.

Level 2 is Verbal Guidance. At this level, you are on the periphery of the play area, verbally guiding the children to set the stage for directing their own play activities. By posing leading questions, commenting on activities, and offering suggestions, you can guide the children to negotiate and collaborate in play routines. Your questions, comments, and suggestions help to guide the children to recognize play initiations, select play

LEVEL 1: MODELED AND DIRECTED PLAY
Look, Sandy (expert player), Monica (novice player) is holding the doll's hair brush.
It looks as though Monica wants to play dolls!
Sandy, why don't you give Monica the doll?
Monica, let's show Sandy how we brush the doll's hair together.
Now you both can brush the doll's hair together, and I'll watch.
Look what we have here, beautiful clothes for the dolls!
Now you can dress the doll together.
Maybe you can dress these two dolls and take them shopping?

LEVEL 2: VERBAL GUIDANCE
Jerry (expert player), what do you think Eddy (novice player) wants to play?
What can you do to let Eddy know that you want to join him in playing cars?
Jerry, do you think Eddy understood your message that you want to play cars with him?
What else can you do to let Eddy know that you want to play with him?
Since you tried different ways to invite Eddy to join you and he didn't respond, why don't
you try playing beside each other for a while.
Is that okay with you, Eddy?
Now you guys are playing side by side with the cars, maybe you can build a roadway for the
cars to travel on together.
Eddy, you like to race cars on the roadway. Why don't you show Jerry how you build a road-
way?

LEVEL 3: NO SUPPORT

themes, organize and arrange play materials, and assign roles and partners.
By reframing the play events and giving subtle reminders, you enable the
children to learn to reflect on their own actions and experiences. Table 8.2
portrays the sort of verbal guidance you might provide to engage children
in mutually enjoyed play activity.

Level 3 is No Support. At this level, the children no longer require your
support as they independently mediate their own play activities. You withdraw yourself, remaining silently on the periphery of the group. A good
indication that adult guidance is no longer required is when all the children are so obviously absorbed in play that they appear almost oblivious to
your existence. You nevertheless stay within close range so that the children can check in with you when they need to.

Social-Communication Guidance.   Social-communication guidance is
another feature of guided participation. Focusing primarily on promoting
the social dimension of play, the strategies help the children establish a
mutual focus by recognizing and responding to initiations in play. By interpreting the subtle verbal and nonverbal cues of novice players as meaningful and purposeful acts, experts learn to nourish play interactions. By the
same token, interpreting by breaking down the complex social cues of

expert players allows novices to better understand and fully participate in the play context. Directed to both experts and novices alike, social-communication guidance strategies foster attempts to do the following:

1. INITIATE by enlisting a peer to play
2. PERSIST in initiating by enlisting a reluctant peer to play
3. RESPOND to cues or initiations of a peer
4. MAINTAIN or expand an interaction with a peer

To guide these social exchanges, present the children with simple logical sequences of nonverbal and verbal strategies. For purposes of integrated play groups, we designed posters and corresponding cue cards depicting picture-word combinations of what the children can do and say to elicit and sustain another child's attention in play. Table 8.3 illustrates.

Introduce these strategies when natural occasions arise in play groups. For instance, if you see a peer is calling the name of a novice player who has not yet learned how to respond, you can encourage the peer to stand close to the other child, say the child's name, touch the child's arm, and ask, "Do you want to play?" These types of cues are especially useful to start an interaction. Once the interaction is in progress, children may look to the cues as a way to fill in the blanks when they feel uncertain about what to say or do next. The intent is for children to incorporate these strategies naturally into their repertoire and no longer rely on your guidance or the presence of visual posters. Naturally, the strategies may need adaptation to accommodate different ages, developmental levels, modes of communication, and styles of learning. As with joint activity routines described in Chapter 7 and social stories described in Chapter 9 of this text, some children may find scripted sequences of play events frequently encountered in play groups helpful for organizing and regulating play activities.

Play Guidance.   A critical feature of the integrated play model is that children are *fully immersed* in the total group-play experience. Rather than presenting play as discrete subtasks, children engage in the whole play experience, even if active participation is minimal. Novices may partially participate in larger play themes organized by more experienced players. Play guidance offers a set of strategies to expand on each child's existing

▶**TABLE 8.3**

Examples of Social-Communicative Guidance

What to Do	What to Say
Look	Name [of playmate]
Stand close	Do you want to play?
Tap shoulder	What do you want to play?
Take hand	What are you doing?
Point	Can I play with you?
Give [toy]	Whose turn is it?
Take turns	Can I have a turn?

play repertoire while he or she is fully immersed in play. Play guidance involves fostering increasing participation in play activities that reflect emerging play skills. Children participate in activities and carry out tasks that they may not yet fully comprehend. For example, a child who has a particular inclination to manipulate objects through ritualistic banging may incorporate this into a larger play theme of constructing a building with blocks. With the assistance of more capable peers, the child may take the role of a construction worker and hammer the blocks with a play tool. By building on play initiations and encouraging participation in activities that are just slightly beyond the child's present abilities, you may help a novice begin to explore and diversify existing play routines. The following strategies can be adapted to any number of different play scenarios and events.

1. Orienting Strategies. Some children with autism have a difficult time tolerating close proximity to peers. As a first step in play groups, you might encourage a novice player to simply observe the other children in play while maintaining distance from them. You might suggest to the other children that they play with something of particular interest to the novice as a way to elicit the child's attention.

2. Mirroring Actions. Many children with autism are very responsive to the mirrored actions of their own behavior by others. This is a fun way for a peer to attract the attention of a child who is preoccupied in a repetitive activity. This type of mirror play often generates curiosity leading the child to purposefully alter a play routine.

3. Parallel Play. While some children enjoy watching and being close to other children, they may nevertheless resist direct contact. Encouraging children to play independently beside other children in a parallel fashion may serve as a temporary alternative. Parallel play fosters children's awareness of one another's activities as they play with similar materials in the same play space. During such occasions you may comment on the children's activities, suggesting they watch one another and show one another their materials.

4. Joint Focus. As children attend to different aspects of the same play activity and materials, they develop a common focus in play. When this occurs, you can encourage them to actively share materials and informally take turns in play. For instance, you can propose that children exchange doll clothes and accessories while they play with different baby dolls.

5. Joint Action. Once children establish a joint focus on the same play activity and materials, they often seek ways to coordinate their actions. To foster joint action schemes, you can guide the children to formally take turns while actively manipulating the same objects or participating in the same game. For example, you can naturally suggest that children take turns putting one building block on top of the other while constructing a tower.

6. Role Enactment. Role enactment involves portraying real life activities through conventional actions. Hammering a block tower, feeding a doll with a spoon, pushing a shopping cart, and stirring a pot on the stove are all role enactment in which children can take part. Children who have not yet reached the stage of advanced pretense can enact roles within the context of sophisticated play themes organized by more experienced peers.

7. Role-playing. Role-playing includes advanced forms of role enactment that extend beyond simple pretend acts. Children take on pretend roles and use objects in imaginary ways while enacting complex themes and scripts. A child who is pretending to feed the baby doll can take on the reciprocal roles of mother and baby. You can guide the child to talk to the baby as would a mother and to respond as a baby would by crying. This role play can be integrated into a larger theme of playing house.

Designing Supportive Play Environments

The social and physical ecology of play conditions can have a significant impact on the play development of children with autism. To bring about most competent forms of play, we must pay particular attention to designing play environments that foster both interactive and imaginative play

▶**TABLE 8.4**
Guided Participation in Integrated Play Groups

I. MONITORING PLAY INITIATIONS
  • Recognizing object-, self-, and other-directed play acts
  • Interpreting conventional and unconventional play acts as initiations
  • Responding to independent and supported play initiations

II. SCAFFOLDING INTERACTIONS (adjusted levels of adult support)
  • Level 1: Modeled and Directed Play
  • Level 2: Verbal Guidance
  • Level 3: No Support

III. SOCIAL COMMUNICATION GUIDANCE (verbal and nonverbal cues)
  • Initiate by enlisting a peer to play
  • Persist in initiating by enlisting a reluctant peer to play
  • Respond to cues or initiations of a peer
  • Maintain or expand an interaction with a peer

IV. PLAY GUIDANCE
  • Orienting strategies
  • Mirroring actions
  • Parallel play
  • Joint focus
  • Joint action
  • Role enactment
  • Role-playing

---

experiences. For purposes of integrated play groups, we developed some general guidelines for organizing play opportunities for children with autism and peers and/or siblings.

There are a variety of natural integrated settings suitable for setting up play groups. We define a natural setting as a location where, given the opportunity, children would naturally play. An integrated setting refers to a social setting characterized by children with diverse abilities, with a higher proportion of children who are socially competent to children who require extensive social support. Inclusive schools, integrated school sites, after-school programs, recreation centers, neighborhood settings, and home environments are all appropriate settings for play groups.

A balanced play group limits the number of familiar peers and/or siblings who meet on a regular and consistent basis over an extended period of time. Play groups usually include at least three and not more than five children. Play group members have diverse abilities, with a higher proportion of children who are socially competent to children who require a higher degree of social support. A typical play group might consist of two novices and three experts. Different configurations of group members in terms of age, developmental status, and gender may promote different types of beneficial play experiences. Attempts should be made to include children who complement one another in terms of interests, styles of interaction, and character.

Consistency and predictability are critical features of a supportive and nurturing environment. Our play groups generally meet regularly a minimum of two times a week for thirty minutes over the course of a year. Children who have a difficult time with change and transitions need to know well in advance when play groups are going to take place. Establishing a *consistent schedule and routine* will help children exert a sense of control over the environment as they anticipate future events. Visual schedules or calendars may be personalized for children. Opening and closing rituals such as brief plan and review periods, or a simple song at the start and finish of play sessions can be integrated into the routine.

To promote optimal opportunities for social participation in play, play spaces should be designed with consideration of spatial density and size, spatial arrangements, and organization of materials. Play spaces should be restricted in size while comfortably accommodating small groups of about three to five children. We suggest avoiding large open spaces because they tend to inhibit social interaction, and small overcrowded spaces because they often intensify interpersonal conflict. Play areas should be clearly defined by boundaries on at least three sides. A corner is a logical location because two walls can serve as boundaries. Tall shelves are practical partitions as they can be used to store play materials. Child-size kitchen sets made up of a play stove, refrigerator, and sink are also useful as dividers.

Arranging a play space so that materials are highly visible and easily accessible is also important to consider. Avoid overcrowding a play area with too many play materials and sets of toys that contain multiple little pieces. These tend to get thrown all over the play area, making accessibility almost impossible. You might want to store certain prized toys in a neutral place and make them available on request.

Arranging play materials in a highly organized fashion not only is helpful for children to organize their play, but also facilitates ease in cleaning up after play sessions. Every item should have a specified place. Shelves and containers should be labeled and easy for children to identify. Drawing outlines of containers on shelves and labeling items with picture-word combinations is especially useful.

Play materials and furniture should be arranged logically around specific play themes and activities. A housekeeping area might include a table and chair set. A grocery store might be placed next to housekeeping so that play food can be transferred easily between areas. A carpet might be placed near construction toys and vehicles. Play materials need not be confined to these particular areas.

Selected on the basis of their interactive potential, structure, and complexity, a wide range of constructive and sociodramatic play materials are made available in play groups. When selecting materials for a particular group of children, we also consider age-appropriateness. This refers to play materials that typical children of a particular age group might enjoy if the materials were made available, and does not refer to what is commercially sanctioned or traditionally available in school environments. Toys representing diversity in terms of gender roles, cultural values, and abilities are purposefully included, while toys that are overtly violent or discriminatory are excluded.

We tend to stress toys that can be used in both social and imaginative ways. While puzzles, board games, and computer or video games may be useful in other contexts, we do not recommend them as standard items in a play area. Most of the play materials we prefer tend to be very plain and simple such as European-style toys. These have the appearance of being handcrafted and are generally made of plain or painted wood and some durable plastics. We try to avoid toys made of cheap plastic, especially commercial toys that display TV or cartoon characters. Dress-up clothes are the one exception in terms of extravagance. One of my favorite play areas boasts a dress up corner filled with 1940s-vintage dresses, hats, high-heel shoes, purses, suits, and ties. Table 8.5 lists some suggested play materials for integrated play groups.

SUMMARY

Peer play experiences can be altogether perplexing for many children with autism. The highly social and symbolic nature of play makes it especially difficult for these children to comprehend. Since we understand play to be

▶ **TABLE 8.5**
Suggested Play
Materials for
Integrated Play
Groups

Child Sized	Miniatures
Baby dolls	Mini race cars
Baby-doll clothes and accessories	Mini garage
Baby bed	Ramps and tunnels
Baby carriage	
	Doll house
Stove	Doll furniture
Refrigerator	Multicultural/ethnic doll families
Sink	Dollhouse accessories (e.g., dishes, blankets,
Dishes, pots and pans, utensils	telephone)
Household accessories (e.g., play vacuum,	
toaster, telephones, camera)	Medium Sized
Occupational sets (e.g., tool set, doctor kit)	Barbie/Ken-size dolls
	Barbie/Ken-size clothes and accessories
Grocery store	Puppets
Shopping cart and baskets	Cars and trucks
Cash register	Ramps and tunnels
Play money	Road signs
Grocery items (cans and boxes, play foods,	Train and track
fruits, and vegetables)	Wooden building blocks
Dress-up clothes and accessories	Miscellaneous
Mirror	Play-Doh, cookie cutters, rolling pins
Makeup and hair brushes	Beanbags and baskets
	Large sheet (for hiding under or making
	a tent)
	Large boxes (for hiding and crawling in)

the very fabric of childhood culture, we must make play a priority in the lives of children who fail to play spontaneously. Peer play is an especially important vehicle for normalization. This chapter offers a number of methods to enhance play in children with autism. Many of the strategies derive from the integrated play groups model. Theories of play and development help to give us a perspective on the nature of the problem in autism. Over the course of childhood, typical children make sense of the world through shared experiences in play. Without these experiences, children with autism may not acquire the social knowledge necessary to pretend and coordinate play with peers. Thus a major goal of integrated play groups is to provide natural opportunities for children with autism to learn to play in the company of experienced players. A social support system for peer play is achieved through guiding participation within carefully designed play environments. As novices endeavor to join experts in play, we must pay particular attention to their subtle initiations. Acting as interpreters, we exploit the children's natural proclivities to explore and construct meaning in collective activity.

REFERENCES

American Psychiatric Association. (1987). *Diagnostic and Statistical Manual of Mental Disorders III Revised.* Washington DC: Author.

Baron-Cohen, S. (1987). Autism and symbolic play. *British Journal of Developmental Psychology, 5* (2), 139–148.

Baron-Cohen, S., Leslie, A. M., & Frith, U. (1985). Does the autistic child have a theory of mind? *Cognition, 21,* 37–46.

Bergen, D., & Oden, S. (1988). Designing play environments for elementary-age children. In D. Bergen (Ed.), *Play as a medium for learning and development.* Portsmouth, NH: Heinemann.

Boucher, J. (1977). Alternating and sequencing behaviour, and response to novelty in autistic children. *Journal of Child Psychology and Psychiatry, 18,* 67–72.

Bretherton, I. (Ed.). (1984). *Symbolic play: The development of social understanding.* Orlando, FL: Academic.

Bruner, J. S. (1986). *Actual minds, possible worlds.* Cambridge, MA: Harvard University Press.

Bruner, J. S., & Sherwood, V. (1976). Peek-a-boo and the learning of role structures. In J. S. Bruner, A. Jolley, & K. Sylva (Eds.), *Play: Its role in development and evolution.* New York: Penguin.

Cohen, D., & MacKeith, S.A. (1991) *The development of imagination: The private worlds of childhood.* London: Routledge.

Corsaro, W. A., & Schwarz, K. (1991). Peer play and socialization in two cultures. In B. Scales, M. Almy, A. Nicolopoulou, & S. Ervin-Tripp (Eds.), *Play and the social context of development in early care and education.* New York: Teachers College Press.

Dodge, K. A., Schlundt, D. C., Schocken, I., & Delugach, J. D. (1983). Social competence and children's sociometric status: The role of peer group entry strategies. *Merrill-Palmer Quarterly, 29,* 309–336.

Fenson, L., & Schell, R. E. (1986). The origins of exploratory play. In P.K. Smith (Ed.), *Children's play: Research developments and practical applications.* New York: Gordon & Breach Science.

Frith, U. (1989). *Autism: Explaining the enigma.* Oxford, England: Blackwell.

Gardner, H. (1989). *To open minds.* New York: Basic Books.

Garvey, C. (1977). *Play.* Cambridge, MA: Harvard University Press.

Glickman, C. D. (1984). Play in public school settings: A philosophical question. In T.D. Yawkey & A.D. Pellegrini (Eds.), *Child's play: developmental and applied.* London: Lawrence Erlbaum.

Harris, P. L. (1989). *Children and emotion: The development of psychological understanding.* Oxford, England: Blackwell .

Hartup, W. W. (1983). Peer relations. In M. Heatherington (Ed.), *Handbook of child psychology.* New York: Wiley.

Hartup, W.W., & Sancilio, M.F. (1986). Chidlren's friendships. In E. Schopler & G. B. Mesibov (Eds.) *Social behavior in autism.* New York: Plenum Press.

Hay, D. F. (1985). Learning to form relationships in infancy: Parallel attainments with parents and peers. *Developmental Review, 5,* 122–166.

Hobson, R. P. (1989). Beyond cognition: A theory of autism. In G. Dawson (Ed.), *Autism: New perspectives on diagnosis, nature and treatment.* New York: Guilford.

Leslie, A.M. (1987). Pretense and representation: The origins of theory of mind. *Psychological Review, 94,* 412–426.

Lever, J. (1976). Sex differences in the games children play. *Social Problems, 23,* 478–487.

Lewis, V., & Boucher, J. (1988). Spontaneous, instructed and elicited play in relatively able autistic children. *British Journal of Developmental Psychology, 6* (4), 325–339.

McCune-Nicholich, L. (1981). Toward symbolic functioning: Structure of early pretend games and potential parallels with language. *Child Development, 3,* 785–797.

Mundy, P., Sigman, M., Ungerer, J., & Sherman, T. (1987). Nonverbal communication and play correlates of language development in autistic children. *Journal of Child Psychology and Psychiatry, 27,* 657–669.

Nicholich, L. (1977). Beyond sensorimotor intelligence: Assessment of symbolic maturity through analysis of pretend play. *Merrill-Palmer Quarterly, 23* (2), 89–99.

Park, C.C. (1967) *The siege: The first eight years of an autistic child.* Boston, MA: Little, Brown.

Parker, J. G., & Gottman, J. M. (1989). Social and emotional development in a relational context: Friendship interaction from early childhood to dolescence. In T. J. Berndt & G. W. Ladd (Eds.), *Peer relationships in child development.* New York: Wiley.

Parten, M. (1932). Social play among preschool children. In R. E. H. &. B. Sutton-Smith (Eds.), *Child's play.* New York: Wiley.

Piaget, J. (1962). *Play, dreams, and imitation in childhood.* New York: Norton.

Putallaz, M. (1983). Predicting children's sociometric status from their behavior. *Child Development, 54,* 1417–1426.

Putallaz, M., & Gottman, J. M. (1981). An interactional model of children's entry into peer groups. *Child Development, 52,* 986–994.

Ricks, D. M., & Wing, L. (1975). Language, communication, and the use of symbols in normal and autistic children. *Journal of Autism and Childhood Schizophrenia, 5* (3), 191–221.

Ross, H. S., & Kay, D. A. (1980). The origins of social games. In K. H. Rubin (Ed.), *Children's play.* San Francisco: Jossey-Bass.

Rubin, K. H. (1980). Fantasy play: Its role in the development of social skills and social cognition. In K. H. Rubin (Ed.), *Children's play.* San Francisco: Jossey-Bass.

Rubin, K. H., Fein, G. G., & Vandenberg, B. (1983). Play. In E. M. Hetherington (Ed.), *Handbook of child psychology: Socialization, personality, and social development.* New York: Wiley.

Schuler, A.L, & Wolfberg, P.J. (1992). *Integrated play groups project final report* (Contract # HO86D90016). Washington DC: Department of Education, OSERS.

Sigman, M., & Mundy, P. (1987). Symbolic processes in young autistic children. In D. Ciccheti (Ed.), *New directions in child development: Symbolic development in atypical children.* San Francisco: Jossey-Bass

Sigman, M., & Ungerer, J. A. (1984). Cognitive and language skills in autistic, mentally retarded, and normal children. *Developmental Psychology, 20,* 293–302.

Singer, D. G., & Singer, J. L. (1990). *The house of make-believe.* Cambridge, MA: Harvard University Press.

Smilansky, S. (1968). *The effects of sociodramatic play on disadvantaged preschool children.* New York: Wiley.

Smith, P. K., & Vollstedt, R. (1985). On defining play: An empirical study of the relationship between play and various play criteria. *Child Development, 56,* 1042–1050.

Smith, P. K., Takhvar, M., Gore, N., & Vollstedt, R. (1986). Play in young children: Problems of definition, categorisation and measurement. In P. K. Smith (Ed.), *Children's play: Research developments and practical applications.* New York: Gordon & Breach Science.

Sorce, J. & Emde, R.N. (1981). Mother's presence is not enough: Effect of emotional availability on infant exploration. *Developmental Psychology, 17,* 737–745.

Stern, D. (1974). The goal and structure of mother-infant play. *Journal of the American Academy of Child Psychiatry, 13,* 402–421.

Tiegerman, E., & Primavera, L. (1981). Object manipulation: An interactional strategy with autistic children. *Journal of Autism and Developmental Disorders, 11* (4), 427–438.

Tilton, J. R., & Ottinger, D. R. (1964). Comparison of toy play behavior of autistic, retarded, and normal children. *Psychological Reports, 15,* 967–975.

Vandell, D. L., & Wilson, K. S. (1982). Social interaction in the first year: Infants' social skills with peers versus mother. In K. H. R. &. H. S. Ross (Eds.), *Peer relationships and social skills in childhood.* New York: Springer Verlag.

Vygotsky, L. S. (1978). *Mind in society: The development of higher psychological processes.* Cambridge, MA: Harvard University Press.

Watson, J. S. (1976). Smiling, cooing, and "the game." In J. S. Bruner, A. Jolley, & K. Sylva (Eds.), *Play: Its role in development and evolution.* New York: Basic Books

Westby, C. E. (1991). A scale for assessing children's pretend play. In C. Schaefer, K. Gitlin & A. Sandgrund (Eds.), *Play diagnosis and assessment.* New York: Wiley.

Williams, D. (1992). *Nobody nowhere: The extraordinary autobiography of an autistic.* New York: Times Books.

Wing, L., & Attwood, A. (1987). Syndromes of autism and atypical development. In D. Cohen &. A. Donnellan (Eds.), *Handbook of autism and pervasive developmental disorders.* New York: Wiley.

Wing, L., Gould, J., Yeates, S. R., & Brierly, L. M. (1977). Symbolic play in severely mentally retarded and autistic children. *Journal of Child Psychology and Psychiatry, 18,* 167–178.

Wolfberg, P.J. (1988). *Integrated play groups for children with autism and related special needs.* Unpublished masters thesis, San Francisco State University.

Wolfberg, P.J., & Schuler, A.L. (1993). Integrated Play Groups: A model for promoting the social and cognitive dimensions of play. *Journal of Autism and Developmental Disorders, 23* (3), 1–23.

APPENDIX 8.1   Play Preference InventoryY

RECORDER:

DATE(S) OF OBSERVATION:

	NOVICE PLAYER 1	NOVICE PLAYER 2	EXPERT PLAYER 1	EXPERT PLAYER 2	EXPERT PLAYER 3
Play Materials What toys or props does child most often use or prefer? Describe features if applicable. (E.g., prefers round objects that can be spun, toys that move, realistic toys.)					
Interactions with Play Materials How does child interact with toys? (E.g., prefers to spin objects, lines up toys, conventional use of realistic objects.)					
Play Activities What play activities does child prefer ? (E.g., rough-housing, quiet play, hide and seek, constructive play.)					
Play Themes What play themes does child prefer? (E.g., familiar routines as grocery store or house, invented stories, fantasy play.)					
Peer Play With whom does the child prefer to play? (May be no one or more than one person, and may depend on the type of activity.)					
Additional Observations					

© Intetrated Play Groups, 1992

APPENDIX 8.2   Profile of Individual Play Characteristics

NOVICE PLAYER'S NAME:
RECORDER:

OBSERVATION DATE:

OBSERVATION DATE:

CHARACTERISTICS	DESCRIPTIONS	CHARACTERISTICS	DESCRIPTIONS
SYMBOLIC DIMENSION No interaction Manipulation Functional Symbolic/pretend		SYMBOLIC DIMENSION No interaction Manipulation Functional Symbolic/pretend	
SOCIAL DIMENSION Isolate Orientation Parallel/proximity Common focus Common goal		SOCIAL DIMENSION Isolate Orientation Parallel/proximity Common focus Common goal	
COMMUNICATION Functions Means		COMMUNICATION Functions Means	
PLAY PREFERENCES Materials Activities Themes Peers		PLAY PREFERENCES Materials Activities Themes Peers	
ADDITIONAL REMARKS		ADDITIONAL REMARKS	

© Integrated Play Groups, 1992

CHAPTER 9

Teaching Children With Autism to "Read" Social Situations

Carol A. Gray

Children with autism have unique perceptions of people and events that result in behaviors their parents, teachers, and peers may find hard to understand. The children are impaired in their ability to understand and interpret social cues accurately (Wing, 1988). To children with autism, the gestures and expressions that are an integral part of human communication are confusing and hold little relevant meaning (Frith, 1989). In social situations, the children may falter at predicting what someone will do next. To keep things understandable, they invest energy and determination to ensure that routines and schedules are adhered to strictly. They have difficulty identifying what others think and feel (Dawson & Fernald, 1987). While a frustrated parent or professional concludes, "I just don't understand . . ." when describing the behavior of a child with autism, from the child's perspective his or her response makes perfect sense.

The challenge in teaching social skills to children with autism is that you and the child are working from two *equally valid but different perspectives*. Those working with children with autism need techniques that help them understand the child's perceptions of a given situation. At the same time, children need help in identifying what is important, and *why*. In addition, they need to learn social skills relevant to their own experiences, with information presented in a way they can most effectively understand. They need help "reading" social situations and determining what is expected of them. This chapter describes Social Reading, an approach to improving a child's understanding of social situations through visual instructional materials.

SOCIAL READING

Social Reading is a broad term given to instructional materials and techniques that use situations from a child's actual experience to visually present social information and teach social skills. Reading and written materials are often a major part of each activity, making an understanding of a child's ability to read, comprehend, and write central to the effectiveness of this approach. Basic reading and communication skills are helpful, though not required. If a child is unable to read, modifications of some activities can be made.

The Social Reading approach focuses on the skills a child needs in a variety of social contexts. To assist children in learning more effective skills in social situations, this approach first seeks to understand the child's perspective. Based on that understanding, and without discrediting the child's perceptions, accurate social information is presented to the child. In addition, social cues and expected skills are clearly identified, using individualized materials and instructional techniques a child can comprehend. The result is improved social skills through improved social understanding.

Steps of Social Reading

Social Reading is divided into three areas of instructional activities: Social Stories, Social Review, and Social Assistance Activities . These three areas are used individually and in combination to gain insight into a child's perceptions of a situation while introducing and supporting new social skills. *Social stories* are short stories written by parents or professionals to describe social situations and identify desired social skills (Gray & Garand, 1993). Social stories are applicable in a variety of settings and may be used to teach a variety of social skills. *Social review* is an instructional process that uses videotaped sequences to informally assess a child's perceptions of a social situation, presents accurate social information, and assists and supports a child in developing effective social skills. *Social assistance activities* are materials and activities that can be implemented for a child with autism in any classroom to provide support for new social skills a child is learning, skills often identified in social stories or through the social review process.

The three areas of Social Reading differ in their use of instructional materials and techniques. Still, they follow four basic steps: targeting a situation or social skill; gathering information; sharing observations; and supporting new social skills (Table 9.1.).

First, a target situation is identified that often results in negative or problem behaviors. A target situation may be one that continues to present difficulty for a child despite traditional interventions or environmental accommodations. Specific social skills may also be targeted for Social Reading interventions.

Next, information is gathered regarding the target situation. For Social Reading to be effective, detailed information is required. Before a Social Reading activity is initiated, the child is observed in the target situation and in other settings if possible. Additional information is gathered through discussions with the child, parents, school staff, peers, and/or other relevant individuals regarding the target situation.

Third, observations are shared with the child after all information is gathered. Social Reading provides an opportunity for a child to compare his or her understanding of a social situation with yours. Those perspectives, yours and the child's, are regarded as equally valid. Social Reading activities structure and simplify how social information is presented to a child. Information is shared through the use of visual materials. For example, when using social review, your perception of a situation is presented verbally and in writing immediately following the child's interpretation of the target situation. Social stories, on the other hand, use guidelines developed for writing for children with autism to share accurate social information. Social assistance activities use written cues to share social information with the child.

▶**TABLE 9.1**
Basic Steps of
Social Reading

I. TARGET A SOCIAL SITUATION
- Look for situations that often result in negative or problem behavior.
- Look for situations that continue to present difficulty after implementation of social skills curriculum and other positive interventions.
- Anticipate situations that are new for a child or contain changes in routine.

II. GATHER INFORMATION
- Gather information regarding a child's interests, abilities, impairments, and factors that may be motivating current responses.
- Observe the targeted situation for factors you can and cannot see.
- Use information to try to assume child's perspective.
- Use information to determine the focus of shared information (social stories).
- Through review of selected videotape sequences, the child identifies and writes lists of objects, people, and conversations in targeted situation (social review).

III. SHARE OBSERVATIONS
- Consider the child's perspective while identifying relevant cues and presenting your perspective.
- Use descriptive and perspective statements and consider characteristics of autism (social stories).
- Review the child's observations and "read" the situation back to the child using the child's observations as a guide (social review).

IV. IDENTIFY AND SUPPORT NEW SOCIAL SKILLS
- Child identifies new responses and social skills on his own.
- New social skills are identified for the child .
- Support for new social skills are provided using individualized visual materials.

Finally, new skills are identified and supported. Support for a child practicing a new social skill is based on individualized visual materials and instructional techniques. For example, new skills identified through social review may be supported with a social story, or information presented to a child for the first time in a social story may be reinforced with social assistance activities. The identification and continued support of newly acquired social skills is a critical component of all three areas of Social Reading.

Each area of Social Reading follows the four basic steps just described. The steps formally structure social review and social stories activities. Social assistance activities informally follow these steps. We turn now to a detailed description of how the basic steps of Social Reading translate into materials and instructional techniques within each area.

SOCIAL STORIES

Social stories are written by parents or professionals to describe social situations that are difficult and/or confusing for children with autism. Each story identifies and describes relevant social cues and desired responses to a target situation and is written with consideration of a child's abilities and learning style. A social story is not limited to words on paper; a variety of materials and instructional methods can be used to make it understandable. In this section, guidelines for writing and implementing social stories are presented to enable you to develop an effective story based on your understanding of an individual child.

Social stories are applicable to school, home, and community settings—any situation that may occur in these environments is a potential social story topic (Gray et al., 1993). Social stories are useful for identifying relevant social cues, introducing new routines and rules, and/or positively defining desired social skills. In addition, social stories in the school setting can prepare a child for unexpected situations such as substitute teachers, fire drills, or school closings. At home, parents may decide to write a social story to prepare their child for an upcoming event, such as a visit to a relative or a family vacation, or to introduce a new daily routine. In a community setting, social stories identify naturally occurring cues and events to provide structure to a situation that is otherwise overwhelming to a child. In any setting, social stories introduce the possibility of unexpected occurrences in such a way that variation is a part of any routine or situation. Whatever the situation they describe or the social skills they address, social stories are written to assist a child in more accurately understanding and responding to a target social situation.

Writing effective social stories is a structured art and should be done according to the following guidelines.

Target a Social Skill

Determine the topic of the story. Usually it will be a social situation resulting in problem behavior that continues to present difficulty after social skill curricula and other positive interventions have been implemented. Other topics will be social situations that are new for a child or contain changes in the routine.

Gather Information

A critical factor in writing an effective social story is your ability to describe a situation in writing objectively and realistically. This will require at least one careful observation of the target situation. The assessment should include two components: what you see, which will result in the objective information you need, and what you don't see, which will provide the realistic information for the story.

The first step is to record objectively what you actually observe. You are looking for as many details as possible. Identify when and where a situation occurs, who is involved, routines and rules, social cues, signals for the start and finish of an activity, and other observable information. Look for related and extraneous activities that are a part of the target situation. For example, if you are writing a story to assist a child with successfully standing in lines and walking in lines throughout school, observe the class for information needed to write the story. Look for posted schedules or rules that apply to the target situation. When the children are asked to form a line, do they put their work away as part of the routine? Do all the children follow the routine independently, or do some children continue to work on an assignment? Observe for details, recording the situation and the variety of activities that surround it.

The second step is to consider and record those aspects of a situation that you do *not* observe. Look for aspects of a situation that may change the situation or alter the basic routine. Since you will not be able to observe the situation every time it occurs, you will need to ask a lot of questions as part of your observation. Chances are the children are asked to stand in lines several times each day—to go to lunch, recess, and the bus; occasionally each week—to go to gym, art, the library, and music; and at other times on an irregular basis—for assemblies, rehearsals, and special occasions. Ask about changes in expectations: Is there a difference between how the children prepare to line up for gym and how they line up for lunch or to go home? What if there is a substitute teacher? Is gym *always* on Tuesday at 9:30, or do teachers sometimes switch time slots or cancel gym altogether? Is there a bell that rings to signal recess? If so, what does it sound like? How is it decided which child is first in line? You will use this information to identify and describe the target situation thoroughly.

The third step is to assume the child's perspective. The most critical factor in writing an effective social story is your ability to consider and incorporate the perspective of the child with autism with regard to the target situation or skill. You will learn quickly that there are many different ways to describe a given situation. Knowing where to start and exactly what to write may be difficult. That's where the perspective of the child becomes important. The more accurate your understanding of a child's perceptions, feelings, and behavior, the better able you will be to provide accurate information that is useful to that child. The perspective of the child determines the focus of a social story, helping you decide which aspects of a situation take priority as you begin to write.

Information to improve your understanding of the child's perspective may be gathered from a number of sources in addition to your observation. If a child is able to communicate, discussing the situation with the child is a good first step. Center questions around relevant cues ("What does your teacher say when it is time for recess?") and responses to those cues ("What do the children do when the teacher says, 'Line up'?"). Ask also about what happens in the situation ("What happens when the children stand in line?"). Often a child with autism will be unable to communicate with you effectively about the target situation. In this case, talk to the child's parents, school staff members, and possibly peers. Ask them about how the child responds to the target situation, and get their opinion as to what motivates his or her current response. As you observe the child in the target situation, begin to incorporate all the information you have gathered about the child.

Target Situations

Chad is a first-grader who seems frightened to stand in line, but you notice he's okay when walking in a line. His parents and teachers report that Chad is very sensitive to touch and that he often complains that people are always hitting him in line, though this has not been observed by staff or students. Close observation of the classroom situation reveals that the children do touch one another in line, sometimes to get the one another attention, but more often unintentionally as they stand close together. Currently, the solution is for the teacher to allow Chad to be first in line, which is creating jealousy among his classmates. His parents note that Chad has difficultly standing in line in other settings, and this is limiting their tolerance for family outings. Others will have different theories to explain Chad's responses. His teacher believes that standing in line is so uncomfortable for Chad it is physically unreasonable to ask him to do it without accommodations. His parents recognize that Chad is very sensitive to touch, but feel he lacks an understanding of why lines are necessary and why other people touch him in that situation. Keep their theories in mind and begin to determine the focus of Chad's social story.

As you observe, imagine you are Chad standing in a line of impatient young children who touch you without warning as they wiggle and squirm while involved in interactions you don't fully understand. In writing your story for Chad, you will need to explain why children often touch one another when standing in line, as well as let Chad know the situation lasts only a short time. You will use the information you have gathered to describe the procedure for standing in line, focusing on how it feels to stand in line, and why (see sample social story in Appendix 9.1).

Another child with autism, Jessica, does not seem afraid of lines but often looks confused and has difficulty following directions that are given to the class. When the teacher announces, "Time to line up!", the teacher must walk Jessica through the process, or ask a classmate to assist her ("Rick, please get Jessica . . ."). Despite their assistance and support, Jessica is learning little about how to follow directions in class, or how to get in a line independently.

Though Chad and Jessica both have difficulty with lines in school, their social stories will have a different focus. Jessica's story will focus on following directions in class and the steps involved in standing and walking in lines at school. Chad's story based on the same situation will describe how it feels to stand in a line, with assurances the situation, though uncomfortable, does not last forever. In this way, the perspective of the child with autism provides direction for developing a social story.

Share Observations

Children with autism need assistance to understand social situations, the perspectives of others, and how they should respond. For this reason, social stories are comprised of three basic types of sentences: descriptive, directive, and perspective. An awareness of each type of sentence and the purpose it serves in a social story will provide you with the tools you'll need to develop a story that directly addresses the goal you have in mind for a child.

Descriptive sentences explain what occurs and why; they paint the backdrop of the social story. Descriptive sentences point out the relevant features of a situation, rendering unmentioned factors irrelevant. The most common mistake in writing social stories is using too few descriptive sentences. Descriptive sentences indicate how well you have visualized the situation and the factors that will be most relevant to the child with autism. Descriptive sentences are often used to begin a social story, stating basic information about a situation: "My name is Chad. I go to Lincoln

▶**TABLE 9.2**
Basic Types of Sentences in Social Stories

I. Descriptive sentences
- explain what occurs and why, "painting the backdrop" of a story
- point out the relevant features of a situation
- often are used to begin social stories

II. Directive sentences
- individualized statements of desired responses
- often begin with "I will . . ." or "I can . . ."

III. Perspective sentences
- describe the reactions of others in the target situation

Elementary School. I am in the second grade. There are 24 children in my class. My teacher is Mrs. Johnson. Sometimes Mrs. Johnson takes the children to other parts of the building. We walk in a line."

Directive sentences are individualized statements of desired responses or social skills. They often follow descriptive sentences, telling a child what is expected as a response to a given cue or situation. Directive sentences often begin with "I can . . ." or "I will . . .". For example, following the descriptive sentence "We walk in a line," may be a directive sentence or two: "I will walk in the line. I can follow the person in front of me."

Perspective sentences describe the reactions of other people in a target social situation. They may relay the feelings of others depicted in a social story: "Mrs. Johnson is proud when the children walk quietly." They may also describe the motivation for a response: "The children should walk quietly so they don't disturb people in other classrooms." Perspective statements should be honest, avoiding overgeneralization of a typical response: "Some children have fun in gym class," not "All the children love to go to gym."

The relationship between the three types of sentences in a story will partially determine the influence of the story on the child. If most of the sentences in a story are descriptive and perspective sentences, with few directive sentences, there is greater opportunity for a child to determine his or her own new responses to a situation. For some children, though, a highly descriptive story will be confusing, leaving them unsure of how to respond or what is expected in a given situation. Directive sentences provide structure for children who need stories that clearly define expected behaviors. You may wish to begin by initially writing a story comprised mostly of descriptive and perspective statements, adding directive statements as needed.

Children with autism need assistance in recognizing and interpreting social cues. For this reason, social stories explain "why" people do what they do. An accurate description carefully attends to the social insights and information we easily and readily assume, assumptions that are at the core of the social impairment in autism. For example, if you are writing a story about standing in line for Chad, assume that he may not know why he is often touched by other children. Explain the behavior of other children. You may indicate that children may need to fix their shirts, or scratch their heads, or move around in anticipation of the line starting to walk down the hall. In addition, explain why certain rules and routines are necessary: "Walking in a line is a safe way to move 24 children from one part of a building to another. That way, other people can walk in the hall, too." Define when a situation begins and ends by citing visual cues if possible.

Children with autism need assistance adjusting to changes and may rely on rigid interpretations of sequences and events. Continually write flexibility into the events in a story, mentioning the possible variations that may occur in the target situation. In this way, you are establishing the unexpected as simply part of the routine. For example, "When I stand in line I can see the person in front of me. It might be Mrs. Johnson, Peter, Gretchen, or someone else." While you cannot write about *all* possible variations, address those you have determined may be most relevant to the child.

Children with autism give literal and often rigid interpretations to language. As you write, use terms like *usually* or *sometimes* instead of *always*. *"We may"* is more accurate than *"we will."* Functionally define terms that are ambiguous. For example, if writing about "taking turns," describe what that means in the target situation, "We take turns being first in line. When I am 'Student of the Day,' I am first in line. Other children are first in line when they are 'Student of the Day.' I can look at the chalkboard to read who is 'Student of the Day.' We take turns." Use statements that are accurate regardless of their interpretation. Instead of "I will not move when standing in line," use the more realistic and positive "I will wait quietly in line." Read the finished social story over to check for literal meanings.

The children may give literal interpretations to illustrations or may become distracted by irrelevant features of an illustration. If an illustration of a child raising his hand in class depicts a child seated in the second row and wearing a blue shirt, a child with autism may give a literal interpretation to the illustration, believing he should request assistance only when he wears a blue shirt and is seated in the second row. Or a child may become

▶**TABLE 9.3**
Considerations
When Writing
Social Stories

I. *Children with autism have highly individual abilities and impairments.*
  • Consider attention span, abilities, interests, and learning style.
  • Use vocabulary and print size consistent with reading level .

II. *Children with autism have difficulty interpreting social cues.*
  • Explain people's motives and actions.
  • Include detailed social information.

III. *Children with autism need assistance to adjust to changes.*
  • Write flexibility into a story.
  • Mention variations and changes in routine.

IV. *Children with autism give literal interpretations to vocabulary and events.*
  • Use terms like *usually* or *sometimes* instead of *always*.
  • Closely define a phrase such as *usually once a week*.

V. *Children with autism have difficulty asking "wh" questions.*
  • Use questions as titles or subtitles.
  • Answer "wh" questions in the body of the story.

---

fascinated by an irrelevant detail in the illustration: for example, the shoes children are wearing. For these reasons, illustrations and/or photographs are not necessary in most social stories.

Photographs are effective in some stories, particularly those where the overall situation is overwhelming. A story about recess or describing "learning center time" in a classroom might include photographs of the different activities that occur simultaneously. The photographs "take apart" the target situation, making the overall situation less threatening and easier to understand.

Often, children with autism have difficulty asking and answering "wh" questions. To assist them in understanding the relationship between questions and answers, titles to some social stories may be stated as questions ("Can You Tell Me About Lines?") with subtitles ("Why Do Children Walk in Lines at School? "Why Do Children Always Touch Me in Line?" "What Are the Rules for Lines at School?").

Finally, because children with autism are highly individual, consider these characteristics of autism as well as a child's attention span, ability, interest, and learning style when writing a social story (see Table 9.3).

The materials and methods used to present a social story to a child are as individualized as the story. As with writing and development, the materials and instruction should be appropriate for the child's abilities, challenges, learning style, and interests. In addition, consideration should be given to the setting in which the social story will be used and others who may be affected by its implementation. These factors collectively impact on how a story is presented to a child. There are three basic methods for presenting social stories: as basic printed stories, as stories with accompanying audiocassettes, and on videotape.

For children who possess independent reading and comprehension skills, presenting a printed social story may be all that is required. A variation of a printed story may be used for a child fascinated with computers, in this case reading the social story on the computer screen with the option of printing it out. When introducing a story to a child, sit at the child's side with the child holding the story and turning the pages. Read the story with the child a few times to ensure comprehension before decreasing adult involvement.

For children who are unable to read independently or who enjoy audio tapes, a printed social story with an accompanying audiocassette may be effective. A story with audio may also be helpful for children who need modifications to attach meaning to verbal requests or information, tying information to written words which are easier for the child to understand. Record the story onto an accompanying audiocassette, using a bell to signal when to turn the pages. This is similar to the format used with many commercially available children's stories. Sound effects or the voices of individuals familiar to the child can be incorporated as part of a social story with an audiocassette; however, keep the story simple and easy to understand.

Another approach combines some of the components of social review with social stories and may be useful for children who are unable to read, or who enjoy videotapes and television. Read the social story aloud onto videotape, filming one page at a time. Videotaped sequences of the target situation may be edited into a story as realistic, moving "illustrations" of the written material. If a child requires assistance with reading, videotaped stories are presented with the volume *on*; a child who reads independently may watch a story with the volume *off*.

Support New Social Skills

Reading a social story may be listed as a "first step" of a positive behavioral plan or intervention, followed by a sequence of additional steps to assist the child in learning a new social skill. Develop a consistent review schedule for a story, one that ensures it is read frequently enough to provide review without needless repetition. Use the Social Story Implementation Plan form in Appendix 9.2 to ensure that everyone understands how the social story will be presented and incorporated as part of the child's educational program.

Share the story with relevant people to increase the awareness and involvement of others. These are people depicted in the story or affected by the child's success. If possible, maximize the child's involvement in sharing the story. The child can carry the story, approach others with it, and hear them read it aloud. In this way, the child learns each person has the same information, and others become aware of their role and the roles of others in a child's ultimate success at learning a new social skill.

As the story is implemented, people will play an important role in helping the child practice a new social skill. They may "cue" the story, making a reference to the story in general ("Remember the story . . .") or reciting a key phrase from the story at the appropriate time. A child may be provided with "story notes" in the target situation, a 3" X 5" card with a list of critical phrases from the story. Stories may also be read with a child immediately following the target situation, encouraging a child to compare his or her perceptions and responses to those in the story.

Once a social story is part of an instructional strategy, it is important to closely monitor the child's response. A child's response to a social story is often immediate, with improvement apparent within a few days. Other stories will result in a more gradual improvement of a child's behavior. Observations of the child in the target situation may provide clues as to how a story should be revised to be more effective. For example, one child with autism had difficulty following the morning routine of putting his things away and taking his seat in the classroom. A social story was immediately effective, except each day he would take his seat with his hat still on, requiring a verbal reminder to place it with his other things. This was confusing to the staff, as they were sure the hat was mentioned in the story along with the rest of the routine. Checking the story, however, it was discovered the hat had never been mentioned. A quick rewrite of the story, including a step to put the hat away, resulted in immediate success the following day. While the need to revise a story is not always this obvious, careful observation and monitoring of the impact of each story is critical to its effectiveness.

Once a child is demonstrating a new social skill, it is time to gradually fade use of the social story by rewriting, revising the review schedule, and/or decreasing verbal cues to the story. To fade by rewriting the story, gradually decrease the number of directive sentences, leaving the descriptive and perspective statements. Rewriting may also be used to expand the impact of a story while fading, encouraging a child to generalize newly learned skills to other environments. To do this, write stories describing other situations in which the new skill or behavior is applicable, including directive sentences in the new stories while decreasing them in the original. To fade by revising the review schedule, increase the amount of time between the child's reading of the story and the target situation's occurrence each day. If the child continues to maintain the new skill or behavior, gradually decrease use of the story. To decrease verbal cues to a story, share the child's progress with others who are also a part of the target situation. Encourage them to wait for longer periods of time before cuing the story.

Whether a story is faded from use entirely is an individual decision. Stories may be kept accessible to the child in an individual social story notebook. In this way, a child may review a story at any time. Individual social story books provide social support for children with autism by their very presence and are a personalized encyclopedia of social situations (and accomplishments) that provide a quick and easy reference and review.

Social Story Variations

Several techniques may be used to further tailor a social story to an individual child and situation. In addition to providing a child with accurate social information, a story may be written to reinforce and rehearse targeted social and academic skills.

Fill-in-the-blank stories are used to describe a situation to a group of children, while addressing the specific social skills each child is learning. To do this, write a story for the given situation, using descriptive and perspective statements. Describe the cues or events that are relevant to all the children in the group. For example: "We will have an assembly at 1:00. An assembly means all the children in the school will be in the gymnasium. Our class will sit together. A person will play the violin for all the children at the same time. He will play the violin for me and everyone else. He will want each child to listen to him play the violin. Most of the children will listen to the violin." Follow the description of the situation with an open-ended sentence completed with a priority social skill for each child: "I will _____ when I am at the assembly," or "Here is a list of things I should do at the assembly." These stories can be read aloud and discussed as a group, with the individualized section of the story reviewed with each child just prior to the target event.

Checklist stories teach new routines. To write a checklist story, write one step of the routine at the bottom of each page, using only one side of each paper. The last page is a checklist listing the steps of the routine. The child completes this checklist after reading the story. The child may use the checklist as a guide to completing the routine in the target situation. Once he or she is performing the routine independently, the child may complete the checklist when the entire routine is completed. Forgetting a step of a routine may be difficult for a child with autism. Checklist stories can be used to teach a child to ask for help in response to a missed step. The adult removes one or two pages of the story. Completing the checklist at the end of the story, the child is helped to identify the forgotten step(s) of the routine and encouraged to ask for help in returning the missing pages or steps. The child uses the story to rehearse an effective response to a missed step (asking for help) in a setting removed from the confusion of the target situation.

Curriculum stories teach social skills while demonstrating the functional application of academic skills a child is learning. Beginning with a target situation from the child's own experience as a backdrop, selected academic skills are incorporated into the story. To build curriculum into a social story, begin with a story written one step or concept to a page. A story describing recess, for example, uses photographs to illustrate the variety of activities. "These boys are playing on the jungle gym. They like to climb on the bars." Pages drawing a child's attention to related academic skills are inserted into the story. "Count the boys on the previous page. There are _____ boys on the jungle gym." Or "I can write the word *boys* here: _____." Considering social stories are often read by a child several times, changing curriculum insert pages keep the story interesting while reviewing the targeted social situation.

Judgment stories provide a child with functional and/or visual cues to make a needed judgment effectively. To write this type of story, describe abstract terms with several functional definitions. For example, "I will keep my volume low when I sing in the school choir. I will sing so I can hear the person singing next to me. I will watch Mr. Geiger's hands. If he moves his hands down, I will sing more quietly." Repeat the functional definitions a few times in the story, for example: "We will sing 'Silent Night.' I will keep my volume low. I will sing so I can hear the person singing next to me." To generalize and reinforce the functional definition of volume in the story, repeat references to visual and functional cues after indicating each song title the choir will sing. Judgment stories provide functional and visual definitions for abstract terms, repeating those definitions as they apply to several variables .

Skill stories may describe a target social skill instead of a social situation, generalizing the skill to other environments. Begin these stories with an accurate and detailed description of the desired social skill, and the reason(s) why the skill is important. In the same story, or through a series of related stories, describe the social skill as it applies to a variety of settings.

Fear-reducing stories, written in response to a child's fears, are highly descriptive. To write this type of story, use careful observation and discussions with others to identify possible causes (factors) for the child's current response. Using these as a guide, describe each factor in the story. For example, if a mechanical item is suspected to be the cause of the child's fear, briefly describe how it works and why people use it. Approach each factor by first describing it, then describing others' typical reactions or responses to it. If possible, identify visual cues that indicate how long the situation will last and when it will be over.

Stories written in response to a child's fears should be written with extreme care. These stories should not contain sentences that discredit the child's perception(s). Avoid statements like "There is no reason to be afraid of . . . , and use few, if any, directive sentences such as those beginning with "I can . . ." or "I will. . . ." The child's perceptions are accurate from the child's perspective, and you want simply to and provide another accurate point of view. Keep in mind there is a reason, or perhaps several reasons, for a child's fearful responses; and while the child knows those reasons, you are only guessing what they may be. Overall, social stories with carefully selected aspects of a situation and/or responses of others, described through an accepting, unassuming, and accurate perspective have the best chance of effectively addressing fear in a child with autism.

SOCIAL REVIEW

Social review is an instructional process that informally assesses a child's understanding and perceptions of a social situation, presents more accurate information, and assists and supports a child in learning effective social skills. Here, the basic steps of Social Reading provide a structured format for recording and sharing a child's perceptions of a given situation with your own. Together, you will take turns "reading" and recording your observations of a videotape of the target situation, finally sharing your observations and identifying new responses. Once familiar with using social review, you will find it a flexible activity that can be modified to address a child's specific abilities and various kinds of target situations. (Table 9.1).

Social review is most applicable to higher-functioning upper-elementary-grade children with autism. Minimally, a participating child will need the ability to communicate either verbally or with other communication systems, the ability to understand and respond to basic questions regarding what he or she sees and hears, and, if possible, basic reading and writing skills. This activity is paced in accordance with a child's attention span.

You will "read aloud" an observed situation simply and objectively, much as a radio announcer reports the action on a baseball diamond or football field (minus the interpretation or references to pregame interviews and insights, of course). Initially this process may feel a little awkward, so experience in "reading" social situations is recommended prior to using social review with a child with autism. To gain this experience, watch a videotaped television show or newscast with the volume turned off, and report the activities of people and observed events using simple sequential statements. Practice pausing between statements, stopping the videotape if needed. Avoid the inclination to report how you believe people feel unless stated as observed behavior ("The woman is smiling. She looks happy.").

Social review is completed in a setting removed from the target situation. You will need a short one- to three-minute videotaped segment that represents the target situation, a video player and monitor, and writing materials (a large display tablet is ideal). Set the tape to run a few moments before the most critical segment of the target situation appears. This will allow you and the child time to become acquainted with each step of the process before responding to the target situation. You and the child will be working together, requiring a small room with a relaxed atmosphere.

Target a Situation

Like the development of a social story, the social review process begins with the identification of a target situation that is difficult or confusing for a child. Let's imagine you are working with Bennett, a sixth grader who has difficulty remembering to raise his hand and wait his turn in class. He continually interrupts lessons, speaking right out despite repeated reminders to "not interrupt." Bennett's parents report he often interrupts conversations at home. Bennett can read at approximately a fifth-grade level, and comprehends what he reads at a third-grade level. You have observed the situation first hand and have prepared a representative two-minute segment of videotape of Bennett in the target situation for social review. In this videotape Bennett is participating with his classmates in a math lesson on fractions. While his classmates are excitedly raising their hands to answer Mrs. Clark's questions, Bennett is calling the answers out of turn. His responses are immediate. A frustrated classmate turns to Bennett and says, "Aw, c'mon Bennett! Give us a chance . . . ."

Gather Information

An important step in social review is gathering information. The goal is to learn as much about the child's perceptions and interpretations of the situation as possible. Be cautious of the tendency to direct a child's attention to relevant events or prematurely provide the child with more accurate information. Follow the child's lead while structuring the direction of the activity. You will be asking the child to identify the setting, objects, people, events, gestures, and conversations he or she sees and hears on the videotape. Provide structure for the child to respond without providing answers or solutions.

During this step, pause the videotape several times to allow the child time to respond. Wait about a minute for the child to answer your questions or to comment, which may feel slightly longer than seems reasonable. Considering the communication impairment associated with autism, the child may need additional time to listen, observe, and respond to a given situation. Someone does not always have to be talking; silence is a valuable educational tool. Begin by sharing the purpose of the activity and briefly describing step by step what you and the child will be doing together. Identify if there will be a break and when the activity will be completed: "Bennett, we are going to be watching a video of Mrs. Clark's class. We're going to watch this video together and talk about what we see. We'll write down what we see on this tablet. We will take a break at recess, and we will be finished before the lunch bell rings."

Next, identify the setting and situation depicted in the videotape. With the volume *on*, watch the target situation. Briefly identify the setting and/or the situation, recording it as a title on the display tablet. If a child is able and willing to write, have him record the information. If not, have the child dictate his responses. You may play the tape and ask, "Where is this?" with Bennett responding, "My class," or "That's Bennett in Mrs. Clark's class."

Review the videotape with the volume *off* several times, each time directing the child to observe a different aspect of the situation. Begin by asking Bennett to list all the objects he sees in the classroom. Remind him to write down only those things he can see. Help Bennett stay focused on the relevant items.

View the videotape again, this time directing Bennett to list the people in the room. List them on the left-hand side of the paper—by proper name, if possible, or by their role or relationship to the child. Ask what key people are doing, and write the activities opposite their names on the list. Play the tape again, asking if anyone's movement or facial expression suggests that he or she is telling the others something. Record these observations opposite the names of people on the list.

In our example, suppose Bennett identifies Mrs. Clark and himself in the room and writes, "talking to Bennett" opposite Mrs. Clark's name. When asked if anyone else is in the room, Bennett shakes his head "no." When asked a second time if others are present, Bennett repeats that "Mrs. Clark and Bennett" are the only people in the room. When asked what he is doing, Bennett replies, "Talking to Mrs. Clark." Bennett adds that Mrs. Clark is "smiling and moving her hands."

Now, review the videotape with the volume *on* to bring the child's attention to what people are saying. As in all the steps involved in gathering information, try not to give the child cues or direct attention to important communication. Quickly list a few words opposite the names of the people on the list, or list names and conversation in sequential order separately.

**Share
Observations**

Review the child's observations and share your perspective of the target situation. In your review, first focus your attention on the child's list of observations. Do not disagree with the child's description of the situation or indicate the child has made a mistake. You might begin with "Let's see what you wrote about . . .," proceeding with a brief review of key points.

Next, "read" the situation to the child to share your perspective of the situation. Put into practice the skills you rehearsed earlier when "reading aloud" newscasts and television shows. With the child's written observations posted close by, record your observations on a new sheet of paper. Follow the same sequence of reporting as the child: identify the setting, objects, key people, gestures, and conversations. Focus first on areas where your observations are in agreement with the child's. For example, "Bennett, I see the chairs, desks, and pencils, too. I see you and Mrs. Clark. You are both talking about fractions."

Continue your review by focusing last on those areas where your perceptions or interpretations of the situation are different. For example, consider Bennett's observations as you begin to formulate your comments. Since he did not list classmates in the room as part of his observation, Bennett may not recognize their social significance. Bennett may not realize Mrs. Clark is talking to everyone in the class simultaneously, or that other children are competing for Mrs. Clark's attention. Therefore the concept of "interrupting" or the teacher's past requests for Bennett to raise his hand to speak may hold little meaning or seem unnecessary to him. To present your observations that are different from Bennett's, focus on visual cues, "I see Brenda, Angie, Juan, and Matthew, too." Involve Bennett in confirming anything you visually observe that is relevant to your perspective. "Do you see them, Bennett?" Still writing as you talk, describe what the other children are doing, and check for confirmation from Bennett, "I see the children raising their hands. The children are doing what?" Last, explain the motivations of the other children through visual cues, "I think they are raising their hands because Mrs. Clark is talking to them about fractions, too. They want to be called on to answer her questions. I think that is why they are saying, 'Mrs. Clark!' and 'I know!' when they raise their hands."

**Support New
Social Skills**

You and the child will be identifying more effective responses to a situation based on the information gathered in the previous steps. Support for these new skills will be provided through a variety of visual activities, many which can be implemented on a continuing basis in the following weeks. The identification of new responses and related social skills will depend on the child and situation. A child may identify a new response on his own. For example, on hearing your perspective of the situation, Bennett might conclude, "I can raise my hand, too, before I answer." More often, the child will need assistance to identify the new response. If this is the case, you have a variety of options. If you feel the child is close to independently identifying a new response to the situation, have him or her read your

observations back to you, as you did when you reviewed the child's observations. Or you can repeat the activity at another time using the same
videotape or a new videotape of a similar situation. Some children will
need you to identify the response. If this is the case, emphasize why it is
the response of choice. For example, "Bennett, Mrs. Clark needs to give
everyone a turn to answer. You can help by raising your hand. We'd like
you to try that." Involve Bennett as quickly as possible. "Show me how you
can raise your hand."

After the identification of a new social skill, help the child understand
the details of its application. Keep in mind that beginning to use a new
social skill is like buying a new car: the child needs to know how to use it,
as well as its advantages and disadvantages. Honestly sell the response.
Describe the steps involved. Bring attention to what the child may have
overlooked. In Bennett's case, imagine him raising his hand in class for the
first time. What should he realistically expect? On a new sheet of paper
titled "Hand Raising," involve Bennett as you write the steps and implications of hand raising in Mrs. Clark's class and in other classes such as art
and music. List details Bennett may not be aware of: "Wait for the teacher
to call your name." "She may not say your name every time." "If she
doesn't say your name, you can try again." "Teachers know it is their job to
give everyone a chance to answer." "There may be whole days when you
are not asked to answer a question, and that's okay." Indicate positive outcomes, listing how Mrs. Clark will feel about Bennett raising his hand.
If the child is on a positive behavior-modification program, list rewards
that apply.

Support for new social skills begins with the child sharing the result of
social review with relevant individuals. If possible, the child writes a note
to those most directly impacted. This note is one or two simple statements
that describe the new response. Bennett might write, "Mrs. Clark, I will
raise my hand for a turn to answer." Bennett shares the note with Mrs.
Clark on return to the classroom.

Continuing support for a child practicing new social skills incorporates
a variety of visual materials. Social stories may be used to describe the
steps and implications of a new social skill, clarify concepts that may be
confusing for a child, or identify how a child can secure help. In Bennett's
case, a social story discussing what is meant by interrupting or the implications of raising his hand would be helpful. In addition, social assistance
activities, can be incorporated to support a child in the target situation. We
will examine social assistance activities next.

SOCIAL ASSISTANCE ACTIVITIES

Social assistance activities provide support for new social skills a child is
learning and at the same time increase the child's independence. They may

reinforce information and skills presented through social review and/or social stories. The ideas listed here are either modifications of materials found in almost any classroom, or new activities to incorporate into the daily routine. All of these ideas can assist a child with autism in understanding school routines and activities. Many will benefit other children in the classroom as well.

Often, through the process of targeting a situation and gathering initial information, it will become apparent that a child can be assisted with the independent use of these activities, making social review and social stories unnecessary. Social assistance activities often provide the minor modifications or supports that make a critical difference in the success of a child in school.

A posted classroom schedule is a part of any classroom. A typical posted schedule may indicate "Monday—Art Class, 10:00; Tuesday—Gym Class, 2:15." For a child with autism, include an additional statement at the top of the classroom schedule, "Usually we have . . . ." with the schedule listed below. This introduces the possibility of variations in the routine as part of the schedule.

A "why" list of classroom rules reminds children why each rule is necessary. Classroom rules are posted in many classrooms. Often these are developed as part of a classroom activity, with children contributing ideas for rules to ensure their classroom is a safe environment where everyone can learn. Include in this discussion, and as part of each posted rule, statements explaining why each rule is listed ("We whisper during work times so others may finish their work."). Social stories may be written for a child with autism to further explain the implications and functional application of each rule.

A direction board lists simple instructions that are part of the classroom routine. Occasionally the teacher uses the board to direct the class, giving them experience following written instructions, or a child is selected to point to the appropriate direction to instruct the class. To involve the entire class in the selection of the correct response, the teacher may point to incorrect instructions, asking the class, "Is this next?" A variation of this board may be laminated to use with an erasable marker to write the cue that will introduce a new or special activity ("Time for the class party!"). This gives the child with autism advance notice of an upcoming event and the cue that will be used to announce it.

Computer conversations are, as the name implies, conversations between you and a child with autism at the computer. They are useful when the conversation is of critical importance, giving the child both auditory and visual feedback of the conversation. In this way, it may be easier for a child to "keep track" of both sides of a conversation. Sitting with the child at the computer, talk while simultaneously typing your conversation, using a format similar to a script for a play. Keep your phrases short. For example:

MRS. JOHNSON: Steven, we are going to talk about recess. I am going to type everything we say. We will be finished before you need to go to gym class.

Type the child's responses. For example:

STEVEN: I'm not going out to recess anymore. I hate it out there.

While you "talk," follow the child's lead to determine his or her perceptions. Answer the child's concerns and describe events he or she may be misperceiving. Identify solutions together. The child is given the printed version of the conversation at the close of the activity.

Social Reading folders are useful when the target situation or behavior relates to seat work, and the child needs reminders to practice a new skill. Create a folder with one solid half and the other half cut as a 2-inch border. A child's assignment is inserted into the folder so the border surrounds it. On the top border is a written reminder to the child: "It's okay if I make mistakes. That's how children learn." A statement on the bottom border may direct the child where to place the completed assignment. These written reminders may be taken directly from a social story, serving as cues to the story and providing support for the child in the target situation.

Social Reading bookmarks are similar to the folders, providing the child with a simple written reminder. On a bookmark a short statement is written ("I will raise my hand before I talk."). The bookmark is inserted into the child's textbook. This provides the child with a written cue as it helps locate the lesson for the day.

"Keep me posted" notes inform children in advance of changes. Children with autism may be asked to leave the classroom to meet with other professionals. Where many children look forward to the opportunity to leave the classroom and perhaps an unfinished assignment, the child with autism may react quite differently. By placing a note on the child's desk in the morning to inform her or him of such a transition, the child will be less surprised and more prepared to respond appropriately.

A reminder sign may be used when a child is not the only child having difficulty with a given behavior. A bright sign with the word "Reminder" is the teacher's silent cue to the entire class to make an extra effort to practice a specific skill during a critical period of time. If for example, a child with autism continually interrupts in class, speaking out over the other children without raising a hand, the teacher may consider that many children occasionally interrupt and thus introduce the reminder sign, explaining that when it is displayed they must work extra hard to listen quietly, or raise their hands, or wait their turn. The teacher draws the attention of the class to the fact that the reminder sign is displayed, describing and writing the specific desired behavior on the chalkboard near it: "Please listen quietly."

Social calendars are motivating for some students and are a beginning step toward learning self-evaluation. Social calendars may be especially effective with students who determine their own new responses to a situation based on descriptive information in a social story, or as the result of a Social Review activity. At the top of a calendar of each month, a priority social skill is stated as a goal ("I will finish my work."). At the end of each day, either the student, the teacher, or both write "YES!" to signify the response was achieved that day, or "Maybe tomorrow!" if it was not.

SUMMARY

Children with autism have unique perceptions of people and events, which result in responses that may seem unpredictable or inappropriate to others. These children have cognitive impairments that effect their understanding of communication, interaction, and social situations. Efforts to teach children with autism social skills should include accurate information regarding what people do and why. This information must be relevant and based on a child's actual experiences, presented with materials and instructional techniques designed to be most easily understood by the child.

All three areas of Social Reading either formally or informally follow four basic steps. First, a situation difficult for the child is targeted. This is a priority situation that often results in negative responses. Second, detailed information is gathered concerning the situation, the child's abilities and interests, and possible motivation for the child's current responses. Third, observations are shared with the child, providing the child with accurate information regarding the target situation and expected responses. Finally, new responses are identified, functionally defined, and supported using individualized materials.

Social Reading is an approach based on efforts to improve not only a child's understanding of the events and expectations that surround him or her, but also others' understanding of the child's perceptions and responses. It is hoped that the activities described in this chapter will improve understanding and effectively assist children with autism to become productive and contributing members of their communities.

REFERENCES

Dawson, G., & Fernald, M. (1987). Perspective-taking ability and its relationship to the social behavior of autistic children. *Journal of Autism and Developmental Disorders, 17,* 487–498.

Frith, U. (1989). *Autism: Explaining the enigma.* Oxford, England: Blackwell.

Gray, C., Dutkiewicz, M., Fleck, C., Moore, L., Cain, S.L., Lindrup, A., Broek, E., Gray, J., & Gray, B. (Eds.).

(1993). *The social story book.* Publication of the Jenison Michigan, Public Schools.

Gray, C., & Garand, J. (1993). Social stories: Improving responses of students with autism with accurate social information. *Focus on Autistic Behavior, 8,* 1–10.

Wing, L. (1988). The continuum of autistic characteristics. In E. Schoper & G. Mesibov (Eds.) *Diagnosis and assessment.* New York: Plenum.

APPENDIX 9.1   Sample Social Story

The Lines of Children at School

My name is Chad. I go to Lincoln Elementary School. I am in the second grade. There are 24 children in my class—there's me and 23 other children. My teacher's name is Mrs. Johnson. Sometimes the children in my class get in a line.

The children know when to get in a line. Sometimes in the classroom Mrs. Johnson will say, "Line up at the door," or "Let's line up row by row," or "Time to line up, class!" The children line up. I can line up. When the children are outside for recess, they line up when they hear the bell ring. The bell rings, the children line up. The bell rings, I can line up.

There are different kinds of lines at school. There are standing lines, there are walking lines, and there are slow lines.

Standing lines stay in one place. Usually we wait in a standing line. Sometimes we wait for everyone to line up after recess. Sometimes we wait for all the children to be quiet. Sometimes we wait for all the children to get their gym shoes. We wait in standing lines for other reasons, too. Sometimes I will wait in a standing line.

Children stand close together in a standing line. Sometimes they touch one another. Children may touch one another when they scratch their head, or tuck in their shirt, or tie their shoe. This can make standing lines feel a little crowded and squishy. Standing lines are not squishy for long—usually they become walking lines.

A walking line is a safe way to move 24 children from one place to another at school. That way, other people can walk in the hall, too. Each person gets where they are going safely. I will get where I am going safely.

Sometimes Mrs. Johnson takes our class of 24 children to other rooms in Lincoln School. We walk in a line. I walk in the line. Mrs. Johnson safely moves many children from one place to another.

Sometimes I am the first person in the line. Sometimes I stand in the middle of the line with children in front and in back of me. Sometimes I am the last child in the line. Sometimes, when I am the last child in the line, I will hear Mrs. Johnson say, "Chad, turn out the light!" That means it's my job to turn the light off in the classroom.

Slow lines are standing lines that move a little now and then. The lines of children in the cafeteria are like this. The children wait. I can wait. One at a time, each child has to get their lunch. I will have my turn to get my lunch, too. Each child stops to pay for their lunch. Each child needs to have their turn. I can wait for my turn.

APPENDIX 9.2   **Social Story Implementation Plan**

Name:_____ Date_____

Title of Story_____

Story format: Printed story _____ Story and audiotape _____

                    Story on videotape_____

Suggested Implementation: Begin implementing story on ____/____/____

1. To introduce the story_____

_____

_____

_____

2. Review schedule _____

_____

_____

_____

3. Monitoring new skills_____

_____

_____

_____

Progress Review Dates: ____/ ____/ ____; ____/ ____/ ____; ____/ ____/ ____

Suggested Fading Procedure: _____ Fading by rewriting

                                    _____ Revising review schedule

                                    _____ Decreasing verbal or other cues

                                    _____ Other

Support Materials and Activities:

_____ Revise posted classroom schedule   _____ Story bookmark(s)

_____ Revise, modify written classroom rules   _____ Reminder sign

_____ "Keep me posted" notes

_____ Computer conversations

_____ Story folder

_____ Social calendar/goals

_____ Other

Describe:_____

_____

10

Environmental Supports to Develop Flexibility and Independence

Nancy J. Dalrymple

As children grow up they are expected to become increasingly independent and free from the influence of others while at the same time taking responsibility for their own conduct and obligations. They learn to be flexible, to make decisions, to react to numerous and ever-changing stimuli in socially appropriate ways. We value self-reliance, independence, self assurance, and responsibility, and we expect cooperation, interdependence, and caring about others.

Most children conform to the standards and images adults set for them because they follow the usual developmental sequences. Most children (1) want to please people who are important to them; (2) cooperate more with adults who reason with them; (3) model their behavior from the people they love, admire, and see rewarded; (4) learn to understand others through empathy, perception of social cues, role-taking, and communication; (5) develop autonomy through many successful experiences; and (6) develop embarrassment, shame, and guilt when they fail to be like others or as others want them to be (Dalrymple, 1989; Konner, 1991).

However, when a child is impaired in his or her ability to socially interact and communicate, has many sensory needs, and processes and organizes information differently, the foundation for learning independent and responsible behavior is also impaired. Children with autism may (1) relate better with objects than with people; (2) fail to understand social cues, (3) be confused by the stimuli around them, (4) have difficulties understanding verbal language, and (5) have limited means of expressing their wants, needs, and thoughts (American Psychiatric Association, 1987; Courshesne, Akshoomoff & Townsend, 1990).

The purpose of this chapter is to demonstrate how concrete environmental supports help children with autism learn to change and become more flexible as well as grow in independence. Various types of supports are described along with ways to use them effectively.

RATIONALE FOR THE USE OF ENVIRONMENTAL SUPPORTS

Children with autism usually have to rely on others to help them make sense of their world. Adults try to provide supportive environments that consider each child's special learning needs. Environmental supports are materials that assist the individual children, taking into account their sensory needs, their need to understand the passage of time, their modes of learning and strengths, and their need for accurate, reliable information. Teachers and parents have to learn to see the world through the eyes and experiences of children with autism to effectively help them learn and grow up to be productive adults in their community. Effective teaching involves providing the various environmental supports that each child needs (Dunlap & Robbins, 1991).

For the purposes of this chapter, environmental supports refer to aspects of the environment other than interactions with people that affect the learning that takes place. Therefore location, sequence, and type of stimuli are considered as they impact each child and as the child relates to them.

Frith (1989) suggests that the common denominator that underlies all features present in individuals with autism "is the inability to draw together information so as to derive coherent and meaningful ideas. There is a fault in the predisposition of the mind to make sense of the world" (p. 187). Further, she suggests that "a meaningful stimulus is meaningful because it belongs as a member of a set. It is already organized as to its place in memory" (p. 97). Frith postulates that a weakness of coherence in central thought process keeps children with autism from operating with a central drive to derive meaning from segmented stimuli.

Frith has developed this hypothesis about the nature of the intellectual dysfunction in autism:

> In the normal cognitive system there is a propensity to form coherence over as wide a range of stimuli as possible, and to generalize over as wide a range of contexts as possible. It is this capacity for coherence that is diminished in autistic children. As a result their information-processing systems are characterized by detachment (1989, p. 101).

Children with autism may produce what they hear verbatim, or what they see exactly, rather than understand the gist or global meaning of an event. Frith reports that children with autism do better on tasks requiring isolation of stimuli and poorly on tasks requiring connection of stimuli. Therefore part of the job of teaching children with autism is to attach meaning to connected stimuli and then to retain meaning and understanding when one segment of a sequence is changed.

Stokes and Baer (1977) have discussed the limited generalization of children with autism. The children who were studied could not generalize their experiences across environments unless explicitly taught to do so. In addition, a common characteristic of children with autism is perseveration. Perseveration involves emitting a single response or responding to a single stimuli instead of sampling other responses or stimuli (Koegel, Rincover, & Egel, 1982). Planned environmental supports allow meaning to be established between concrete stimuli and can teach the child varied response patterns and generalization.

Courshesne et al. (1990) have demonstrated that children with autism have problems with attention. They take longer to shift attention, both to engage and disengage; therefore they have problems understanding information that requires constant shifts of attention, particularly shifts from one modality to another. The responses of children with autism are significantly different from those of normal subjects to unexpected changes in auditory stimulation, yet responses to unexpected changes in visual stimulation are similar across the two groups. Concrete, visually coded environmental supports can help the child with autism better predict events and improve recall and attention.

▶TABLE 10.1 Environmental Supports	I. ARRANGEMENT OF STIMULI WITHIN THE SETTING
	II. LOCATION OF CHILD WITHIN THE SETTING
	III. PLANNED VISUAL INFORMATION • Pictured • Pictured and written • Written • Objects/activities for specific situations
	IV. ELECTRONIC TECHNOLOGY • Computers • Audio tapes • Programmed messages • Videotapes/movies (with or without audio)

THE PURPOSE OF ENVIRONMENTAL SUPPORTS

Children with autism are vulnerable to constant correction as they try to make sense of their confusing worlds. Sometimes they become excessively rigid about routines, room layouts, routes that they travel, and their own belongings and space (Smith, 1990). As they struggle to comply to the adults in this confusing world, they may grow dependent on verbal cues and adult presence to direct them, and they become quite upset if they make a mistake (Handleman, 1992). Carefully designed and individualized environmental supports help the child understand his or her world better, accept change easier, and become more independent (Simpson & Myles, 1993).

Because the ability to utilize sensory input to apply meaning to segmented stimuli is impaired in children with autism (Frith, 1989), parents and teachers become the primary sources to organize environments and learning sequences so a child can learn by association and respond appropriately. Of necessity, this requires intervening more directly than with most children. "Children with autism will learn more easily, express more interest, and have fewer behavior problems if there is predictability to their daily and weekly routines" (Olley, 1987, p. 414). They are less anxious when they accurately know what to expect.

Growth of Flexibility

Children with autism have problems with stimulus overselectivity (Goldstein & Lancy, 1985; Koegel, Egel, & Dunlap, 1980). The slightest change may make a situation appear different to the child. Entering from another door, getting help with a coat or sometimes not wearing a coat, the teacher being there or having a substitute, needing to use the bathroom, carrying something, or the TV being on or off—all create different sequences of environmental stimuli. Most children can adapt to such changes easily and be directed by verbal information; but often the child with autism is so strongly influenced by environmental stimuli that his or her whole chain of behaviors is modified by one changed variable.

Since variables do change and flexibility is essential, it is important to determine what key environmental supports will help the child with autism learn the behaviors needed in each and every situation. It might be necessary to plan a consistent "entering school" routine that does not rely on random changes in people or time of day. The child needs to know which door to enter every morning and exactly where to go after entering. Whether they ride on the bus or come with dad, the routine needs to be the same once they arrive at school. If children wait outside or in a gym before school, the exact rules that govern these events need to be clearly stated and presented to the child with autism so that he understands. Even rules such as "Stay outside on sunny days" have to be presented to the child concretely.

The fact that routines and schedules vary has to be specifically taught. Because the child with autism depends so heavily on past experiences, and because spoken words are seldom sufficient, it is best to plan and practice ahead of time. This is especially true when the child is in the middle of a situation and/or anxious. If there are classrooms or places the class visits often, teach the routine for "visiting" each time you go there and label it the same way, then "visiting" behavior will be learned. This routine might be to carry a chair and place it at the back of the room, then sit down; or it might be to walk beside another child and sit on the floor by him or her. Entering unfamiliar environments often creates anxiety and confusion, therefore extra attention needs to be given to the way expectations are conveyed.

Although all this planning sounds as though it is very time-consuming, it requires much less time than leaving the learning to chance. Too often the environmental cues that tell children with autism what to do are not clear and precise. The problems of overselectivity and generalization may cause them to miscue, and the inability to shift attention may create a confusing learning situation for them. Without planned teaching strategies, children with autism learn miscues and incorrect associations, and either become anxious and unable to elicit appropriate behavior or emit inappropriate behavior and then must "unlearn" the incorrect association.

With this emphasis on order and predictability, it might seem odd to suggest that environmental information can also help the child with autism learn to be more flexible. Certainly, a degree of flexibility is necessary to live and interact with other people. Events, people, and environments are constantly changing, sometimes quite rapidly. With help, the child with autism can learn to be more adaptable and make transitions. Support in the form of clear, understandable information provided ahead of time helps the child predict what is going to happen; thus equipped, he or she can adapt and become more flexible (Orelove, 1982; Powers, 1992).

When the child expects to go to the library each Friday or expects to have hamburger, french fries, and coke at McDonalds because past experience has told him to expect this, he will need preparation to understand that there is to be a change. It is easier to make the change as clear and concrete as possible if a picture or written information about the change is available. The change can then become participatory by removing one piece of information from a visible schedule and substituting another. The sequence of events can also be lengthened in this way. For instance, if a child with autism expects the school bus to follow a certain route, but today two new children are added and the route varies, the child may scream or refuse to get off the bus. If gym class can't be held today because voting machines are in the gym, then the child needs to know this. These types of schedule changes can be explained to the child by concretely inserting the activity card/picture/word that represents the change. For example, it might help to show the child what a voting machine looks like, once he or she knows there is a change and understands the situation.

It is always necessary to look for factors in the environment that might be contributing to a particular behavior problem. By analyzing them carefully, many environmental stimuli can be adjusted, changed, or explained in a way the child understands. For example, the child who yells and screams when asked to leave the classroom to go to a school convocation may be confused. From his perspective, he wants to finish his work or needs to know what is going to happen. He needs prior information about the convocation (i.e., new experience) in written, picture, or video form. He needs to "experience" a convocation slowly. He may need to leave his classroom after everyone else and watch from a distance. The next time he will need to know where he will sit and how he can ask to leave. Gradually he will gain success with convocations. Many other children are not bothered by the change, since they sense the excitement and can gain information verbally and relate it to previous experiences.

Because children with autism might react to changes by becoming agitated and upset doesn't mean that they can't learn to accept change. The important factors are to identify what environmental stimuli a child relies on for stability, to provide accurate information about the change prior to the event, to offer choices about alternatives to the change when possible, and to elicit the child's involvement in the change when appropriate.

Always consider the environmental needs of the child. Eventually, children with autism will and can learn to function in a variety of environments, but they need careful introduction and desensitization to environments that require adaptation to constantly changing and challenging stimuli. The children must succeed at their own pace.

Growth of Independence

Many children with autism become dependent on adult presence and adult prompts to know what to do or to perform correctly. Much of this dependence comes from the manner in which learning sequences have been taught. Because a child may have been distractible, overly stimulated, unable to perform motorically, or uneven in performance, an adult may become part of the activity by providing ongoing prompts and cues that tell a child what to do next. Verbal cues often are difficult to fade, thus requiring the teacher to be present. Teaching children to respond to environmental supports develops more independent behavior.

For instance, some children never learn to toilet alone because someone has verbally cued them through each step. Fading verbal prompts and chunking steps together can eventually be accomplished through a pictured/written sequence that is rehearsed ahead of time and posted in the bathroom. Colored tape on the faucet might help the child know how to regulate the water, a timer might let the child know when sitting time is over, and a special toy might be used while sitting. Completion will need to be made clear through following a set, learned sequence. Perhaps turning the water off, getting a towel, drying, and throwing the towel away signals the end of the bathroom routine.

Environmental cues also help with independence in doing chores. For example, there are many ways to go about setting a table. Matching the place mats to the number of chairs around the table, matching the place settings to a model, or a drawn imprint on each place mat leads to independence. Consider whether it's necessary to count out the correct number of spoons or whether the learner can take a handful and match one to each place setting, then return the remainder or get another one or two if needed. If counting is desired, it might be necessary to use a jig to match the correct number before taking the stack to the table. Children with autism need a consistent sequence that is planned from the beginning to meet their learning needs and help them become as independent as possible. Completing the entire sequence independently will help a child feel a sense of responsibility and pride.

An ordered environment is a great comfort to children with autism and adds to independent behavior. For example, if a child's coat is always put on the hook by him or her, it will always be there when he or she needs it. If the child always empties his or her book bag when arriving to school and puts it in a cubby, that's where it will be. Even though these same principles apply to anyone, they are *essential* for the person with autism. Living in an environment that is disorganized, or where people make constant changes and do not respect the needs of the child, is frustrating and impedes learning.

TYPES OF ENVIRONMENTAL SUPPORTS

For purposes of this discussion, there are four general categories of environmental supports: temporal, procedural, spatial and assertion. *Temporal supports* are used to organize sequences of time and time frames. *Procedural supports* are used to organize the relationship between steps of an activity or relationships between objects and people. *Spatial supports* are used to provide specific information regarding the organization of the environment. And *assertion supports* are used to help the child with autism initiate and exert control.

Temporal Supports

Temporal supports are used to organize sequences of time for the child. There are a variety of temporal suports, including schedules, completion guidelines, waiting supports, and strategies for accepting changes.

Schedules.   Schedules may give information about part of a day, an entire day, a week, a month, or a year. They may also sequence the routine within a specific time frame. These supports help the child with autism have a better perspective of the order of events and how they relate to one another.

The world becomes easier to understand with concrete, visual schedules in the form of pictures and/or written words that sequence events in the order that they will happen. Connecting clock times to events that occur at specific times sometimes helps a child become more independent. However, it's important not to attach specific times to events that don't occur consistently at specific times. It might even help to have a range of time when the event might start. For instance, reading group starts between 10:15 and 10:30. Another way to introduce flexibility into the schedule is to build in some free choice times in which the child will learn to do a variety of familiar activities. These time fillers are very useful when the bus arrives any time within a fifteen-minute period, when the child finishes assigned work, or when an emergency arises.

Some children insert their own time supports by relating their daily schedule to TV programs or other dependable time-oriented events. One preschooler knew it was time for school after a certain TV program; another had to watch the early morning news that showed the skyline of the city to start each day. Yet another child watched "Wheel of Fortune" after dinner every night. Many children with autism seem to know instinctively when it's time for daily activities. Although they often don't relate well or understand the words that denote time relationships and passage of time, they seem to need to order their days through certain events. Since TV shows, meals, and class lessons are usually predictable, they use them. They also may relate time to the actions of people—for example, when the classroom assistant takes a break or when another child goes to speech group. It is useful to consider the events that occur regularly in the child's day and provide accurate, consistent information in a concrete, visual form.

Completion Guidelines.   Completion or finishing depends on the situation, who is judging, and previous expectations. For example, the child who is supposed to color the paper and makes two strokes is told to finish. He makes two more, and is told to finish. Is there a model to show him completion, or is it ten strokes? The signal that a meal is finished could be "when all the food is gone from the plate," "when the person next to you gets up," or "when the bell rings." Many children with autism become quite confused when they want to leave the table because they don't want to eat any more, but are told to "finish." Sometimes a child looks at an activity and decides it is so overwhelming that he or she will not even try it, since there seems to be no way to finish it. Sometimes when a child is doing well he is required to do an activity over and over again, but on a day when he is not doing so well he has to do it only once. Sometimes a lesson ends with one activity, sometimes it ends with another; sometimes lesson materials have to be put away, sometimes they don't. Sometimes a child watches a videotape to the end; other times a videotape is used as a short filler activity, and the child refuses to leave until the tape is completed. Environmental supports can be useful in defining completion specifically and understandably, always considering the child's perspective of the situation.

The following are some examples of supports that help a child see completion more clearly.

1. Use timers in the form of digital countdowns, hourglasses in the form of sand or oil bubbles, or timers that turn.
2. Specify amount to be done rather than a time frame: match the number done to a jig, mark each item completed on a card, put a certain number of chips in a jar, use a counter, or complete the exact number set out.
3. Set cues for finishing a particular activity; for example, a certain song means the end of music, putting materials away signals the end of the lesson, or the teacher standing up means the end of eating. Take care to choose cues that will always mean completion. One child was totally lost when a classmate who was his model for returning his tray in the cafeteria was absent.
4. Supply a concrete model or a demonstration

Waiting Supports. Waiting is an abstract time concept. Waiting in line, waiting for an appointment, waiting for others to get ready, waiting for a bus, waiting for dinner, waiting for someone to pay attention, or waiting to go to the bathroom all require different strategies and behaviors, yet the child usually receives the same verbal direction for all situations. Supports to help the child understand what behavior is expected require both time information and concrete information. Time information involves the length of the wait; therefore the strategies described for understanding completion are applicable. Additionally, teaching the child an activity to do while waiting can translate into "waiting behavior." If the waiting activity is versatile and can be transported, a specific cue can be taught that indicates "it's time to wait"; that is, it's time to do the waiting activity. Some examples of waiting activities are looking at a comic book or picture book, listening to a tape on a Walkman, playing a hand-held computer game, using a visual toy like a spinner or Koosh ball, or playing with a deck of cards. The waiting activity should be used only for waiting times.

Additional environmental supports for waiting help the child to learn to stand in line and move forward, learn to do something while someone else is engaged, or learn where to stand or sit while waiting. In other words, waiting behavior is complex and really must be learned as it applies to each situation.

One mother reported that her son learned what waiting meant by playing T-ball. He had to "wait" on first base and paced around the perimeter of the base. He learned a strategy that involved staying in a small space and used this same behavior in other waiting situations. Another mother reported that her son learned to wait by sitting in church services; so to him waiting involved sitting. As this necessary concept is taught, all the visual supports possible need to be in place; then the entire waiting strategy is taught by practicing in each situation.

Learning to stand in line is often taught by pairing the child with a specific peer. A line that is short and that has a reward such as food is sometimes easier to manage than a line at the bank. However, a line at a bank might be easier to understand since there are often ropes to delineate where to stand in line. Knowing the outcome at the end of the line often helps the child be more patient about waiting. If the skill required after the wait is anxiety producing like ordering food by oneself or making complex choices, then the waiting in line behavior might need an external reinforcer.

Strategies for Accepting Time Changes.   When concrete information is in place about the day's or week's events, it is far easier to explain change than having to rely on verbal explanations alone. Often when change is explained verbally, the child with autism repeats it over and over or asks endless questions. If he doesn't have a way to ask, he may proceed as if the change is not going to occur. For instance, if the child usually goes home on the bus, but today Uncle Bob is picking him up, he needs to participate in seeing the bus crossed out or picture put away and Uncle Bob's picture, name, and/or car put in its place.

Sometimes parents and teachers say that the child knows his or her schedule, therefore he or she doesn't need a visual schedule. However, the child usually has an internal script of exactly what past experiences have told him or her will happen. Verbal explanation alone seldom changes this script. Seeing it changed visually and participating in the change helps the child understand and accept the changes better.

The same strategy can apply to explaining changes that can't be planned ahead of time, as when someone is late or sick, when the ice rink or swimming pool is closed, when a sudden stop has to be made, or when the cafeteria runs out of chocolate milk. If at all possible, a substitute needs to be put in place before the child becomes upset. If the child is in control, a choice can be offered. Dwelling on the change seldom does much good, but supporting the learner to understand the change by giving information about what is happening visually and putting information about the change right into the daily sequence helps to get everything back on track. One college student with autism managed a change when he had a class canceled. At first, he was so upset that he could not proceed with the rest of his day. But after discussing and writing down various alternatives he decided that the strategy that would make him feel most comfortable would be to sit through the class in the empty classroom so that his day could proceed in the expected sequence. Strategies that are established for certain situations are useful, but regardless of how many are learned, there will always be unexpected changes. When there is a way to solve the problem with visual supports, there is a greater chance that the change will be accepted with less anxiety.

Procedural Supports

Procedural supports are used to clarify the relationship between steps of an activity or relationships between objects and people. Procedural supports can include clarification about routines, personal possessions, or privacy.

Routines.   Routines are supports that explain the order within an activity. For instance, it is easy to learn to go through a cafeteria line because all the visual supports are in place to give cues for the next behavior. It is easier to choose because you can see what is available. In contrast, the sequence for making cinnamon toast or a sandwich, for taking out the trash, or for taking a note to the office might not be as clear from environmental cues. Therefore organizing the sequence with visual cues, such as using all the materials for each step as it is completed and using the environment to give cues for the next step, is helpful in building understanding and independence.

Doing a task alongside someone also provides naturally occurring environmental cues. The sequence is provided by a direct model. However, dependence on the model's presence may prevent the person from doing the activity alone. Learning set routines from visual and environmental cues and learning through repeated experience doing the activity in exactly the same predictable way helps the person with autism learn more quickly.

Possession.   Personal property, common property, property belonging to someone and not available to anyone else, shared property, property that is loaned or given, stolen property: explaining the complex nature of possession requires teachers and parents to consider the way children with autism view the environment. The following are just a few samples of questions that need to be answered precisely and clearly:

Is a toothbrush shared or is the blue one always Jim's?
When a new one is purchased does the red one then become Jim's?
Are the french fries mine or can you take some?
Can I take some of yours?
Does the computer at school (the chalk, the paints) belong to you, to me, or to whom?
If this is my work, then why can someone mark all over it?
Why does my lunch box have to stay up on the shelf? Maybe I won't see it again.

Ordered environments that teach clearly and concretely about possession help the child with autism learn these concepts. Specific rules that govern use of property and are posted with visual supports help convey clear meaning.

Privacy.   Children with autism may not know much about private behavior in private places. Remember that they are just beginning to learn about interaction with others. Teaching private behaviors such as toileting in set routines and incorporating them into the natural learning environment from the beginning is important. For instance, the cue to undo one's pants should be given when the bathroom door is closed, not in the hallway. Beginning early to use environmental cues to reinforce and teach specific private behaviors in private places helps the child practice appropriate behavior later.

Spatial Supports

Spatial supports are used to provide specific information regarding the organization of the environment. Spatial supports include information about the location of objects, can assist the child in becoming comfortable with a situation that is overstimulating, can clarify places for keeping personal belongings and help the child understand his or her spatial relationship to others.

Location.   Knowing where things are located, seeing pictures/words on the outside of closed spaces such as drawers and cupboards, or having see-through containers and drawers helps the learner with autism know how to access what he or she wants. An ordered, planned environment helps the child organize his or her world and function better. For example, putting all the items needed for a lesson in one container, then later having the items pictured or written for the child to gather together before the lesson helps teach the organizational process.

Supports for Sensory Overload.   Noise, visual distractors, open space, movement, depth perception, smells, and touch annoyances or needs all must be considered when planning the learning environment. A child who must sit in the cafeteria with his hands over his ears is not comfortable. Being in a gym class with many other children is often overwhelming. Smelling the food being cooked or having to wear uncomfortable tights may throw the child's whole day off. Children with autism can often be desensitized to sensory problems in their environments with supports over a period of time. They can learn to tune some stimuli out by focusing on other stimuli. Learning the routines and the layout sometimes helps the child with autism become familiar and less anxious in the situation. However, sometimes it's necessary to provide alternatives to such sensory bombardment. One kindergartner became physically sick in the cafeteria. After she had become comfortable in school and her mother packed her favorite foods for lunch, the cafeteria was reintroduced in a planned way. She was able to accept the environment with the planned supports in place. She visited the cafeteria, it was pictured on her schedule, and she knew where she sat and how long she stayed. Knowing what would happen after lunch also helped her be less anxious.

Most children with autism are such good visual learners that they need the whole picture to understand the sequence and relationship of the parts. Using environmental supports that are adaptable to various learning styles and being creative in using them aids both the teacher and the learner.

Personal Space.   These types of supports are the same as those for privacy, but deal more with the place for keeping personal belongings. Learning that there is a specific place for personal belongings and learning to take the responsibility for transporting personal property and returning it helps the child with autism keep his or her environment ordered and reliable.

Relationship to Others.   Spatial cues and supports that give children information about how close to stand while in line, who can be touched and where, who can be hugged and when, how to greet people, and the other protocols that are followed in school, home, and society is quite complex. One child with autism asked his teacher, "When can you hit on the playground?" The teacher was a bit surprised and stated that the rule was that you never hit on the playground. The child persisted by explaining that other children do hit on the playground. He did not have the other part of the rule that most children learn from one another: "You can hit on the playground when the teacher is not around." Learning rules that apply to certain locations and learning how to relate to others in specific environments is very complex. However, visual reminders, rehearsals, and practice help children with autism learn. When there are conflicting rules or when the rule is not followed consistently, children with autism need additional supports to help them understand the deviation.

Assertion Supports

Assertion supports are used to help the child initiate and exert control. Assertion supports assist in the child in making choices and maintaining self-control.

Making Choices.   Visual supports in the form of objects, pictures, or written information help a learner with autism exert choice. Information provided only verbally is often confusing and misunderstood. Limiting the number of choices, understanding how the child makes a choice, and encouraging that he or she follow through with the choice helps the child make real choices. A verbal child may verbally echo "Do you want a drink?" to mean that he wants a drink, or may repeat both choices from a verbal choice of two. A choice-making routine with visual supports is a skill the child can use the rest of his life. Choice also involves refusal. The child must have a way to refuse and know that it is an option that will be respected. Visual means can be in place to teach refusal and to convey that it is a choice.

Self-Control.   Having a place to go to be alone or being able to ask for space and time alone can be built into a child's educational plan. If the child isn't allowed or shown how to incorporate this request in a concrete way, he or she may use a previously learned alternative behavior such as having a tantrum or using the bathroom to escape. Learning to pair a relaxation routine with a "quiet place" leads to self-management and self-control.

CHARACTERISTICS OF ENVIRONMENTAL SUPPORTS

Although environmental supports can be used for a wide range of purposes, it is most essential that the design of supports for any child be individualized, socially validated, consistently used, age appropriate, and adaptable.

Individualized   Each child with autism and each situation needs to be carefully analyzed and interpreted from the child's perspective. For instance, it's usually not enough to have the class schedule on the board. This is often general and the child doesn't use it as his or her personal piece of information. One child accepted his daily schedule on a wipe-off board on his desk, another learned to change his schedule on the computer, and still another had words attached to a small strip of Velcro on his desk. A made-to-order purse, a fanny pack, a book bag, or a notebook might attract the interest of a specific child. Whether in the form of pictures or written words or objects such as books, charts, or flip cards—and whether it provides choices, information, or reminders of completion—each support must be designed to meet the needs of the individual.

The position of the child with autism in relation to the environment can be either supportive or distracting and detrimental. Individualization must come from knowledge of specific learning styles. One child may do better sitting near the back and to one side. Another may do better right in the front in the middle. One may need to sit across from the teacher, while another may do better beside the teacher. One may need to sit away from the windows or shiny surfaces; another may need to be away from the door and the flow of traffic.

Some children want to walk behind another person so they can see where to go by following the feet in front; some want to be in front so they have a clear vista. Some children want to be first in line at school, some want to be beside a certain child. Some become quite upset walking in the halls when there is noise and lots of movement, but do better either walking alone or with a few children. Consider what adaptations need to be made to help each one with his or her particular need. Often space, depth perception, noise, lights, and movement create varying environments.

What we perceive as being exactly the same as yesterday, may in fact be quite different to the child with autism because of a slightly changed environmental stimuli.

Socially Validated

Sometimes teachers and parents are reluctant to use environmental supports that they feel may single the child out as being different. Perhaps we need to view the supports from another perspective. Most people are able to choose their own ways to obtain environmental supports. They arrange their bookshelves, their wallet, their calendars, their phones, their closets, and their cars in ways that enable them to function in an organized, stress-free manner. When one of these supports fails, when a wallet is lost or keys are misplaced, a person usually becomes quite anxious.

Children with autism need help with this organization and need help to take increasing responsibility for it as they grow older. The support from the environment should be individualized and meet the child's needs in a way that is helpful and as natural as possible. However, providing visual schedules that can be changed through use of Velcro or plastic sleeves is similar to providing glasses or hearing aids to other children. These supports are *necessities* for children with autism to function in settings that are confusing to them. As the child grows older the supports should not disappear, but should be age, individual, and situation appropriate.

Consistently Used

Children with autism have to rely on adults and peers to help and to provide information in formats that are understandable. Consistency in cues and stimuli is something that is absolutely necessary to make an environment or an activity understandable. If the child is accustomed to a personal schedule and someone forgets or decides he or she no longer needs one, the child may not be able to advocate for him or herself, and may display behaviors that interfere with learning. The child may not be able to tell someone that he or she is upset when lunch is late, when the bus is late, when the teacher is not there, when the computer isn't working, or when he or she doesn't know what to do in the art room. Consistent use of carefully planned environmental supports is absolutely necessary to the learning of children with autism. Inconsistent use impedes learning and adds to anxiety.

The supports must be part of the environmental organization. The child can't be expected to keep track of the supports without lots of experience. A picture/written schedule may need to be on the child's desk at school and on the refrigerator at home. If there is something the child is carrying from place to place, the method for transporting must be carefully analyzed, and the cues to help him or her remember should be built into the plan.

Age Appropriate

Sometimes we provide for young children supports and adaptations that are quite difficult for them to give up or change as they become older. Most children, who receive encouragement and gain experience with new and more age-appropriate objects are able to make a change. The social pressure from peers often is not as great a factor in establishing age-appropriate supports for children with autism as it is for other sociable children. Therefore it becomes necessary for parents and teachers to teach the child using age-appropriate activities and adaptations. However, each individual child's needs must be considered. Trying to mold a child with autism into our idea of what is age appropriate may be destructive. We are not looking for conformity, but rather for learning and growth.

For instance, if a child eats his hamburger by taking it all apart, it will be more socially appropriate when eating out to learn to eat it as a whole. This can be taught using visual supports and modeling. If a child flips every piece of string he finds, he may eventually need to be taught to flip just one short string that he carries in his pocket and further be taught when it is appropriate to do the flipping. If a child understands the passage of time by relating to holidays, and looks forward weeks ahead to Halloween, he will need to be told through visual supports and rehearsal if change from his past Halloween experience will occur. If this year there will not be a dress-up party at school or he will not participate in trick or treat, he needs to know exactly what he will be doing. All too often a child with autism learns a specific sequence of events to a given cue and becomes extremely upset when that sequence is altered without prior understanding about the change.

Adaptable

Adaptability should be considered as environmental supports are being designed. It takes time to make and organize these supports, as they usually are implemented across settings and people. They have to be able to expand and change easily and stand up to rigorous use. Sometimes teachers overlook very simple ways to provide support in favor of complicated, fancy means. Computers, Velcro, wipe-off boards, chalkboards, marks on the floor or faucets, timers, see-through boxes, and calendars offer quick ways to provide supports.

Room arrangements, school adaptations, and even community adaptations often require prior planning. When the VCR doesn't work and a child refuses to get his coat on to go home because he has not seen the video, the teacher needs an adaptation to let him know that he will be all right. If there is a visual suport in place, it becomes much easier to "cross off" video and put a very short alternative activity in its place. No words can provide the information as clearly as visual representation to the child at this time! One 5-year-old became very upset when learning to print letters because the *g* went below the line. All the other letters she had learned to print, *a–f*, had been above the line. She probably could have profited from seeing the whole alphabet before she began to learn to print letters or to see the alphabet as a whole in front of her. In this way the rules for printing letters could have been visually explained by choosing and grouping letters that go under the line and ones that go above the line. Sometimes we try to break the learning sequence into steps without the child understanding the whole.

IMPLEMENTING ENVIRONMENTAL SUPPORTS

When implementing environment supports, one should consider where the supports would be useful and when to use the supports.

Where Supports Are Useful

Environmental supports are useful everywhere. They provide information that the child needs and help the child become competent across settings, people, and stimuli. Environmental supports enhance the child's ability to participate in activities with others and to be included in a variety of settings. Having a place to go to relax and be alone in a classroom full of other children, or knowing what part of the playground is safe and fun, helps a child with autism cope with difficult environments. Expecting a child with autism always to be part of a group and to handle new and constantly changing situations without environmental supports that provide accurate information just invites failure.

School. With supports like visual schedules, an organized school day, and a means to control the environment when it becomes too difficult, the child with autism can experience success. One school turned off the bells until the child with autism could adapt to the school, learn the meaning of the bells, and become desensitized to the sound. Another school put colored stripes in the hall to designate the path to various places, while yet another designated the library as the quiet spot for the child with autism to go in free time.

Inclusion into community activities can also be successful when everyone understands the needs of the child with autism. Going out to McDonald's may sound quite routine, but if the child is used to getting a Happy Meal from McDonald's and he goes with his class and is given only the choice of a soft drink, he may become quite confused and upset. This confusion may also occur if he goes at 10:00 A.M. and can't order a Happy Meal. He also may have learned from past experiences that going to McDonald's means going through the drive-through window and may not be able to wait in a line of three people without being taught. So even though most children with autism can identify the McDonald's golden arches rather early, the particular meaning to them comes from their direct experience. When the routine associated with the symbol and word changes, the child becomes confused and anxious, often resulting in interfering behavior.

In order to ensure success, the teacher should know a great deal about the prior experiences of the child with autism, when possible. Always work from the assumption that accurate information must be provided in a way that the child with autism understands. Making the child conform to rigid time frames without time to observe, feel comfortable, and "experience" the environment contributes to failure. Understanding the child's needs for environmental supports and then providing the supports contributes to successful inclusion.

Community.   When ordering food in a fast-food restaurant or any restaurant, everyone uses visual supports. Some restaurants provide picture menus. The child with autism needs to know the ordering procedure and needs to know what his or her choices are. When the child goes to McDonald's for breakfast, the breakfast menu and the time need to be paired. Breakfast foods have to be taught as a concept through pictures, objects, written and verbal words, and experience. If the child is learning to run laps, he or she may need to remove a loose wristband at the end of each lap to know exactly how many to run. To understand completion when shopping, a pictured or written sequence can be provided.

Using a YM/WCA, going grocery shopping, going clothes shopping, or attending a sports event can all be supported through environmental cues and information provided ahead of time. This requires planning, but once supports are in place, they enable everyone to be more successful. Use the natural cues that are in place by making the child aware of them and their meaning.

Home.   Because home is less structured in time sequences, it can be the perfect environment to encourage choice making and organization of time into sequenced activities. Providing an ordered home environment with rules that are applied as consistently as possible will help the child be more successful. The home environment offers endless ways to provide organized materials, visual supports, and schedules to help the child learn. Bedtime and morning routines can be pictured and/or written to provide information, explain change, and enhance independence. Specific environmental choice boards are helpful for eating and leisure activities. They tell the child specifically what the options are for today.

Children with autism need environmental support for most changes. Involving the child in the rearrangement of the living room helps him orient to the change. There is a better understanding of space and location by being part of the move. Sometimes the child may do better with a major change than with a small one. For instance, moving to a new house many not be as difficult as moving to a new bedroom in the same house or moving a bed from one side of the room to another.

Work. Even in elementary school it's important to consider the environmental supports that help the child perform jobs as independently as possible. Whether the task is washing dishes, vacuuming, setting the table, or carrying a message, specific environmental supports will help the child be successful. Growth of competence and independence will help the child with autism work successfully in the community some day.

When to Use Environmental Supports

Environmental supports are used by everyone all the time. Too often children with autism connect one meaning to a cue or connect their own personalized meaning rather than connect stimuli together to make sense. For instance, sometimes a class goes outside after eating lunch. It depends on the weather. A child with autism associated taking his coat to the cafeteria to mean that he was going out. When it started raining during lunch one day and he couldn't go out, a major problem arose. To solve such a problem, one teacher used a sign on the classroom door that was checked by each child after lunch to know whether to go out or stay in; a symbol for the classroom door along with the words "In? Out?" was added to the autistic child's personal schedule. Another child learned to self-initiate using the toilet when this activity was added into the pictured sequence of his day. Getting a backpack can be the signal that school is almost over, the male-female figures on doors let children and others know which rest rooms to use, and lights turned off may signal quiet time.

It's wise to anticipate using a variety of environmental supports with every child who has autism. The personalized supports should be passed from teacher to teacher with explanations. They should be constantly updated with the child and his parents included in the planning. Often, a child rejects a type of support or appears to no longer need it when the knowledge is part of his or her repertoire. Assess whether another form of the same support is needed, whether a schedule may be needed only to explain change, or whether the information is so well known that it's important only to make sure all personnel know the same information. Sometimes a simple note pad or small wipe-off board can substitute for the more specific supports to be available when other methods aren't working. Too often teachers aren't aware that a child with autism can read, and therefore they fail to use this quick, available way to give information. Appendix 10.1 provides guidelines for determining the type of environmental support needed for the child and steps to evaluate its effectiveness.

Giving information accurately so the child with autism can predict expectations and situations accurately and avoid the correction mode is a major reason for environmental supports. Build them into all instruction. Individualize them when necessary. If they are imbedded in the classroom in some way for everyone, the child will be further included as part of the group. Always, the unique perspective of the child with autism must be considered in designing individualized supports to ensure that his or her needs are met.

SUMMARY

This chapter has discussed the use of environmental supports to enhance the ability of children with autism to be more adaptable in accepting change and to be more independent. Temporal, procedural, spatial, and assertion supports were described, although supports have infinite application. The characteristics of environmental supports and considerations for implementation were discussed, including individualized, socially validated, consistently used, age appropriate, and adaptable. The discussion concluded with some ideas for expanding their use.

As educational systems and communities move toward inclusive environments, all environments must consider the perspective and needs of each child and provide the individualized supports needed for success. Considering the special needs of children with autism will enhance successful inclusion for everyone. Children with autism are often not able to express their needs directly and therefore rely on others to help organize their environmental supports. A team approach to assess, design, and evaluate environmental supports will produce the most reliable supports and lead to the greatest success for each child with autism and those who teach them.

REFERENCES

American Psychiatric Association. (1987). *Diagnostic and statistical manual of mental disorders* (3rd ed., rev.). Washington, DC.

Courshesne, E., Akshoomoff, N. A., & Townsend, J. (1990). Recent advances in autism. Current opinions in pediatrics. *Current Science*, ISNN 1040–8703.

Dalrymple, N. (1989). *Learning to be independent and responsible*. Bloomington, IN: Institute for the Study of Developmental Disabilities.

Dunlap, G., & Robbins, F. R. (1991). Current perspective in service delivery for young children with autism. *Comprehensive Mental Health Care 1*(3).

Frith, U. (1989). *Autism, explaining the enigma*. Worcester, England: Billings.

Goldstein, G. I., & Lancy, D. F. (1985). Cognitive development in autistic children. In L. S. Siegel & F. J. Morrison (Eds.), *Cognitive development in atypical children*. New York: Springer-Verlag.

Handleman, J.S. (1992). Assessment for curriculum planning. In D. E. Berkell (Ed.), *Autism: identification, education, and treatment*. Hillsdale, N.J.: Lawrence Erlbaum Associates.

Koegel, R. L., Egel, A. L., & Dunlap, G. (1980). Learning characteristics of autistic children. In W. S. Sailor, B. Wilcox, & L. J. Brown (Eds.), *Methods of instruction with severely handicapped students*. Baltimore, MD: Brookes.

Koegel, R. L., Rincover, A., & Egel, A. L. (Eds.). (1982). *Educating and understanding autistic children*. San Diego: College-Hill.

Konner, M. (1991). *Childhood*. Boston, MA: Little, Brown.

Olley, J. G. (1987). Classroom structure and autism. In D. J. Cohen & A. M. Donnellan (Eds.), *Handbook of autism and pervasive developmental disorders*. New York: Wiley.

Orelove, F. P. (1982). Developing daily schedules for classrooms of severely handicapped students. *Education and Treatment of Children, 5*, 59–68.

Powers, M. (1992). Early intervention for children with autism. In D. E. Berkell (Ed.), *Autism: Identification, education, and treatment*. Hillsdale, N.J.: Lawrence Erlbaum Associates.

Simpson, R. L., & Myles, B. S. (1993). Successful integration of children and youth with autism in mainstreamed settings. *Focus on Autistic Behavior, 7*, 1–12.

Smith, M. D. (1990). *Autism and life in the community*. Baltimore: Brookes.

Stokes, T. F,. & Baer, D. M. (1977). An implicit technology of generalization. *Journal of Applied Behavior Analysis, 10*, 349–369

APPENDIX 10.1   **Guidelines for the Use of Environmental Supports**

I. TO DETERMINE THE TYPE OF SUPPORTS NEEDED, ANSWER THE FOLLOWING:

Does the child:
- understand all the verbal directions in the setting?
- attend to the verbal directions in the setting?
- have trouble accepting changes in his/her schedule?
- have trouble accepting changes within a routine?
- have trouble accepting changes in personnel/people?
- have trouble accepting changes in the environment?
- have trouble accepting new changes?
- have trouble accepting changes he/she doesn't understand?
- depend on verbal cues or gestures to do activities?
- depend on verbal cues or gestures within activities and routines?
- depend on set environmental cues? Which ones? Where?
- depend on adult presence to perform?
- exhibit the need to locate him/herself in certain places?
- become upset in certain places?
- know completion cues in each activity?
- understand the passage of time?
- know how much to do in a time frame?

II. TO DETERMINE INDIVIDUAL NEEDS, ASSESS THE FOLLOWING:

- What sensory needs does the child have?
- How does the child learn best?
- How much desensitization to an environment does the child need?
- How much observation time does the child need?
- How much does the child need to experience the whole environment before concentrating on a single activity?

III. TO EVALUATE THE USEFULNESS OF SUPPORTS, DETERMINE THE FOLLOWING:

- Are the supports socially valued or can they become socially valued?
- Is there consistent use across environments?
- Do all people, including peers, use the supports?
- Even if the child doesn't initiate or ask for the supports, are they available?
- Are the supports easily transported?
- Are the supports individualized?

APPENDIX 10.1   (continued)

- Are the supports age appropriate?
- Can the supports be adapted to a number of situations easily?
- Do the supports help the child?
- Do the supports increase the child's independence?
- Do the supports help the child be more flexible in accepting changes?
- Do the supports help the child know what to do in natural settings?

11

Solving Social-Behavioral Problems Through the Use of Visually Supported Communication

Linda Quirk Hodgdon

Communication difficulties constitute one of the principal deficit areas in the syndrome of autism. Behavioral problems and atypical social skill development are other characteristics of this disorder. It is common to associate the syndrome of autism with behavioral problems. There is increasing professional acknowledgement of the relationship between the communication difficulty experienced by children and behavioral problems they may display. As more is learned about autism, it appears that challenging behavior may not be a specific characteristic of the disorder so much as a result of certain other characteristics: difficulty establishing and maintaining attention, interpreting verbal communication, and developing skills such as sequencing and organization. Reactions to typical life demands are affected by the child's style of taking in information, processing it, and then formulating responses to situations as Adriana Schuler points out in Chapter 1 of this book.

Most discussion about the communication abilities of children with autism centers on their expressive skills (Paul, 1987), with comparatively little research or writing directed toward their ability or inability to take in and make meaning of the communication stimuli that surround them. The focus of this chapter will be on the autistic child's difficulty understanding the communication demands in his environment. Identifying the disorder in receptive communication will lead to a discussion of environmental supports and teaching strategies designed to reduce or eliminate many social/behavioral problems, followed by some methods to teach skills that should result in more appropriate social behavior.

THE RELATIONSHIP BETWEEN SOCIAL-BEHAVIORAL PROBLEMS AND COMMUNICATION

Although many approaches to behavioral intervention have taken a clinical view of behavior and treated it as an isolated entity, current approaches tend to identify a need to view behavior in the environmental context in which it occurrs. Not only is there acknowledgment that antecedent and consequential events directly affect a child's behavior; there is also increasing recognition that a direct relationship exists between children's displayed behavior and their ability or inability to use other means to adequately communicate their intent in a situation. The behavior is considered to have a communicative function; it is an attempt to send a communication message (Donnellan, Mirenda, Mesaros & Fassbender, 1984). This recognition has focused on the communicative functions of aberrant behavior, identifying socially inappropriate or unacceptable behavior as a means (albeit an inefficient means), of letting people know something. The child's inability to communicate his wants and needs through more socially or communicatively acceptable means has thus been targeted as an area for training. Looking at behaviors in the context of communication has produced some teaching objectives that have resulted in long-term improved functioning for children.

The behavior-as-a-form-of-communication approach effectively attacks an aspect of the communication problem. It focuses on the child output to be remedied, giving more attention to the antecedent events and less attention to how the form of input and resultant processing affect the end result—the acceptability of the child's social and behavioral skills.

Using visually coded environmental supports to enhance the communication to the child and to provide a framework for life's demands has significantly affected many autistic children's overall behavior and management of social expectations. Used as a means to enhance communication-loaded activities such as giving information and teaching routines, environmental supports have produced some dramatic changes in child participation (Hodgdon, 1991).

Defining Social-Behavioral Problems

Undesirable behaviors exhibited by children can range from aggressive or self-injurious episodes, to noncompliance and perseverative or annoying interludes. Identifying a behavior as a problem is subjective. What is responded to as a severe problem in one environment may be considered acceptable in another setting or with different people. What is perceived as annoying or intolerable to one person may be interpreted as a form of communication to another caregiver. It can a refer to patterns of ritualistic responses, chains of actions or routines that cannot be interrupted, perseverations, or other reactions to life demands that are characteristic of autism. Difficulties beginning or terminating activities, transitioning to new activities, changing locations, or changing expected routines are classic potential problem areas. The child's ability or inability to handle home, school and community routines with independence also falls within the realm of "behavior." For the purpose of our discussion, behavioral problems will refer to those actions or behaviors that have been targeted to change due to their negative impact on the child's social environment or educational accomplishment.

Identifying Communication Difficulties

Caregivers of children with autism and those experiencing severe communication difficulties make observations about the child's ability to understand verbal information. It is not uncommon to hear evaluations that include "he is really inconsistent," "he understands everything I say but he is just being bad," "he just does what he wants," or "he manipulates everyone." A more careful observation of these children reveals many of them experience significant difficulty understanding and using language information effectively. Their comprehension of the demands in their environment is based more on piecing together gestural cues, other environmental cues, and expected routines than on understanding specific verbal messages (Prizant & Schuler, 1987). Their lack of cooperation or lack of independence may actually be the result of not understanding fully what is expected of them or what is going to happen. They may be interpreting only fragments of the communication message accurately.

Current research suggests that children with autism experience difficulty smoothly and accurately controlling the shifting and reestablishing of attention (Courshesne, 1991). Their ability to modulate sensory input is thus affected. Early acquisition of social-communication skills requires the ability to interpret the rapid and dynamic ebb and flow of social interaction quickly; however, children with autism lack this capacity, resulting at least in part in the early aloof and nonengaged behaviors and the auditory inconsistencies described by researchers of autism. Children with autism display preference for things that are more invariant and more predictable (Courshesne, 1991).

Communication modes such as speech, manual signs, and gestures are transient; they remain visible for only a short period of time and require a rapid rate of processing. Tasks that require the sequential processing of transient information constitute an area of weakness in autism (Schuler, 1995). The children demonstrate comparative strengths with tasks that involve interpretation of nontransient stimulus (i.e., visual) that is processed in a gestalt fashion. The term *gestalt* suggests interpretation of the message as a whole rather than through analysis of its component parts (Prizant & Schuler, 1987).

It is important to consider the implications of a child who experiences difficulty shifting attention and trying to capture the essence of a transient auditory message. The transiency of the auditory message combined with the child's attentional deficits creates an inefficient system for understanding the environment. A spoken message may be completed before the child is focused enough to receive it. Conversely, the presentation of visual (nontransient) communication messages provides an opportunity for the child to engage his attention before the message disappears. The stability of the visual message allows the element of time necessary for the children to disengage, shift, and reengage attention. As a result, many of these children appear to understand what they *see* better than what they *hear*. In addition, the visual message can remain visible to enable the child to focus on it long enough or return to it as needed to establish memory of the message that has been communicated (Schuler, 1995).

Using visual environmental supports to mediate communication interactions and support understanding provides a nontransient foundation essential for more effective communication. It builds on children's strengths rather than placing more demands on their area of greatest difficulty. When visual supports are used to give these children information and directions, child comprehension increases *significantly*. For many children with severe communication difficulties, the use of visually supported communication is more effective and efficient than just talking to them.

The implementation of visually supported systems and strategies as a part of autistic children's communication system has proven to significantly reduce various behavioral problems and increase functional effective communication interactions for most children (Hodgdon, 1993). The techniques discussed in this chapter can be adapted to support most basic behavioral programs that have been developed to meet child needs. In many instances, once a visually supported communication system has been developed to accommodate specific needs, it becomes a behavioral program in itself, and other, more elaborate behavioral tools become unnecessary.

Identifying Goals

There are two main goals when addressing child social-behavioral problems from the viewpoint of communication: create a supportive environment, and develop alternative skills.

Creating an environment that makes the social-behavioral difficulty less likely to occur is accomplished in part by developing a system of visual aids to support communication, focusing particularly on giving information. When analyzing situations where undesirable behaviors occur, it becomes obvious that many of them are the result of a child not understanding what is happening in his life. It is common to assume the child understands. In reality, many times he or she doesn't. Educational methodology suggests teaching predictable routines and establishing a regular schedule: changes and transitions from the familiar are common potential problem times. All of the strategies outlined in this chapter have been part of programs that have successfully reduced or eliminated a variety of social-behavioral difficulties. The purpose of using visually supported communication is to enhance the child's understanding of what is happening in his life and what is expected of him. Once the child understands, he or she is more likely to comply with the demands of the setting. It does not matter whether a child is verbal or nonverbal. The primary purpose of these strategies is to support communication to the child, to give information and structure.

In addressing the second goal, developing skills that make unacceptable behavior less likely to occur, again it does not matter whether a child is verbal or nonverbal. The presence of visual aids helps children focus their attention, handle transitions, accept change, communicate choices, follow procedures, and develop many other skills that lead to a reduction of behavioral difficulties. Visual aids can be used to teach steps to activity routines or responses to specific situations, enabling the children to behave in more acceptable ways.

When developed effectively, visual supports will transcend environments so their application for home, school, and community settings will become obvious. The use of visual aids will become a part of the child's comprehensive communication system.

CREATING ENVIRONMENTS TO SUPPORT UNDERSTANDING

Do you carry a calendar or daily planner? Do you write yourself notes and lists? How about using menus and schedules? These basic tools can be translated into endless numbers of visual aids to support children's comprehension. Many teachers use a few visual aids to organize their classrooms. Clocks, signs, posters, labels, furniture arrangements, and other visual signals give children information if they understand how to get the information from them. The first step is to teach children with autism to accurately interpret the visual communications that already naturally exist in their environments. After tapping the naturally occurring cues, you can create additional supports to target specific problem areas or give support for more independent functioning.

Creating environmental supports increases child understanding, which results in reducing or eliminating social-behavioral problems. As children understand more clearly what is happening or what is expected, they are more able to comply with expectations. It is helpful to think of the purposes of tools when investigating what supports to consider for meeting the needs of a specific child. This chapter will highlight three specific types of supports: tools to *give information*, tools to *give directions*, and tools to *communicate rules*.

TOOLS TO GIVE INFORMATION

A major function of communication is to give information. In the typical environment, a majority of the information given is transmitted verbally. It is not unusual to assume that the child already knows or remembers information. That assumption may result in the information not being given at all, or at least not given in a way that the child can understand and remember. That is what happened to Byron. Byron was confused. Some days when he got home from school his mother was there to meet him. On Thursdays his father was there instead. In addition, a babysitter met him after school one or two days a week. The changes in his schedule created much anxiety for him. This resulted in questioning his teacher dozens of times each day about who was going to be home today. Every day he was told what would happen, but his anxiety indicated he needed more support. Byron needed a better way to understand the changes in his life. The teacher created a small calendar to display Byron's daily happenings. Putting the information in a visual form to help answer Byron's questions about his caregiver routine was significant in helping reduce his anxiety. When he began to question about his schedule, his teacher was able to refer him to the calendar to get the information. Eventually Byron learned to answer his own questions by looking at the calendar independently.

Schedules, charts, calendars, signs, lists, and an endless list of visual aids can be developed to give children information (see Dalrymple, this volume for more detail). The two tools to give information that will be discussed here are the use of schedules and techniques for communicating the meanings of "NO."

Schedules

Providing children with a schedule of daily events will produce one of the greatest returns for the effort when setting up a smoothly running classroom. There are many benefits in understanding and cooperation when the schedule clearly informs children what is going to happen.

Sam is one of those children with autism whose overall communication skills are quite limited. It is especially gratifying to observe him enter the classroom and proceed directly to the schedule that is posted on the board. He stands there looking for quite a while each morning. One morning after looking at the schedule for several minutes he walked over and took off the picture of bowling (a less favored activity) and replaced it with music (a favored activity). Communication! Not only was Sam understanding very clearly what was supposed to happen, he was using the same system to express his own desires.

Schedules are an extremely effective tool for conveying a variety of information:

1. What is happening as a part of the regular day
2. What is happening that is new or different
3. The sequence of events
4. What is not going to happen that the child would normally expect
5. What is changing or going to be different (changes in we plans or unexpected events)

The main daily schedule helps to guide the child through major segments of his day. It is too cumbersome to include every single activity in that main schedule. Minischedules are practical and convenient systems to supplement the daily schedule. Minischedules may be directed toward more individual needs, guiding the choices or sequences of activities during a particular time segment or activity period.

Figure 11.1 is a sample morning schedule that lists the general activity segments for the class. Two students, Paul and Mary, each have some minischedules to guide them through selected routines. When he arrives at school in the morning, Paul wants to go to his favorite chair and listen to his radio. He needs support to help him remember the sequence of steps to follow as he transitions into the classroom, so his minischedule helps him remember what to do. Mary does not experience difficulty remembering her routine, so no additional support is necessary. Academics, snack, and cooking are all time slots where the specific activities for each child may vary from day to day. Each child has an individual minischedule to direct them through those time sequences. The individual jobs or activities may be planned by the teacher and organized beforehand, or the child may make choices to be accomplished during that time. Grooming is another time where a specific routine is followed. Again Paul needs support and Mary does not.

Creating the tools is only a part of the process. It is essential to use them consistently to gain the most for the effort. The more the use of schedules is integrated into the routine, the more they will support positive child behavior. It is helpful to review the day's activities in the morning, use the schedule during transition times, and refer the child back to the schedule when he or she is choosing an action or behavior that is inappropriate at the time.

Have the children participate as much as possible in the preparation of the schedule at the beginning of the day. Have them assemble it, copy it, or develop their own personal version in some way. Use this as a time to talk about what will happen. Include a review of rules or other related information the child needs to remember. The more visual supports used in this review, the better. For example: Today is gym day, but there is a substitute gym teacher. Pictures of the regular teacher and the sub can be used to prepare the children for the change.

▶ FIGURE 11.1
Minischedules
Include Specific
Routines or
Individual
Activities That
Occur During
Larger Periods
of Time on the
Main Classroom
Schedule

Schedule and Minischedule Format

MAIN SCHEDULE

		Paul's MINISCHEDULE	Mary's MINISCHEDULE
8:30	Arrival	Coat / Lunchbox / Bathroom	
8:45	Greetings		
9:00	Academics	Make shopping list / Work on computer	Make shopping list / Cut coupons / Get money ready / Bathroom
9:30	Snack	Set table (cups, napkins, knife) / Clean up dirty dishes / Listen to radio	Make juice / Put away food
10:00	Shopping		
11:00	Cooking	Make french toast	Set table / Get out condiments / Put fruit in serving bowl
11:30	Lunch		
12:15	Grooming	Take medication / Bathroom / Brush teeth / Wash face / Comb hair	

Refer the children back to the schedule when it is transition time. Many children benefit from a physical representation (cross it off, turn it over, take it down, etc.) that one activity is completed and another is about to begin. This is particularly helpful for children who do not easily terminate one activity to begin something else. Since the schedule is established as the "great authority," you can tell the child, "The schedule says . . . ." Whereas he or she might argue with you, it is harder to argue with the schedule.

Refer children back to the schedule when they choose actions or activities that are inappropriate at the time. For example: Paul is supposed to be working at the computer. Instead he gets up to retrieve his radio. Use the schedule to tell him it is computer time. Show him on the schedule when he will be able to listen to the radio. Once he understands concretely that there will be a time for him to use the radio, he will be more apt to redirect his attention successfully. Whenever he is doing something he should not be doing, the schedule can be enlisted to direct him back to task.

Communicating the Meanings of NO

In the context of giving information, NO is a powerful word. Most children with autism have received more than their share of this exhortation. The way it is communicated can significantly affect how they will respond to it.

The word NO is used to convey a variety of concepts. Imagine the child who frequently hears NO in the context of "Don't do what you are doing, you are being bad." He develops a pattern of acting or reacting to that word. Then when he is told "No—there isn't any more," he may respond as if he were told "No—you were bad and you can't have any." Not being able to have or do what they desire or what they expect significantly affects the behavior of children with autism.

The use of the concept of NO can create much confusion or misunderstanding. Figure 11.2 lists the surprising variety of meanings we convey with that simple word.

When communicating any of the concepts suggested in Figure 11.2, terminology is important. Telling a child that his favorite snack is "all gone" might produce a different response from answering "NO you can't have any." Informing a child that "we will do it later, after aerobics" should have a more positive effect than "NO—not now ."

Along with well-thought-out terminology, visual tools can assist in communicating the concepts of NO in more concrete ways that help children understand. It is just as important to be able to give them information in a visual form about what is not available or what is not an option as it is to give them choices. Understanding that something can occur later this afternoon is different from thinking it will never happen again in their lifetime.

Techniques for Indicating NO

This is an opportunity to use your creativity. It is important to develop systems that make sense to the children. The goal is to have activities, choices, and other information represented visually so the negation can be superimposed on the existing format.

One option is to use the international NO sign, the familiar circle with a line through it. This symbol can be placed on cabinets where children may not go, on doors they may not exit, or on rule charts to emphasize behaviors that are not acceptable. That symbol has a strong appearance that children easily identify. It is particularly effective for indicating firm NOs.

A second technique is to cover things up. When something is not available, it seems logical to simply remove the choice (i.e., on a choice board).

▶ **FIGURE 11.2**
The Word NO
Communicates
a Variety
of Meanings

MEANINGS OF NO		
NO	Stop	Don't do what you are doing That behavior/action is not permitted
NO	That is not a choice	You cannot choose that now You cannot choose that ever
NO	Not the right time	You can't have/do it now, but you can have/choose it later
NO	Time to terminate	We aren't going to have/do this anymore Finished/all done
NO	No more	There was some and you had it, but now there isn't any more You can't have any more
NO	Nonexistent	There isn't any
NO	You are not permitted	You can't open this You can't go in/out of this location
NO	You lost the privilege	You did what you shouldn't do You didn't do what you should do
NO	Adult's choice	I don't want you to You already had some You already did it You already had a choice
NO	My preference	I don't want it I don't want to I don't feel like it

The problem is that the simple removal of an item does not ensure that the child will understand it is unavailable. Children may perseverate on a request for an item removed from a choice board because they remember the item was there. Give children an opportunity to *participate* in creating the communication. For example: If the record player breaks, have the child assist in covering up the picture of the record player on the choice board with a NO symbol. When the item is still there it is easier to communicate about it, and the visual symbol over it helps you explain the lack of availability.

Another strategy is to use additional visual tools to explain the concept. Schedules and calendars can help explain negation in relation to time. Something that will happen at a different time can be indicated to show the child when it will occur. Use whatever visual cues or objects will help convey the concept. Any objects or visual representations that "tell the story" or explain the consequences can be used as communication tools to explain to or remind the child of the negation. For example: A child loses the privilege of coloring because he has deliberately broken crayons. A NO symbol is placed on the picture of crayons on the choice board. When the child requests crayons he is shown the NO symbol and the broken crayons as a part of the communication that he has lost his coloring privilege and must choose a different activity.

Using visual ways to give children information can help reduce confusion and enhance their understanding. Other forms of visual tools can give such information as what is changing, what the choices are, what is not a choice, when new choices are available, where we are going, who is here, who is not here, who is coming at another time, how long we will be on vacation, when we will go swimming again, and more. As children understand more about the events in their lives, they display less anxiety and more willingness to comply with variations and changes. This results in a reduction of verbal reminders and the avoidance of many difficult behaviors.

TOOLS TO GIVE DIRECTIONS

A major challenge when working with children with severe communication impairments is giving instructions and directions in ways that facilitate a smooth flow of activity through the day. Those with more severe learning needs earn reputations of needing one-to-one individual attention, a commodity that is frequently more easily stated than provided. They can require multiple repetitions of directions and considerable redirection to stay on task to complete the requirements at hand.

Scott is one of those children who has difficulty attending to the task at hand. An example of his typical performance occurred while he was part of a group doing a cooking activity. The teacher asked Scott to get an egg from the refrigerator. Scott got up, walked to the washing machine (in the opposite direction) and twirled the dials, and then watched a fan as he took the long route to the refrigerator. Then he opened the door, grabbed a gallon of milk, and brought it back to the table. Not only does Scott experience difficulty focusing on the task at hand, but his diversions can cause classroom management problems.

Teaching a child like Scott to be dependent on constant adult intervention or supervision is not desirable. One educational goal for all special needs children should be to give them the structure and skills necessary to function as independently as possible. The more they are able to successfully follow the requests and routines presented in their environment, the more independent they become. Visual aids used to support teacher directions do the following:

1. Help gain and maintain a child's attention
2. Ensure that children get complete instructions
3. Help refocus a child's attention
4. Clarify instructions
5. Support child performance to completion
6. Reduce the intensity of adult support needed

When communications to targeted children are supported visually, their participation is more like that of the other children. To accomplish these goals, we will examine two types of aids to support classroom instruction: classroom management aids and task organizers.

Classroom Management Aids

Specifically designed to help the teacher communicate more effectively to the children, classroom management aids support various routine and novel communications that the teacher uses in the course of daily activities. The focus of classroom management aids is to support those teacher communications that provide directions to children and basic instruction.

When children are not on task it is easy for the teacher to increase the amount of verbalization in attempting to manage them. By employing visual strategies, including gestures, physical prompts, visual tools, or other nonverbal prompts, a teacher can retain the child's attention and comprehension without bombarding him or her with more verbal input. The extra verbalization used for child management can distract not only the child with autism, but also the other children, from the intent of the original communication.

Significant numbers of children with communication handicaps require less, not more, teacher verbalization. Although enlarging and expanding the verbalization is a strategy frequently recommended to build children's linguistic comprehension, that technique often proves ineffective with autistic children. *Reducing* the language used—that is, uncomplicating the auditory environment—produces positive results for many. Make directions very clear and concise. The process of creating classroom management aids helps teachers weed out wordiness and focus on those communications most essential for effective classroom management. Putting the communications in a visual form encourages simplicity and supports continuity among the variety of people interacting with or directing those children.

In addition, encourage simple, routine communications. It is not uncommon to say the same thing in many different ways. Communication consistency can benefit many children. This does not mean everyone in the child's life needs to speak from a script; however, attaching consistent verbal routines to the performance routines that children are learning will enhance the overall learning process. Labeling the visual tools with the language that goes with them will help accomplish this process.

The development of classroom management aids should evolve around specific identified needs. Visually representing everything said in the course of a day would be an overwhelming task. Luckily, the task becomes simpler once one begins to target one or two challenging situations. A teacher communication book and/or a collection of pictures can assist with the process.

A teacher communication book is the teacher's support tool for talking to the children, a variation of the more common communication board used by children. Look for those few key phrases that can have significant impact across the day. Most teachers can jot down a short list of phrases repeated frequently and regularly throughout the day or week. Some of those may be represented on the visual schedule, or as rules, or in other tools produced as a part of the classroom program. Some, addressed to specific children, may become part of an individual child aid. For a teacher communication book, target communications that occur very frequently, are used during transitions, or are presently not very effective. Try representing some of these in a visual form and putting the pictures in a little photo book that can be carried in a pocket. Hold up the book and point to the visual representation while stating the direction to the child. Although the possibilities are nearly unlimited, the number of visual aids should be small enough to be functional. Examples: five more minutes (before the schedule changes), get your chair, line up at the door.

An alternative strategy is to create a file of pictures of objects and/or steps used for directions given in the course of specific training activities. These can be particularly helpful in situations where the teacher gives different children different directions or when the directions vary from session to session. Show or give a picture to a child when giving the direction. Remember Scott, who was participating in the cooking activity? When Scott's teacher handed him a picture of an egg to accompany the verbal direction to get one, his attention to the task increased. He looked at that picture almost continually as he walked directly to the refrigerator and followed through to accomplish his task correctly.

Task Organizers   Many children have learned how to perform the parts of a job or activity, but they lack the ability to complete the whole task or sequence of steps independently. Perhaps they forget in which order the steps occur, perhaps they get distracted and eliminate steps or leave the activity, or maybe they just can't remember what to do next. These are the times when behavioral difficulties can develop.

Task organizers and cookbooks are step-by-step prompts to help a child complete a task more independently. Just as the chef needs to go to the cookbook to find and follow a recipe, many children need a set of cues to assist them in successfully accomplishing a task. This strategy can be instituted for accomplishing any task that requires a sequence of steps to completion.

A common problem in teaching children with autism is that each teacher or caregiver may use different methods or sequences to accomplish the same task. Even when specific procedures are agreed on, there can be a tendency to personalize them. Some trainers continually vary the methods or task sequences for teaching skills without evaluating the consequences of the changes. Variations in the training procedures can inadvertently lengthen the time necessary for skill acquisition. Visual tools help establish a systematic, organized, consistent way of teaching the steps to completion. They provide the opportunity for error-free learning.

Some children will use the visual tools until they have memorized the procedures or routines and then will naturally cease referring to the tools for support. Other children will continue to use the tools forever to successfully stay on task and complete their goals. Some cooks memorize recipes, others need the cookbook. The support from using the task organizers and cookbooks can greatly affect children's overall social/behavioral appropriateness.

COMMUNICATING RULES

Rules are the guidelines for acceptable behavior or procedures. In a typical environment, it is assumed that the child knows or remembers the rules. If there is doubt about the child's ability to remember, the rules are generally repeated verbally. It is common for children to need to be reminded regularly about the rules. In most environments it is not uncommon for rules to change or be enforced inconsistently. The process of putting the rules in a visual form ensures greater mutual understanding of exactly what the expectations are, resulting in more consistent child behavior. Instruction should include a review of the rules as a part of the routine they involve. For example, classroom rules that are a part of the behavior expected throughout the day can be included as part of the morning routine. Rules for walking in the hallway might be posted on the door and reviewed before the child leaves the room. When a specific behavior is being targeted during a selected activity, a review of the rule can be a part of the routine to begin that activity. Referring to and rehearsing the visually represented rules frequently results in less "management" of children during ongoing activities. When children begin to exhibit behaviors that do not follow the rules, a simple gesture to the rule can refocus their attention while reciting a simple script can often redirect them. Pointing to the visual symbol and telling the child, "The rule is . . ." has a marvelous influence. It is sometimes amazing (or even amusing) how much authority the visual symbols can hold with the children.

Rules can be presented to children with autism in a variety of ways. Children can be told what to do, what not to do, or the consequences of their actions ("if you do that, then this will happen"). Although it is generally preferable to state expectations in a positive manner ("Use a quiet voice, please") it is sometimes necessary or more effective to state the negative ("No yelling!") or to pair positive and negative together ("Use a quiet voice, please—no yelling in school"). It is necessary to be very clear when communicating to children what behavior is expected from them. If the expectations are not clear, the results will not be consistent. The process of putting rules in visual form is an exercise that frequently assists teachers to carefully identify their behavioral expectations and forces them to identify simple, clearly communicated targets.

Although children who experience behavioral difficulties generally have many rules to learn, a sound teaching strategy is to limit the number of new rules for any child. When selecting rules to teach, it is advisable to target those behaviors that are the going to have application across the day. "Listen to the teacher," "Follow directions," "Tell someone when you need help": these are examples of generic rules that will transcend many behavioral variations. Teaching acceptable behavior is a process. Just as aspiring athletes need much practice to acquire their maneuvers, many children need repeated training and support to accomplish their behavioral goals. The visual tools give a structure and consistency to the training process. They can make some fairly abstract ideas about social rules appear more concrete.

When children spend time in several environments, with parents, teachers, and other caregivers sharing charge, it can be difficult to establish consistent behavioral expectations. Visual tools assist the caregivers in establishing consistent procedures and terminology, while they help children demonstrate acceptable behaviors across settings and people. Children with autism benefit from the predictability of clear communication and consistent consequences. One of the classic exhortations for caregivers is to be consistent. Putting guidelines in a visual form helps achieve that goal. Behavior programs are more effective if consequences are clearly determined and understood by all.

The rules format is also effective to give options for handling specific situations the children may encounter (see Figure 11.3). Listing the options puts parameters on acceptable choices, creating a menu from which to choose. This gives the child variety in choices, but it eliminates unacceptable options.

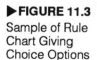
▶**FIGURE 11.3**
Sample of Rule
Chart Giving
Choice Options

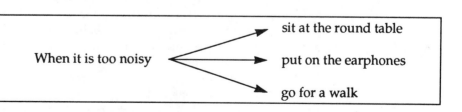

When it is too noisy → sit at the round table

When it is too noisy → put on the earphones

When it is too noisy → go for a walk

Some rules are appropriate for the whole class. Others are targeted for specific children. Both have an appropriate place in the context of a classroom program. Classroom rules may be posted on a board or affixed with velcro so they can move to where they are needed. If they are needed in more than one location, it is advisable to place a copy in each area so they can be referred to easily. Selected rules may be included in the teacher communication book to be transported where they are needed.

Rules established for individual children need to be mobile. Taped to a desk, included in a book that the child is responsible for, or hung up where he can easily refer to them, the rules need to be readily available and visible to serve as a reminder. Surprisingly, a piece of paper with a rule carried in the child's pocket can be enough of a reminder to help him monitor the targeted behavior.

Rules in a visual form serve children as a reminder and tool for self-regulation. Their effectiveness is established by referring to them regularly as part of the classroom routine. It is essential to expose children to the rules and teach what they mean and the routines that they trigger while the children are *not* experiencing behavior difficulties. Then when a problem surfaces, the teacher can redirect the child by referring to the visual rules. Since the child is already familiar with the routine associated with the rule, he or she will be more likely to follow it.

TEACHING ALTERNATIVE BEHAVIORS

When a child develops a pattern of handling a situation in a manner that is not socially or educationally acceptable, it is advantageous to use visual tools to teach a new skill or pattern of handling that situation. Using visual cues to teach behavior sequences has resulted in some remarkable successes. A wide range of social and behavioral routines are taught more effectively when the teaching is supported visually. The visual tools serve to prompt children and help them focus their attention during unfamiliar or difficult times.

When teaching alternative behavior patterns, specifically label or describe the targeted behaviors and identify in a concrete way exactly what actions or alternatives are acceptable. Learning a new routine to handle a social situation can be enhanced by a set of visually represented steps. Rehearsing the sequences or actions, following the symbols on the visual tool, helps a child learn the routines more rapidly. A new routine can be as simple as one step ("Keep your hands in your pockets"), or it can contain several steps ("When you walk into the room, look at Mr. Smith, say 'hi,' and hand him the note").

Using the visual tools as the main prompt or focus when teaching children a sequence of steps to manage their own behavior reduces the caregiver's role in the management process. This can result in a reduction of negative emotional components or unintentional changes in the behavioral expectations. Verbal direction is reduced considerably, and the behavioral expectations are clear and predictable. The result: children who are able to regulate their own behavior more effectively.

Tools to teach new behaviors can change as children continue to acquire more skills. Advanced charts can contain several elements resulting in more information or increasingly sophisticated choices (see Figures 11.4 and 11.5). These invite a script that gives more information.

Formats for Communication Aids

The development of visual tools can be a highly personal and creative process. Although it would be convenient to buy them ready made, that isn't possible. The most successful tools are those that are made to target very specific needs. Although endless varieties of formats are possible, several guidelines can produce effective results.

The goal of using visual communication aids is to support communication exchanges. The tools are typically a combination of picture symbols and words. It is desirable for the representations to be very quickly and easily identified. Picture symbols can be any variety of photos, line drawings, labels from packages, or the like that are appropriate for the targeted need. The symbols should be those most easily identified by the child. It is not necessary for everything to be in the same format. Simple, concrete, realistic representations will be more effective than abstract drawings or language. Label visuals with the exact script or phrase associated with the symbol. Educators have access to scores of picture resources, but they are seldom labeled with the script that will meet the current need. Combining the symbols and words create tools that give the most support and ensure the most consistency.

Once you begin to use a tool it will become obvious when changes are necessary. Adding more elements or taking out parts that are not necessary should be a part of the ongoing refinement process. Making modifications will ensure developing tools that are most effective.

▶ **FIGURE 11.4**
Sample of Chart to Teach a New Behavior Routine

WHEN YOU GET MAD:
1. MOVE AWAY FROM THE PERSON
2. COUNT TO 10
3. TELL HIM WHAT YOU DON'T LIKE
THEN
TELL A TEACHER   OR   GO SIT AT YOUR DESK

▶**FIGURE 11.5** Sample of Chart to Teach New Behaviors

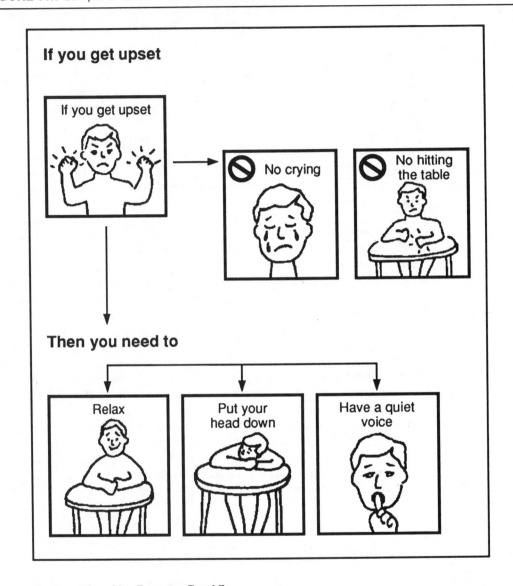

Courtesy of Young Ideas Enterprises, Troy, MI.
Copyright © 1993 by Linda Quirk Hodgdon.

GUIDELINES FOR USING VISUALLY SUPPORTED COMMUNICATION

The Environmental Observation Questionnaire (Appendix 11.1) will assist the process of targeting situations, locations, and activities that may be positively affected when visual aids are used to support the child's communication process and behavioral control. A suitable system of visual supports may evolve more from trial and error in your ongoing observational assessment than from any checklist developed. The most successful systems are the result of observing child behavior, hypothesizing what tools might provide more information or support, and experimenting to determine the child's response.

CASE STUDY

The following case study illustrates how visual aids were used to support a child's understanding of a situation that previously resulted in a severe behavioral disturbance.

Teddy listened as his teacher informed the class what was going to happen for the day. The teacher showed the class a schedule while she told them about the morning activies and a planned shopping trip for half the class. She told Teddy that he was not going to the store and that he would get a turn next week. Today he would go to Miss Timmon's room to work on the computer. When some of the class put on their coats to leave for the store, Teddy began to put his coat on, too. As the teacher directed him to take off his coat and go to the computer classroom, Teddy became agitated. When he entered Miss Timmon's computer room, he expressed his displeasure by throwing a chair across the room. Several other items managed to soar through the air before Teddy's episode was over. Predictably, his agitation did not completely subside until his classmates returned from their shopping excursion.

Within the context of analyzing behaviors for their communicative functions, it is fairly obvious that Teddy's outburst was a form of protest. Even though he is a verbal child, he chose to express his frustration with a series of behav-

iors. He needs to learn to use some more effective, socially acceptable methods to communicate his displeasure. Perhaps the most significant element of this incident, however, is Teddy's *understanding* of the situation. *Why* did Teddy have his outburst? Did it occur because Teddy did not understand the shopping logistics? Did he understand that he was not going to the store today but that he would get a chance next week? Teddy's misunderstanding of the school schedule led to a behavioral situation that might not have occurred if he had understood the sequence of events better.

When looking back at the situation, Teddy's teacher realized that while she gave her class information about the day via a written daily schedule, the *exceptions* to the schedule were communicated to the children verbally. That was not enough for Teddy. Even though she was attempting to implement some basic visual strategies in her classroom programming, she was not providing Teddy with *enough* details.

Teddy's teacher made some additions to her visual aids. During the next weeks when members of the class were going on shopping trips, she included more visual information in the shopping/computer time slot on the schedule. In addition, she created a calendar that helped each child see when his turn to shop was going to be. With the additional visual supports, Teddy understood the schedule variations better; however, he was still unhappy when it was not his turn to shop. The teacher used the schedule preparation time and the transition time (when children were preparing to go out or to the other classroom) as a time for communication training. Visual supports were developed to teach alternatives to his current protest behaviors, suggesting some acceptable things to do when he was mad. Since Teddy could talk, his teacher also established a plan to specifically teach some of the phrases Teddy needed to better express what was happening and how he felt about it. With training that addressed both his receptive and expressive difficulties in this situation, Teddy's overall behavior improved.

SUMMARY

One of the greatest challenges for children with autism is understanding and interpreting the demands of their environment. The development of visual tools to give children information and structure supports that need. Visual aids support socially appropriate behavior by giving children information in a form that they can understand more effectively than verbal instruction alone. This concept enhances the teaching of social skills and management of behaviors necessary for children to function effectively in a variety of environments.

Frequently the successful functioning of children with autism comes from the implementation of a variety of strategies that eventually work together to create an effective communication system. The principle of visually supported communication is simple, yet its impact on the functioning of most autistic children can be profound.

REFERENCES

Courshesne, E. (1991). A new model of brain and behavior development in infantile autism. *Autism Society of America Conference Proceedings*. Indianapolis.

Donnellan, A., Mirenda, P., Mesaros, R. & Fassbender, L. (1984). Analyzing the communicative functions of aberrant behavior. JASH, 9201–9212.

Hodgdon, L. (in press). Successful strategies for improving communication: practical application of visual supports.

Hodgdon, L. (1991). Solving behavior problems through better communication strategies. *Autism Society of America Conference Proceedings*. Indianapolis.

Paul, R. (1987). Communication. In D. Cohen & A. Donnellan (Eds.), *Handbook of autism and pervasive developmental disorder*. New York: Wiley.

Prizant, B., & Schuler, A. (1987). Facilitating communication: Language approaches. In D. Cohen & A. Donnellan (Eds.), *Handbook of autism and pervasive developmental disorder*. New York: Wiley.

Schuler, A. (1995). Thinking in autism. In K.A. Quill (Ed.), *Teaching children with autism: Strategies to enhance communication and socialization*. Albany, NY: Delmar.

APPENDIX 11.1   **Environmental Observation Questionnaire**

Name:_____ Date:_____
Evaluators:_____

What is the expected student activity in the environment?

How does the student know what to do?

How is he given overall information about his time/day/week?

How does he receive directions/assignments/information?

How does he make selections/choices?

How is he given rules/guidelines/correction?

How does he know where to go/what to do?

What cues does the student need?

To follow routines?

To follow directions?

What rules does the student need to follow to be successful in the environment?

What natural environmental cues are already present to give information?

Does the student use the information from these cues efficiently?

What problems or special needs arise?

Who?

When?

APPENDIX 11.1   (continued)

What is supposed to occur?

What does occur?

How is it presently handled?

Do the current intervention strategies work?

Are there predictable parts of the day/routine, locations, or types of activities where students are more likely to have difficulty?

What is the primary communication mode currently used when communicating to the student?

How is the communication modified to accommodate for individual needs?

What causes communication breakdowns?

How are communication breakdowns handled?

How much effort is necessary for students to understand?

©Hodgdon 1993 SUCCESSFUL STRATEGIES FOR IMPROVING COMMUNICATION

CHAPTER 12

Cognitive Picture Rehearsal: A System to Teach Self-Control

June Groden
Patricia LeVasseur

Inclusion of children with autism, mental retardation, and other developmental disabilities in educational programs and community environments has become a national objective for service delivery programs For this philosophy to gain wide acceptance, procedures must be available to assist these children to deal effectively with problematic behaviors that might prevent them from being accepted as full participants in integrated environments and interfere with their chances of enjoying a satisfying way of life.

This chapter will focus on a procedure termed *cognitive picture rehearsal,* which can provide a strategy suited to the characteristics and varying needs of children with autism and developmental disabilities. It combines the principles of learning theory (Hilgard & Marquis, 1968) and the technology of visual supports into a personalized program that has widespread application and can be cost effective. The use of cognitive picture rehearsal allows the learner to experience repeated practice of successful adaptive behavior with immediate reinforcement each time the program is implemented. It does not interfere with normal classroom programs and can eventually result in empowerment of the child by teaching self-control.

Embodied in our concept of teaching self-control is the philosophy that stressful life events can cause people to experience anxiety. This construct of stress and anxiety has pragmatic value in understanding some of the maladaptive behaviors of children with special needs. These events, typically stressful to persons with normal development, are particularly exacerbated in children with autism. They can be happy or unhappy events and are often associated with social relationships, fears, change in routines, and sensory stimuli. If the attribution is made that behaviors such as tantrums, disruptions, or stereotypic behaviors are maladaptive responses to stress, the application of stress reduction procedures can be beneficial (Groden, Cautela, Prince, & Berryman, in press). Therefore stress reduction procedures can be incorporated into the cognitive picture rehearsal format to teach children with autism appropriate coping strategies. When the stressful events occur in the natural environment, children with autism can use these coping strategies to practice self-control.

COGNITIVE PICTURE REHEARSAL

Cognitive picture rehearsal is an instructional strategy that uses repeated practice of a sequence of behaviors by presenting the sequence to the child in the form of pictures and an accompanying script. Although many different psychological procedures can provide the framework for a cognitive picture rehearsal program, the scenes presented in this chapter are based on the positive reinforcement principle of learning theory. This procedure holds that pleasant events following a behavior increase the probability of that behavior occurring again. The combination of this psychological approach to learning with the visual support of pictures prompts results in a unique method of instruction that capitalizes on the strengths of children with autism (Groden, Baron, & Cautela, 1988).

Although it is widely recognized that children with autism have strengths in the area of visualization (see Adriana Schuler's discussion in Chapter 1 of this book), there is very little literature to show its use in therapeutic endeavors with this population. Cognitive picture rehearsal has its roots in the imagery-based procedures described as "covert conditioning" (Cautela & Kearney, 1993). It is based on the assumption that behaviors such as thinking, feeling, and imaging follow the same laws of learning as do observable behaviors (Groden & Baron, 1991). A child imagines performing a desired behavior and then imagines a pleasant event. Covert conditioning and other procedures that use imagery—for example, desensitization (Wolpe, 1990) guided imagery (Leuner, 1969), and emotive imagery (Lazarus & Abramowitz, 1962)—have been used extensively at behavioral medicine and sports clinics to treat a variety of problems ranging from pain and high blood pressure to lagging self-esteem. However, there has been little extension of these procedures to children with disabilities. Adapting imagery-based procedures for use with this population by adding pictures to aid in focusing attention and sequencing led to the development of cognitive picture rehearsal.

SELF-CONTROL AND SOCIAL SKILLS

The long-term goals of cognitive picture rehearsal are to enable the child to acquire a needed skill or response, to recognize when and where to use it, and ultimately to use it independently in the appropriate situations. The major focus is in the development of self-control and the acquisition of social skills (Groden & Cautela, 1988). The scenes that are developed often address these needs simultaneously. If, for example, a child responds to criticism by being aggressive or throwing a tantrum, it is helpful for the child to know the appropriate verbal response, such as "I can change that easily." However, because the child may have a learned behavior of responding immediately with anger, it is also necessary to build into the scene a response such as relaxation, that will reduce the stress of the criticism, allow him to control his angry response, and then make the appropriate verbal response. The scenes in the following pages will serve as examples of how the development of self-control and the acquisition of social skills are closely interwoven. Being taught such skills can enhance the quality of life for the child with autism by expanding his social relationships. In this conceptualization self-control and social skills are sets of responses that any child can learn to make, rather than a higher-level ability that is only possible for those children within a select cognitive range (Groden, Cautela, LeVasseur, Groden, & Bausman, 1991). The following sections will describe the process of development of a cognitive picture rehearsal scene, followed by specific illustrations to enable the reader to create scenes independently.

DEVELOPMENT OF A COGNITIVE PICTURE REHEARSAL SCENE

Once a potential teaching objective is identified, all cognitive picture rehearsal programs should start with behavioral analysis to systematically collect all relevant information about its occurrence, including its frequency, rate, intensity, and its relationship to environmental events as well as its lack of occurrence at appropriate times (Groden, Stevenson, & Groden, 1992). It is beyond the scope of this chapter to detail the use of a sound behavioral analysis; however, a variety of books and articles on this subject are available (Groden, 1989; Kazdin, 1989; O'Neill, Horner, Albin, Storey, & Sprague, 1990; Upper & Cautela, 1977). Obtaining detailed information on the setting events, immediate and distant antecedents, and consequences of any behavior provides us with an ecology of the interaction that allows us to plan behavior change within that interaction. When the objective is to teach a specific social skill, such as playing a board game with a friend, an ecological inventory provides information on when and where it should be used and the natural cues and prompts available. The three basic components are the identification of (1) the target behavior, (2) the antecedents to the behavior, and (3) possible reinforcers.

First you must identify the target behavior. The objective may be learning a new skill, for example, or playing a game with a classmate; or it may be acquiring a skill that occurs at too low a frequency to be functional for the learner. The child who can ask or sign for help but instead waits passively is an example of this. A target behavior may also be one that is incompatible with a disruptive or otherwise problematic behavior, such as using a relaxation response instead of having a tantrum (Groden, 1992).

Using the behavioral analysis and an ecological analysis (Falvey, Grenot-Scheyer, & Luddy, 1987), identify predictable antecedents to the target behavior. Antecedents are events that are stressful to the child, such as medical appointments or going to a party. Responses to perceived stress can be both physiological, (e.g., face turning red or rapid heart rate) and behavioral (e.g., screaming, feeling anger). The objective of the program is to provide the child with an adaptive way to cope with these stressors.

The third component of any plan to change behavior is the identification of pleasant consequences, or reinforcers, that follow the behavior and increase the likelihood of its happening again. There are a number of ways to discover potential reinforcers for children. Observation in the natural environment, asking the child, asking family and friends of the learner, paper and pencil surveys (Cautela, 1990), and sampling procedures can be used. It is best to develop an individualized list of pleasant events for each child. See Appendix 12.1 for an overview of these steps.

Examples of Scenes

Four cognitive rehearsal scenes that we have used successfully with children with severe behavior problems and autism will be described here. Our data show that all four students mastered the self-control strategies they practiced using the cognitive picture rehearsal procedure. The scenes depict the use of cognitive picture rehearsal programs to assist the children in coping with stressful situations in school and at home. These examples were chosen because they illustrate situations that frequently are stressful for students with autism. They focus on classroom schedules and transitions, a bathtime routine, accepting corrective feedback, and the need for assertiveness. Each scene is constructed by describing the antecedent situation followed by the selected target behavior and then the reinforcement. Picture cards are made to correspond to each of these components. The number of cards for each part of the scene can vary according to the requirements of the scene and the abilities of the learner. Following each example, critical elements in its development and implementation will be discussed. Areas of discussion following the first scene include writing the script, the selection and presentation of pictures, reinforcement, implementation, generalization, and specificity. In order to avoid repetition, the discussion following subsequent scenes is limited to the most relevant elements of each.

SCENE 1: CLASSROOM TRANSITIONS

This scene was developed for a 9-year-old boy with autism. The goal was to teach the child to make a compliant transition between routine classroom activities rather than engage in disruptive behavior. Transitions of any type can be difficult for children with autism who may prefer to remain engaged in a familiar activity. Making a change involves a shifting of attention, a neurologically mediated process that can be problematic for individuals with autism (Courchesne, 1992). Transitions also involve the concept of time, an abstract concept if it is not in some way anchored to a concrete representation. Schedule boards with pictures are frequently used to make time concepts and the transitions they symbolize more concrete. In this case the cognitive picture rehearsal program was developed as part of a treatment package that also included the use of an individualized schedule board. In this scene two stressful elements, the transition itself and the additional factor of moving from a preferred activity to a less preferred one, were addressed. Transitions that involved both elements were more difficult for the child and frequently resulted in disruptive behaviors in the classroom.

Writing the Script

This scene demonstrates an example of a simple script consisting of the three basic elements of a cognitive picture rehearsal scene. The antecedents are the teacher's direction and the bell; the target behavior is putting the toy away; the reinforcer is juice. The script is written in direct, straightforward language. For example, our script reads "The teacher . . . says, 'Time to put toys away,'" rather than "The teacher tells the class to put the toys away." The direct quote is a less complex grammatical structure and thus preferred over the latter construction, which is more complex grammatically. Each picture card presented to the child has a corresponding script. The specific situation depicted in this scene was identified from an analysis of data recorded on disruptions in the classroom. To accommodate the attention span of the learner, the scene is brief. Frequent repetition of brief scenes, two or three rehearsals scheduled at least twice a day for example, has been found to work well with children with autism. It provides frequent reinforcement of the behavioral sequence being taught and helps to make the scene part of a predictable routine for the learner. When he rehearses the scene, the child is engaging in a form of self-instruction in which he practices what his behavior will be in a described situation. As he becomes more familiar with the scene, he begins to know what to expect in the real situation. When the child feels comfortable in a social situation, he is less likely to perceive it as stressful. The implementation of each cognitive picture rehearsal scene becomes a structured, predictable interaction in which the child is successful and receives reinforcement. Success and predictability are important considerations in every learning situation for chil-

▶**FIGURE 12.1**
Classroom
Transitions

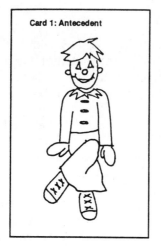

Card 1: Antecedent

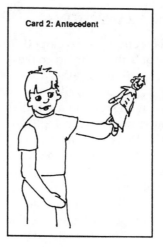

Card 2: Antecedent

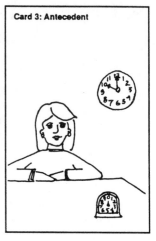

Card 3: Antecedent

*You're having fun
with the blue puppet
at recess.*

*You move the hands
in and out. You move
the head up and down.*

*The teacher rings the
bell. She says, "Time
to put toys away."*

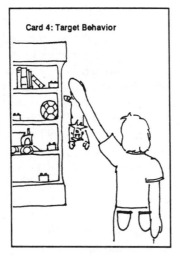

Card 4: Target Behavior

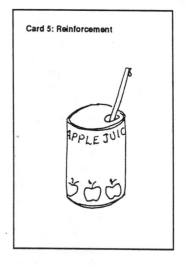

Card 5: Reinforcement

*You pull the puppet off
your hand and put it on
the shelf.*

*Now imagine holding this
cold can of apple juice.
You take a big drink. It
tastes good. You like juice.*

dren with autism. More complex scripts add either more details to the sequence being taught or more steps in the sequence, an accommodation to the individual attention and sequencing abilities of the child.

Sensory detail is incorporated into the script, particularly in the reinforcer description, as a way to enhance the effectiveness of cognitive picture rehearsal programs. By including sensory detail (how something looks, feels, smells, tastes, sounds, or moves), you can make the stimuli clearer and more vivid to the child. Because children with autism sometimes respond with heightened sensitivity to different sensory input, it is necessary to keep individual preferences and idiosyncrasies in mind when writing the script. In this scene we have included the fact that this child enjoys the tactile and visual feedback of moving his hand inside the puppet, as well as the tactile feedback from the cold can of juice.

The language abilities and verbal style of the child are also taken into consideration in writing the script. This youngster has minimal skills in expressive verbal language, but his receptive abilities are better and he does use sign and gesture to communicate. When rehearsing the scene, the teacher uses signs and gestures as well as words. The words and phrases in the scene are ones that are familiar to the child, and the sentence length matches his receptive language abilities.

The Selection and Presentation of Pictures

Simple line drawings with minimal background detail were used in this program. Relevant features were highlighted in color, such as the familiar blue of the puppet. The five picture cards were laid out on the desk from left to right, facing the child. The teacher pointed to the card she was describing as she related the script. When she finished, the child repeated the script, pointing to the appropriate picture and using sign, gesture, and single words with prompting from the teacher as needed.

Reinforcement

A list of five other reinforcers in addition to apple juice was developed for this child. Each day a different one was randomly selected for use in the scene. He often smiled on seeing the chosen reinforcer card; he also displayed physical signs of thinking about the reinforcer, such as licking his lips and swallowing when the picture card was shown.

Implementation

The program is done in a quiet area in a one-to-one instructional format. The teacher or therapist sits either beside or across from the child (Groden, Cautela, & Groden, 1991 [video]). The cards are laid out on the table or desk, facing the child; the script is written on a separate card that the teacher holds. The teacher runs through the entire scene first, pointing to each card in the sequence and checking the child's eye gaze to monitor his attention and participation. The child then repeats the scene. Two or three repetitions can be done in one session.

Generalization and Specificity

The original script used one specific antecedent situation identified in the behavioral analysis (i.e., playing with the blue puppet). A plan for generalization was developed to include other identified antecedents, such as playing with different toys, in subsequent scenes. Picture cards were drawn for each antecedent identified. This is done to increase the generalizability of the appropriate behavior being taught. If it were not done, the child could be expected to make a smooth transition only when he had been playing with the blue puppet.

SCENE 2: ACTIVITIES OF DAILY LIVING

Scene 2 was developed to teach a 5-year-old boy a bathtime routine that would become a comfortable part of his daily living activities. This child's parents reported that bathtime was often the setting for crying, screaming, and other disruptive behaviors. The cognitive picture rehearsal scene created a specific learning experience, incorporating pleasant, preferred toys and activities in a sequence of steps that help make bathtime a predictable and enjoyable event. These steps then became adaptive responses to replace the maladaptive ones he had been using. The scene was practiced several times a day at school; then his parents rehearsed it with him at home. An important advantage of cognitive picture rehearsal programs is that they can be implemented in one setting to effect behavior change in another setting. A set of picture cards is portable, therefore easily moved between environments.

Writing the Script

The child for whom this scene was written had mildly delayed cognitive abilities. By looking at the pictures and pointing to the objects referred to in the script, he could follow the verbal sequence associated with each card. Sensory details such as watching the water run and feeling bubbles on his arm are those that he naturally enjoyed. In this scene the name of the book to be read is left blank so that he can make a choice, thus adding his own personalization and increasing his interest. In this way, too, the reinforcer is varied so that satiation does not occur. If he were to select the same book repeatedly, preselected picture cards of three or four favorites could be presented on a rotating basis for him to make a choice.

The Selection and Presentation of Pictures

Pictures can take many forms for cognitive picture rehearsal scenes, depending on the preferences and responses of the learner. Sketches and stick figures drawn on index cards, photographs, and magazine cutouts have been used. Concrete stimuli have also been used. An example of this is having plastic eating utensils fastened with velcro to individual cards in order to teach eating skills. While some children respond with increased attention to photographs of themselves, this boy attended selectively to irrelevant details of photographs. The problem of stimulus overselectivity

▶**FIGURE 12.2**
Activities of
Daily Living

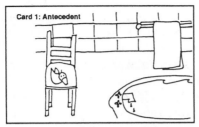

Card 1: Antecedent

It is time to get ready for a bath. You get your towel, your toy, and your pajamas.

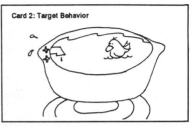

Card 2: Target Behavior

You watch the water go into the tub. You put your toy in and you get into the tub.

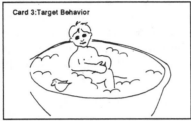

Card 3: Target Behavior

Now you sit in the warm bath with bubbles on your arms. You wash your arms, then your legs, then your chest.

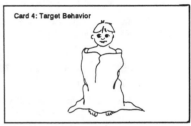

Card 4: Target Behavior

You play with the toy and (mom) washes you. She says, "It's time to get out now." You stand up, get out, and put your towel around you.

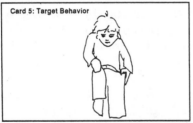

Card 5: Target Behavior

You're all dried off and you put on your pajamas.

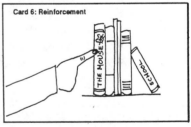

Card 6: Reinforcement

Now you pick a book to read tonight. It is the story of (name of book).

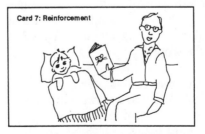

Card 7: Reinforcement

You're in bed with your blanket, listening to the story and looking at the book. You feel happy. You like this time of day.

(Schreibman, Koegel, & Craig, 1977) has been noted in children with autism. It should be considered when selecting the type of picture for a scene so that there are not too many confusing details. Simple line drawings were used in this scene to depict objects and locations with details that the child would recognize, such as his preferred towel and bath toy and his blanket. Children with the ability and the interest can increase their participation in cognitive picture rehearsal programs by drawing or coloring their own picture cards. Once a set of pictures has been made, it can be copied for use in other settings such as at home or riding in a car, and it is easily available to the child for practice before any stressful situation.

For this program, the pictures were bound loosely into a book because this student enjoyed looking at storybooks. This allowed the teacher to make changes in the cards before presenting the scene so that pictures of either Dad (see Figure 12.2) or a baby-sitter could be substituted in Card 7 and in the script as the other person in the routine. If a child tends to become distracted by a number of cards in front of him, the pictures can be held up singly, an adaptation that also allows the teacher to control the pace of the presentation.

Generalization and Specificity

Although the goal of this scene is to teach a routine that will make bathtime predictable and enjoyable, care must be taken that the routine does not become a rigid one. Children with autism often develop routines that appear to help them organize and predict their environment; building in systematic variations from the start can provide flexibility within the routines that are taught through cognitive picture rehearsal. In this scene many elements can be alternated to promote generalization. The color of the bath towel, the type of toy, the adult involved, and the pajamas are a few examples.

SCENE 3: ACCEPTING CORRECTIVE FEEDBACK

The scene in Figure 12.3, developed for a youngster who became upset when he made an error on a class assignment, provides an example of cognitive picture rehearsal used to teach children to accept feedback. Children with autism often become upset when they get an answer wrong. The resulting stress can lead to behaviors that cause disruption in the classroom.

Writing the Script

The goal of this scene was to help the child handle corrective feedback by teaching him a verbal coping statement. The content of the script was taken directly from data recording actual events preceding and following the crying behavior. This script has six cards and it includes language about feelings, an individual adaptation that matches the cognitive and language abilities of this student. It supplements a language program developed to

▶**FIGURE 12.3**
Accepting
Corrective
Feedback

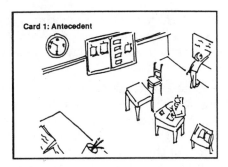

You're at your desk working on addition.

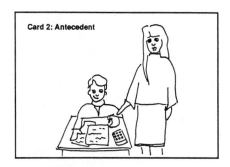

The teacher looks at your paper and says, "Tom, check the last problem. That's not the right answer."

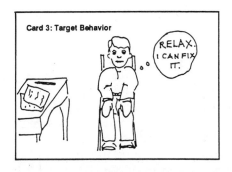

You take a deep breath, relax your arms. You breathe out slowly and say, "No big deal, I can fix it."

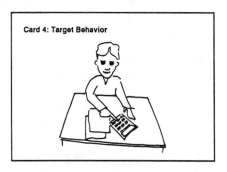

You use your calculator and do the problem again.

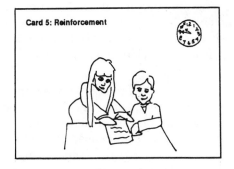

Now you have the right answer; you feel good about that. You tell the teacher.

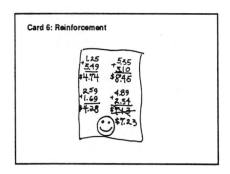

She smiles and puts a sticker on your paper. You're happy. You can't wait to show Mom when you get home today.

teach him to express his feelings. This script also incorporates the use of relaxation (see Card 3), a self-management procedure to reduce stress, that the child has learned and practiced every day (Cautela & Groden, 1978).

The Selection and Presentation of Pictures

Six photographs were used when this scene was presented initially. The child enjoyed looking at pictures of himself and his classmates, and the detail seemed to help him picture himself more clearly in the situation being described. The photographs were put in a six- by nine-inch album, one to a page. The words of the script were written out on the facing page. The specific people, situations, and locations captured in a photograph can limit the generalizability of a cognitive picture rehearsal scene. To make it more abstract and less specific, line drawings were introduced after the child demonstrated some familiarity with the scene. In this case the child did not have any problems with the change in format. If it had been diffi-cult, an alternative approach would have been to take photographs of vari-ous locations and activities and alternate their use when the scene was rehearsed.

Generalization and Specificity

To increase the probability of this coping response occurring in many dif-ferent situations involving feedback, not just when the child is adding prices in his classroom, the same target response of saying, "No big deal, I can fix it" can be rehearsed in a number of different antecedent situations. Different picture cards are used in this stimulus generalization procedure. Variations of Card 1 could depict the child working on spelling, or cutting out pictures, or building a Lego airplane. He could be at a group table, or in the art area, or sitting on the floor. For Card 2 it could be a specific teacher or a parent or peer who points out the mistake to him. Picture cards are made for each situation, and they are randomly changed. Another gen-eralization strategy would be to employ more abstract terms, such as "Someone notices that you made a mistake," or "You're doing an assign-ment." The behavioral analysis provides specific information to develop an initial scene; expanding and varying it are also necessary to maintain its functionality for the child. The coping strategy taught in this scene, using relaxation and a positive statement, can also be extended to vocational situ-ations such as supervisor feedback in the workplace.

Reinforcement

Because this child enjoyed verbal praise from teachers and parents, the reinforcement used in this scene is one that is preferred, natural, and the-matically related to the script. It is beneficial to have a supply of pictures of reinforcers so that different ones can be used at different times. Many chil-dren can choose from an array of reinforcement cards prior to beginning the program. Tangible reinforcement can follow the practice of cognitive picture rehearsal programs to reward compliance and cooperation.

SCENE 4: ASSERTIVENESS

The fourth scene demonstrates the use of cognitive picture rehearsal to address a target in the area of social development. It demonstrates that cognitive picture rehearsal is an effective way to make an abstract concept, assertiveness, concrete for the learner. This scene was developed for a 12-year-old girl with autism, who seldom initiated interaction with peers or teachers. She was usually compliant and worked quickly when given an assignment. The staff reported that she was being teased in subtle ways by classmates who apparently noted her tendency to do whatever she was told.

Writing the Script

A behavioral analysis indicated that working in group settings and eating lunch were two occasions for the occurrence of teasing. In one frequent situation, a classmate would repeatedly touch her foot or leg with his foot under the table. She shifted her feet and became distracted from her work. She was unhappy and stressed because she was unable to complete her work quickly. The functionally equivalent, more adaptive response of telling her classmate to stop kicking her was the behavior targeted to increase.

In this presentation the cards were line drawings, laid out on the table from left to right. This child was able to focus her attention on one card without being distracted by the others. If she had experienced difficulty attending, an alternative method of presentation would have been to hold up one card at a time or to lay the cards out face down, turning over one at a time. This girl was also able to follow a sequence with eight parts, and her receptive language level included understanding compound sentences. The teacher had the words of the script written on a cue card in order to repeat the entire scene to the child. If cards are to be presented by holding up one at a time, the script can be written on the back and the teacher can read from it.

Generalization and Specificity

Applying the concepts of specificity and generalization to this scene results in a number of possible variations. Since lunch time was another identified problem time, an alternate Card 2 could depict the lunch setting. The target behavior, using an assertive statement, would remain the same in this variation. As in other examples, the pleasant consequence, Card 8, would be one of a number of pictures of reinforcers that could be alternated with each rehearsal. The reinforcer depicted in this scene is unrelated to the script.

As inclusion becomes the general practice in schools, children with autism may be faced with being taken advantage of and being teased. Having a learned strategy available to cope with these situations can

▶**FIGURE 12.4**
Assertiveness

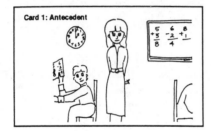

It is quiet in the classroom. The teacher is working with (name of student).

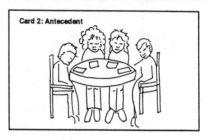

You're doing spelling at the back table with your group.

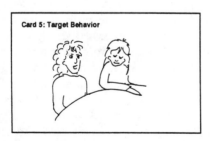

You feel something touch your foot.

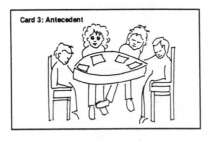

You move your foot. Something hits it again.

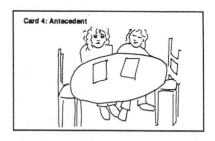

You look up and say, "Please stop that. I don't like to be kicked."

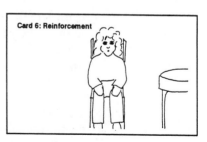

Now you are not being kicked. You take a deep breath and relax. You feel better.

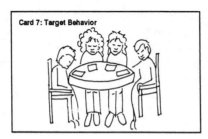

You get back to work on your spelling paper.

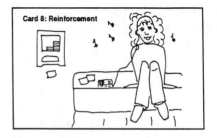

Now, imagine sitting on the couch at home listening to music with your head phones. You like to sing with the radio; you know the words. You feel happy.

reduce the child's stress. This child began to use the assertive response in the rehearsed situation very soon after beginning the program. It was effective and naturally reinforcing because the teasing did decrease. Within a short time she generalized the assertive response by telling a classmate to stop when he tried to get in line in front of her.

GUIDELINES FOR DEVELOPING COGNITIVE PICTURE REHEARSAL PROGRAMS

In this chapter we have described the development of cognitive picture rehearsal through the presentation of actual scenes, and then we have provided comments on variables that affected each particular program. In this section a summary will be provided in the form of guidelines to ensure that critical variables be considered in the development of cognitive picture rehearsal programs. Selecting an instructional target requires setting priorities within a child's behavioral repertoire. Factors to consider include the immediate severity of problem behavior and the child's responses to other treatment strategies. However, issues of social relevance, such as how others perceive and interact with the child as a result of inappropriate behaviors, are equally important considerations. New skills that are alternatives to problem behaviors involve self-control and social skills. They result in more appropriate ways of coping with emotions such as fear, anger, confusion or frustration.

Implementation   To implement a cognitive picture rehearsal program, it is best to chose a quiet area with minimal distraction. It should be scheduled regularly as is done with reading, art, or any other lesson. Cognitive picture rehearsal programs are typically brief, requiring no more than ten minutes; therefore it is possible and strongly recommended to schedule them two or three times daily. For those children with the ability to understand, a rationale for the program is often given. The teacher may talk about how hard the child has tried to perform a certain desired behavior and then suggest this as a new way that may help him to remember it. For the younger child, the program can be introduced as a story time. In both instances the cognitive picture rehearsal scene becomes a routine part of the child's program that is practiced every day. Not until the child demonstrates familiarity with the scene are the cards introduced in the actual stressful situation that has been rehearsed. There are a number of ways to tell that a child has become comfortable with a scene. He may say the words of the script before the teacher does; he may smile in anticipation of a favorite part of the scene; or he may show physical responses to imagined stimuli such as licking an ice cream cone. When a child can reliably show that he is familiar with the behavioral sequence, the cards can be introduced prior to the anticipated stressful situation.

Generalization and Specificity

Cognitive picture rehearsal is a flexible procedure that can be used before, during, and after a problem situation is encountered. If a stressful situation such as a change in plans is anticipated, the child can review the picture sequence that addresses schedule changes just before the actual situation. The pictures can also be used during a problematic incident. In the same example, bring out the cards as the plan is being changed and ask, "Now what can we do?". Review the appropriate responses as illustrated on the cards. After the situation has occurred, the cognitive picture rehearsal program can augment the learning process by practicing it in close proximity to the actual event. Cognitive picture rehearsal programs practiced at these times take advantage of actual opportunities to exhibit self-control as they occur in the natural environment.

The Selection and Presentation of Pictures

Assessments can be done to evaluate the type of picture that elicits the most attention and interest from the learner. Options include line drawings, pictographic symbols, cutouts from magazines, photographs, and real objects. Written words and cartoon drawings can also be used. The more abstract the picture, the greater the generalization. Black and white line drawings without background can often convey enough information for learning to take place, yet not be so specific that they inhibit generalization. In addition to the presentation methods discussed in this chapter, pictures can be displayed in a wallet-style photograph holder; they also can be laminated for durability.

Writing the Script

Individualization can be achieved by matching script variables to the preferences, communication style and ability, attention span, and developmental level of the child. Script variables include the vocabulary, length, sentence structure, use of sign and gesture, and sensory detail. Choices among these variables provide the means to individualize and personalize the cognitive picture rehearsal scene. Using words and phrases that are familiar to the child and that he uses to communicate both increases interest and sustains attention. Children with more severe language deficits require scenes that match their abilities. Cognitive picture rehearsal scenes have been implemented using sign paired with verbalization. Adding picture cues to the sign and word makes the scene part of a total communication approach. In carrying out signed scenes, the teacher presents the sequence first by pointing to each card in order while signing and saying the key word or phrase. When the child repeats the scene, he signs the same word or phrase for each card along with whatever verbal approximation might be possible. A thorough review of the child's current speech and language evaluation can be a good source of information. When the child is repeating the scene, questions can be asked to assist him in imagining himself more clearly in the situation being described. The child whose language development prohibits his understanding of question words can be given simple directions, such as "Show me how you put it on the shelf." As many prompts as necessary are given during the child's rehearsal of the scene. The goal is for the child to imagine practicing the desired behavior successfully, not to memorize words rotely.

Reinforcement

The following principles should be taken into consideration for the reinforcement section of cognitive picture rehearsal programs: (1) the higher the quality of the reinforcement, the more effective it will be; (2) reinforcement should be pictured immediately following the desired response; and (3) rotation of reinforcement is important so that satiation does not occur. It is important *not* to expect quick results, since learning happens over repeated trials, and learning becomes stronger as the number of trials increases. The clinical work of these authors indicates that it takes at least 100 repetitions of a scene to change behavior. It has also been found to take much longer, up to two years, for some children with more severe cognitive deficits. The time and effort have been deemed worthwhile because the results are long lasting.

Self-Control

The goal of this procedure is to develop the child's self-control, which can be accomplished through the following methods:

1. Children can design and draw their own scenes, thereby participating in and choosing their own target behaviors and reinforcers.
2. Children can practice on their own.
3. At appropriate times, teachers, parents or staff can cue the children to use the responses they have practiced in their cognitive picture rehearsal program.
4. Children can learn to identify antecedent events and initiate the use of the appropriate responses, first with the pictures and later without them.

Although it is the ultimate goal to achieve full self-control, there may be some children who achieve only partial independence in using practiced self-control strategies. Lou Brown's idea of partial participation is applicable (Baumgart et al., 1982). If a child can learn partial self-control with the assistance of picture cues or staff cues, it is still preferable to the display of inappropriate behavior.

SUMMARY

Cognitive picture rehearsal addresses the learning strengths of children with autism by providing a visual system combined with structured interactive routines. It reflects an emerging teaching methodology that emphasizes motivating learning experiences, accommodation to sensory sensitivities, and social-communicative needs. By focusing on antecedent events and practicing coping strategies before stressful events occur, it places an emphasis on prevention. Through repeated practice of pictorial scenes, children with autism can learn to identify stressful events and then use learned coping strategies.

It is hoped that the description of these procedures will lead to research in the examination of specific variables that are thought to contribute to their effectiveness. Questions such as "Is it more effective when the reinforcers are relevant to the script?" and "Which presentation style provides the most beneficial results?" can be put to experimental analysis.

Interactive book or video design may promote further interest, increase attention span, and offer more opportunities to expand these concepts. In addition to increasing appropriate behaviors such as daily living and socialization skills, or decreasing maladaptive behaviors, cognitive picture rehearsal can be used to reduce physiological or psychological discomfort. With the expansion in the use of imagery-based procedures in the field of behavioral medicine, cognitive picture rehearsal can provide the means to adapt these techniques to a population with challenging behaviors. The support provided by the visual system allows the expansion of proven therapeutic techniques such as desensitization, flooding, guided imagery, self-instruction, and covert conditioning to benefit individuals with learning and cognitive problems.

Cognitive picture rehearsal offers a strategy to bridge the gap between the ideal of community and school inclusion and the reality of adjustment in these settings. Through these procedures, self-control can be developed to enhance the quality of life for children with autism.

REFERENCES

Baumgart, D., Brown, L., Pumpian, I., Nisbet, J., Ford, A., Sweet, M., Messina, R., & Schroeder, J. (1982). Principle of partial participation and individualized adaptations in educational programs for severely handicapped students. *Journal of the Association for the Severely Handicapped, 7* (2), 17–27.

Cautela, J. R. (1990). *Behavior analysis forms for clinical intervention* (Vol. 1). Cambridge, MA: Cambridge Center for Behavioral Studies.

Cautela, J. R., & Groden, J. (1978). *Relaxation: A comprehensive manual for adults, children, and children with special needs.* Champaign, IL: Research Press.

Cautela, J. R., & Kearney, A. J. (Eds.). (1993). *The covert conditioning casebook.* Pacific Grove, CA: Brooks/Cole.

Courchesne, E. (1992). *Shifting attention impairment in autism: New behavioral, physiological and anatomical evidence of cerebral and cerebellar involvement.* Paper presented at the National Conference of the Autism Society of America, Albuquerque, NM, July.

Falvey, M. A., Grenot-Scheyer, M., & Luddy, E. (1987). Developing and implementing integrated community referenced curricula. In D. Cohen, A. M. Donnellan, & R. Paul (Eds.), *Handbook of autism and pervasive developmental disorders.* New York: Wiley.

Groden, G. (1989). A guide for conducting a comprehensive behavioral analysis of a target behavior. *Journal of Behavior Therapy and Experimental Psychiatry, 20* (2), 163–169.

Groden, G., & Baron, M. G. (Eds.). (1991). *Autism: Strategies for change.* New York and London: Gardner.

Groden, G., Stevenson, S., & Groden, J. (1992). *Understanding challenging behavior: A step-by-step behavioral analysis guide.* Unpublished paper, Groden Center, Providence, RI.

Groden, J. (1992). The use of covert procedures to reduce severe aggression in a person with retardation and behavioral disorders. In J. Cautela & A. J. Kearney (Eds.), *The covert conditioning casebook.* Pacific Grove, CA: Brooks/Cole.

Groden, J., Baron, G., & Cautela, J. (1988). Behavioral programming: Expanding our clinical repertoire. In G. Groden & G. Baron (Eds.), *Autism: Strategies for change* (pp. 49–74). New York: Gardner.

Groden, J., & Cautela, J. (1988). Procedures to increase social interaction among adolescents with autism: A multiple baseline analysis. *Behavior Therapy and Psychiatry, Vol. 19,* 2.

Groden, J., Cautela, J.R., & Groden, G. (1989) *Breaking the barriers: The use of relaxation for people with special needs* [Videotape]. Champaign, IL: Research Press.

Groden, J., Cautela, J. R., & Groden, G. (1991). *Breaking the barriers II: Imagery procedures for people with special needs* [Videotape]. Champaign, IL: Research Press.

Groden, J., Cautela, J., Prince, S., & Berryman, J. (in press). The impact of stress and anxiety on individuals with autism and developmental disabilities. In E.

Schopler & G. Mesibov (Eds.), *Assessment and management of problem behavior in autism.* New York: Plenum.

Groden, J., Cautela, J. R., LeVasseur, P., Groden, G., & Bausman, M. (1991). *Video guide to breaking the barriers II.* Champaign, IL: Research Press.

Hilgard, E. R., & Marquis, D. G. (1968). *Conditioning and learning.* New York: Appleton-Century-Crofts.

Kazdin, A. E. (1989). *Behavior modification in applied settings* (4th ed.). Homewood, IL: Dorsey.

Lazarus, A. A., & Abramowitz, A. (1962). The use of "emotive imagery" in the treatment of children's phobias. *Journal of Mental Science, 108,* 191–195.

Leuner, H. (1969). Guided affective imagery: A method of intensive psychotherapy. *American Journal of Psychotherapy, 23,* 4–22.

O'Neill, R. E., Horner, R. H., Albin, R. W., Storey, K., & Sprague, J. R. (1990). *Functional analysis of problem behavior: A practical assessment guide.* Sycamore, IL: Sycamore.

Schreibman, L., Koegel, R. L., & Craig, M. S. (1977). Reducing stimulus overselectivity in autistic children. *Journal of Abnormal Child Psychology, 5,* 425–436.

Upper, D., & Cautela, J. R. (1977). Behavior analysis, assessment and diagnosis. Section I. Behavioral vs. "traditional" approaches to assessment. In D. Upper (Ed.), *Perspectives in behavior therapy.* Kalamazoo, MI: Behaviordelia.

Wolpe, J. (1990). *Practice of behavior therapy* (4th ed.). New York: Pergamon.

APPENDIX 12.1   Cognitive Picture Rehearsal Guide

Steps	Sources	Comments
I. INFORMATION GATHERING		
1. Identify target behavior	• Behavior reports • Observation • Ask parents, teachers	• Social behaviors to increase • Challenging behaviors to decrease
2. Identify antecedent events	• Behavior analysis • Ecological inventory • Observation • Interview	• Design picture card for each
3. Identify reinforcing event	• Motivation assessment • Reinforcement survey • Sampling procedures • Interview	• Design picture card for each
II. SCRIPT DEVELOPMENT		
4. Sequence the scene	• Language sample • Language assessment • Behavior observation	• Match length and detail to child's ability level
5. Rotate antecedent	• Same as steps 2 and 3	• Practice scene five times daily
6. Decide number of pictures, type of pictures, and method of presentation	• Observation of child's attention and interest	
III. USE OF PICTURE CARDS		
7. Identify precursors	• Behavior reports • Behavior observation	• Present cards before situation
8. Cue child with cards		• Present cards during and after situation
9. Child identifies actual situation to use cards		• Independent use of strategy

Index